Saunders
Medical Assisting
Exam Review

Saunders
Medical Assisting
Exam Review

Deborah E. Barbier Holmes, RN, MLT, CMA-C
Program Chair, Medical Assistant Program
Iowa Western Community College
Council Bluffs, Iowa

Joanna Bligh, MEd, CMA, RT(R) (ret.)
Medical Assisting Adjunct Faculty
Hesser College
Concord, New Hampshire

SAUNDERS
An Imprint of Elsevier

SAUNDERS
An Imprint of Elsevier
The Curtis Center
Independence Square West
Philadelphia, Pennsylvania 19106

Editor-in-Chief: Andrew Allen
Senior Acquisitions Editor: Adrianne Williams
Senior Developmental Editor: Rae L. Robertson

Library of Congress Cataloging-in-Publication Data

Holmes, Deborah E. Barbier.
    Saunders medical assisting exam review / Deborah E. Barbier Holmes, Joanna Bligh.
      p. cm.
    ISBN 0–7216–9566–3
    1. Medical assistants—Examinations, questions, etc. 2. Physician's
assistants—Examinations, questions, etc. I. Bligh, Joanna. II. Title.

R728.8.H65 2002
610.69′53′076—dc21

2001034267

SAUNDERS MEDICAL ASSISTING EXAM REVIEW   ISBN 0–7216–9566–3

Permissions may be sought directly from Elsevier's Health Sciences Rights Department in Philadelphia, USA: phone: (+1)215-238-7869, fax: (+1)215-238-2239, email: healthpermissions@elsevier.com. You may also complete your request on-line via the Elsevier Science homepage (http://www.elsevier.com), by selecting 'Customer Support' and then 'Obtaining Permissions'.

Printed in the United States of America

Last digit is the print number: 9 8 7 6 5 4 3 2

To

Granny and Jon,
My biggest fans and guardian angels

And to

My students,
Who teach me something new
Every day

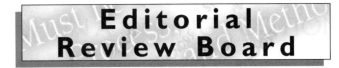

Editorial Review Board

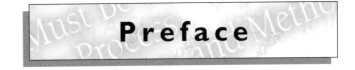

Preface

Skilled. Compassionate. Healer. Competent.

These are words that come to mind when describing the Medical Assistant. As the profession of Medical Assisting continues to change, the Medical Assistant must meet these new challenges. Earning a Medical Assistant credential is the first step.

There are many reasons to achieve this credential. It shows that the student is recognized by the credentialing organization as having met predetermined qualifications. It shows proof of competency, and it shows others a commitment to the profession. This credential will be even more important in the coming years as Medical Assistants become more and more recognized for the versatile allied health professionals that they are.

Saunders Medical Assisting Exam Review was written to aid the student in studying for a medical assisting credentialing exam and was developed with today's busy student in mind. Both the Certified Medical Assistant exam and the Registered Medical Assistant exam are included. The book discusses study tips and test-taking helps.

The book features the following:

■ A single, comprehensive guide. This allows for information to be found easily in one text, and eliminates the need for many big, bulky textbooks and stacks of notes.
■ An easy-to-follow outline format. Information is organized and presented in this format to allow the student to identify key concepts and facts. All subject areas typically included in a Medical Assistant Program are covered.
■ A practice pre-test and post-test, complete with answers and rationales. These may help assess weak and strong areas. Answer sheets are provided. A CD-ROM with different practice exams offers more practice.
■ Simple pictures and diagrams to illustrate the text. These may help to clarify concepts.
■ Study and test-taking tips to help the student be successful. Included are suggestions on how to prepare to study, how to study, and how to take a multiple-choice exam.

As the practicing Medical Assistant moves on in his/her career, this text may be used as a source of reference. It is also useful as a reference for educators in creating lecture material, curriculum, or review courses.

The author wishes the best of luck to all who use this text to achieve their credential. Hopefully it helps make the process a little easier.

ACKNOWLEDGMENTS

I am deeply grateful to the following people who have given me ideas, encouragement, praise, and support.

My students, past, present, and future—they are THE reason for this project. They have been an endless source of ideas, criticism, support, and inspiration.

Adrianne Williams and Rae Robertson at Mosby/Saunders—for supporting, understanding, helping tremendously, and very nicely reminding me that I'm not on schedule. This project started as a discussion at a national convention, and wound up as this book because of them.

Carol Moore, Academic Skills Specialist, Nebraska Methodist College—for providing the test-taking strategies and study skills ideas.

Scott Holmes, typist and spouse—for providing the many, many hours that it took to put my scribbles from legal pads to typed manuscript. He also provided comic relief by his "translation" of anatomy as he transcribed my notes.

David Holmes—for sharing his wonderful gift of words.

David, Robert and Jennifer—the loves of my life.

Deborah E. Barbier Holmes

The idea for this book came to me in 1997 when I was the Medical Programs Director at Northeast Career Schools in Manchester, New Hampshire. At that time I was also president of the New Hampshire Society of the American Association of Medical Assistants, and we had just won an important state legislative battle to defeat Bill 281, which limited the medical assistants' scope of practice in New Hampshire. The Academic Director at Northeast Career Schools, Mary Liponis, was instrumental in encouraging me to submit a proposal for this book to the publisher. Mary felt that, after our successful legislative battle, our cohesive group of medical assisting instructors needed another project. I would like to thank the dedicated medical assisting instructors who inspired this project: Nancy Ouellette, CMA; Barbara Massoni, RN, CMA; and Gayle Farley, CMA. Those who contributed need special acknowledgment and thanks: Carolyn Turner, MT(ASCP), CMA, and Enid Harrington, RN, MSW.

Joanna Bligh

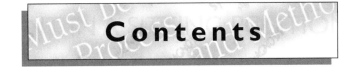

Contents

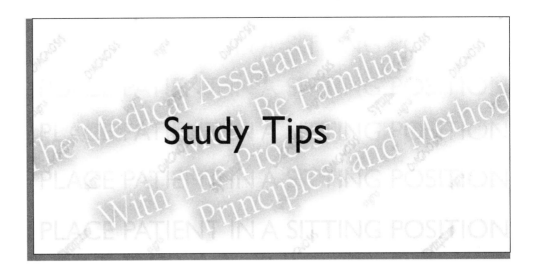

Study Tips

TAKING THE MEDICAL ASSISTANT EXAMINATION

General Examination Descriptions

CMA Exam

The CMA exam is administered on the last Friday in January and the last Saturday in June of each year. Individuals who meet the requirements set by the American Association of Medical Assistants (AAMA) are eligible to sit for this exam. The exam consists of 300 questions in multiple-choice format. Three general areas are covered on the exam, each area consisting of 100 questions. The content of each general area is broken down as follows:

General Medical Knowledge (100 questions)
■ Medical terminology
■ Anatomy and physiology
■ Law
■ Ethics
■ Patient relations
■ Communications

Administrative Knowledge (100 questions)
■ Keyboarding concepts
■ Correspondence
■ Mail
■ Appointments
■ Phone management
■ Filing and records management
■ Banking
■ Bookkeeping
■ Payroll
■ Medical coding
■ Insurance
■ Office automation
■ General office management concepts

Clinical Knowledge (100 questions)
■ Patient interviewing
■ Charting and documentation
■ Physical measurements and examinations
■ Nutrition
■ Physical therapy
■ Radiograph
■ Electrocardiography
■ Surgical treatment
■ First aid
■ Cardiopulmonary resuscitation
■ Laboratory orientation
■ Urinalysis
■ Hematology
■ Chemistry
■ Serology/immunology
■ Microbiology

You are given four hours to complete the exam. All questions are assigned equal weight. Guessing at answers is not counted against you; the exam is scored according to the number of correct answers versus the total number of questions given. An overall minimum standard score of 445 must be attained to pass the exam. On successfully passing the exam, the medical assistant may wear the CMA credential. For more information on taking the CMA exam, visit the American Association of Medical Assistants Web site at www.aama-ntl.org.

RMA Exam

The RMA exam is administered throughout the year at various computerized testing locations across the country. Individuals who meet the criteria set forth by the American Medical Technologists (AMT) are eligible to sit for this exam. The exam consists of 200–210 questions in multiple-choice format, covering the same three general areas as the CMA exam. The approximate percentage of material covered from each section and its content is broken down as follows:

General Medical Knowledge (42.5%)
■ Anatomy and physiology
■ Medical terminology
■ Medical law
■ Medical ethics
■ Human relations
■ Patient education

Administrative Knowledge (22.5%)
■ Insurance
■ Financial bookkeeping
■ Medical secretarial-receptionist

Clinical Knowledge (35%)
- Asepsis
- Sterilization
- Instruments
- Vital signs
- Physical examinations
- Clinical pharmacology
- Minor surgery
- Therapeutic modalities
- Laboratory procedures
- Electrocardiography
- First aid

A minimum scaled score of 70 must be attained to pass the exam. On successfully passing the exam, the medical assistant may wear the RMA credential. For more information on taking the RMA exam, visit the American Medical Technologists Web site at www.amt1.com.

Study Tips for the Exam

Taking the medical assistant certification (CMA) or registration (RMA) examination is an important event in the medical assistant's career. This section will guide you in preparing for the examination by offering study techniques and tips and by describing the exam itself and what to expect when exam day arrives.

A great deal of commitment is required on your part to study for the exam. Your performance on the exam will reflect your study habits. If you give an effort of 100%, you should do well; if you halfheartedly study for the exam, you will not do well. The earlier you begin studying for the exam, the better.

It is up to you to determine what study methods work best for you. Once you have done this, discipline yourself and stick to your plan!

1. **Assess your learning capabilities.** This will help you to determine the amount of time you will need to study.
2. **Request a content outline from your certifying agency.** Review the outline, and determine the amount of time you will need for your own learning capabilities.
3. **Plot a study schedule.** Divide the outline into subjects. Place the subjects into a study schedule. Allow extra time for subjects that are more difficult for you.
4. **Set up a time schedule.** Retention levels are higher when you study in short sessions.
5. **Prepare to study.**
   - Create the environment:
     - Select a place with a desk or table, straight-backed chair, and good lighting. Being too comfortable may encourage sleep.
     - Keep the room temperature comfortable—not too warm or too cool.
     - Avoid interruptions from family, friends, and telephone.
     - Avoid unnecessary noise.
   - Gather study tools:
     - Gather all books, notebooks, and flashcards.
     - Have extra pens, pencils, and flashcards handy.
6. **Commit to study.** You are preparing to take a national exam for your medical assistant credential!
7. **Study!**
   - Study material you do not know. Don't waste time on the material you do know.
   - Take a break halfway through each session.
   - Study the subject you dislike or are weakest in first and the subject you like or are strongest in last.
   - Do not study after a heavy meal.
   - Take your review book, notes, and/or flashcards with you and answer questions at lunch time, coffee breaks, and in your spare time.
   - Attend an exam review class, or join a study group.

The Day Before the Exam

1. Be familiar with the directions and the route to the test site.
2. Review your notes briefly. Do not cram!
3. Go to bed early and get a good night's sleep.
4. Plan to arrive early at the test site. Doors will be locked to late comers after a certain amount of time.
5. Have pencils and supplies ready to take with you to the exam.

The Day of the Exam

1. Eat a light breakfast.
2. Avoid caffeinated drinks. Caffeine can decrease the attention span and can overstimulate the metabolism. This reduces concentration!
3. Dress comfortably in layers.
4. Listen to traffic and weather reports beforehand.
5. Bring your flashcards for a last review while waiting to take the exam.
6. Bring test material, photo identification, admission card, and several No. 2 pencils with erasers.

Taking the Exam

As you sit down to take the CMA or RMA exam, remember these important points.

1. Take a deep breath before starting.
2. Read all directions before starting.
3. If permissible, make notes on the exam booklet.
4. Read each question carefully and analyze what is being asked.
5. Pay attention to words that are emphasized by underline, capitalization, bold, or italics.

6. Concentrate on each question. Don't wander off to other questions.
7. Do not leave any blank answers. Guessing gives you a chance to get it right.
8. Be careful when making answers on the answer sheet so that you don't skip a line or mark an incorrect circle.
9. Check your time periodically. Allow one hour per section.
10. Multiple-choice questions have one correct answer. Do not overanalyze. Give the *best* answer to the question as it is written.
11. If you don't know the answer immediately, start eliminating choices to at least two possibilities. Highlight/mark the question on the test booklet so you can return to it after finishing the rest of the test.
12. After completing the exam, check the answer sheet to make sure it is complete. Check your exam booklet for highlighted questions and return to them.
13. Before handing in the test booklet and answer sheet, make sure your identification information is on the answer sheet and that it is correct.

Multiple-Choice Questions

1. Statements that contain words such as "always," "every," "never," and "all" are usually too broad and often incorrect.
2. If two choices have the same or almost the same meaning, they are both incorrect; eliminate both choices when you select your answer.
3. Be aware of directional words such as "but," "except," and "however." They signal opposite meanings.
4. Try to answer the test question before looking at the options.
5. If you don't know the answer, eliminate the choices you know are wrong.
6. Read the question with the answer you selected to hear how they sound together.
7. To answer a multiple-choice question, you need to:
   a. find the main idea
   b. find and remember details that support the main idea
   c. draw conclusions

Scoring the CMA Exam

As you take the practice tests in preparing for the CMA exam, use the following formula to convert your raw test score (number of correct answers) into a standard test score.

$$(\text{Raw Score} \times 6.2) + 100$$

For example: If you have answered 210 questions correctly (out of 300), your raw score is 70%. Take this percentage and compute your standard score as follows:

$(70 \times 6.2) + 100$
a.) $70 \times 6.2 = 434$
b.) $434 + 100 = 534$
Your standard score is 534 (a passing score).

Note: The above formula is for the purposes of scoring the simulated exams found in this text only and is not promoted by the American Association of Medical Assistants (AAMA).

Scoring the RMA Exam

If you are preparing to take the RMA exam, use the following formula to convert your raw test score (number of correct answers) into a scaled test score.

$$(\text{Raw Score} \times 0.75) + 25$$

For example: If you have answered 134 questions correctly (out of a total 200), your raw score is 67% ($134 \div 200$). Take this percentage and compute your scaled score as follows:

$(67 \times 0.75) + 25$
a.) $67 \times 0.75 = 50$
b.) $50 + 25 = 75$
Your scaled score is 75 (a passing score).

Note: The above formula is for the purposes of scoring the simulated exams found in this text only and is not promoted by the American Medical Technologists (AMT).

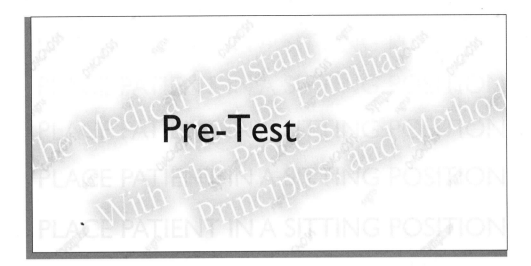

Pre-Test

Directions: Each of the following questions is followed by five possible responses. Select the *best* response by completely filling in the corresponding circle on your answer sheet. Answer sheets are located at the back of the book.

1. An abnormal increase in the size of an organ is
   A. Atrophy
   B. Hypertrophy
   C. Dystrophy
   D. Hypotrophy
   E. Visceral

2. The cell from which bone tissue develops is
   A. An erythroblast
   B. An osteoblast
   C. An osteoclast
   D. A myoblast
   E. A neuroblast

3. The abbreviation for "right eye" is
   A. OD
   B. OS
   C. OU
   D. AD
   E. AS

4. A stethoscope is used to
   A. Measure pelvic width
   B. Listen to breath sounds
   C. Inspect the external ear
   D. Measure eyeball pressure
   E. Palpate a blood pressure

5. A procedure that measures the amount of air that moves in and out of the lungs is
   A. Tracheostomy
   B. Thorocentesis
   C. Intubation
   D. Bronchoscopy
   E. Spirometry

6. Which of the following lab tests would be abnormal for a patient with diabetes?
   A. Serum acetone
   B. BUN
   C. Serum uric acid
   D. Fasting blood glucose
   E. Total cholesterol

7. A patient with leukemia would be treated by which medical specialist?
   A. Oncologist
   B. Cardiologist
   C. Gynecologist
   D. ENT
   E. Pediatrician

8. An abnormal decrease in the total number of WBCs is
   A. Leukocytosis
   B. Leukemia
   C. Leukosis
   D. Leukopenia
   E. Anemia

9. An extremely high fever is called
   A. Pyrexia
   B. Hyperpnea
   C. Hyperpyrexia
   D. Hypertension
   E. Hyperglycemia

10. Which of the following suffixes refers to eating?
   A. -cardia
   B. -phasia
   C. -algia
   D. -phagia
   E. -dipsia

11. A suffix used to denote destruction is
   A. -lysis
   B. -desis

5

C. -pexy
D. -plasty
E. -rrhaphy

12. A KUB is a radiograph of the
    A. Kidneys, uterus, bladder
    B. Kidneys, ureters, bladder
    C. Kidneys, urethra, bladder
    D. Kidneys, ureters, back
    E. Kidneys, umbilicus, bladder

13. Excessive amounts of hair on the body is synonymous with
    A. Alopecia
    B. Myopia
    C. Hirsutism
    D. Vitiligo
    E. Urticaria

14. Another term for swallowing is
    A. Obstipation
    B. Peristalsis
    C. Deglutition
    D. Herniation
    E. Regurgitation

15. A cicatrix in the popliteal area is a
    A. Blister on the shoulder
    B. Polyp on the elbow
    C. Wart on the bottom of the foot
    D. Scar on the back of the knee
    E. Mole on the wrist

16. Fluid may be obtained from a joint by which of the following?
    A. Arthrocentesis
    B. Arthritis
    C. Arthroplasty
    D. Tympanocentesis
    E. Thoracocentesis

17. Adipose tissue is
    A. Lymph
    B. Tendon
    C. Muscle
    D. Fat
    E. Skin

18. A disease process of unknown origin is referred to as
    A. Diastolic
    B. Epidemic
    C. Biologic
    D. Etiologic
    E. Idiopathic

19. The function of the optic nerve is
    A. Hearing
    B. Seeing

C. Smelling
D. Tasting
E. Touching

20. A rhinoplasty is a surgical procedure on the
    A. Uterus
    B. Nose
    C. Cornea
    D. Ear
    E. Knee

21. The study of the diseases and treatment of the male reproductive system is
    A. Nephrology
    B. Oncology
    C. Proctology
    D. Hematology
    E. Urology

22. A diagnostic procedure that internally visualizes the bronchus is
    A. Bronchogram
    B. Bronchoscopy
    C. Bronchial dilation
    D. Cholecystography
    E. Endoscopy

23. A patient with urticaria most likely has
    A. Acne vulgaris
    B. A boil
    C. Shingles
    D. Warts
    E. Hives

24. The membrane that surrounds the abdominopelvic cavity is the
    A. Perineum
    B. Pericardium
    C. Endocardium
    D. Endometrium
    E. Peritoneum

25. Which type of membrane lines cavities that open to the outside?
    A. Cutaneous
    B. Mucous
    C. Synovial
    D. Pleural
    E. Peritoneum

26. The dorsal region of the body is described as
    A. Posterior
    B. Anterior
    C. Medial
    D. Lateral
    E. Superior

27. The body cavity that contains the heart and lungs is the
    A. Abdominal
    B. Pleural
    C. Peritoneal
    D. Spinal
    E. Thoracic

28. Movement of a body part away from the midline of the body is
    A. Adduction
    B. Abduction
    C. Rotation
    D. Pronation
    E. Supination

29. The plane that divides the body into right and left halves is
    A. Transverse
    B. Coronal
    C. Frontal
    D. Sagittal
    E. Horizontal

30. An acute disorder that tends to follow viral illnesses in children is
    A. Muscular dystrophy
    B. Reye's syndrome
    C. Toxic shock syndrome
    D. AIDS
    E. Multiple sclerosis

31. The first section of the vertebral column is the
    A. Cervical
    B. Thoracic
    C. Lumbar
    D. Sacral
    E. Coccyx

32. Which of the following lesions is characterized by asymmetry, irregular borders, and change in color?
    A. Dermatofibroma
    B. Basal cell carcinoma
    C. Keratosis
    D. Squamous cell carcinoma
    E. Melanoma

33. This chronic skin condition is characterized by exacerbations and remissions of patches of scaly skin:
    A. Impetigo
    B. Psoriasis
    C. Scabies
    D. Melanoma
    E. Herpes zoster

34. The bone that makes up the forehead area of the skull is the
    A. Frontal
    B. Ethmoid
    C. Temporal
    D. Occipital
    E. Mandible

35. The peripheral nervous system is composed of how many pairs of cranial nerves?
    A. 2
    B. 5
    C. 12
    D. 20
    E. 31

36. The largest part of the brain is the
    A. Brain stem
    B. Cerebellum
    C. Cerebrum
    D. Thalamus
    E. Medulla

37. Malabsorption of vitamin B12 results in which type of anemia?
    A. Hemolytic
    B. Microcytic
    C. Pernicious
    D. Hemorrhagic
    E. Bone-marrow deficiency

38. Wheezing is a classic sign of which respiratory disease?
    A. Asthma
    B. Bronchitis
    C. Emphysema
    D. TB
    E. Atelectasis

39. Another name for the eardrum is
    A. Stapes
    B. Tympanic membrane
    C. Cochlea
    D. Oval window
    E. Organ of Corti

40. The vein that returns blood to the heart from areas below the diaphragm is the
    A. Subclavian vein
    B. Superior vena cava
    C. Inferior vena cava
    D. Axillary vein
    E. Brachiocephalic vein

41. The pacemaker of the heart is the
    A. Sinoatrial node
    B. Atrioventricular node

C. Cardiac septum
D. Bundle of His
E. Purkinje fibers

42. Which electrolyte is important for the activity of the heart muscle?
    A. Chloride
    B. Sodium
    C. Acid phosphate
    D. Potassium
    E. Bicarbonate

43. Which of the following demonstrates a voluntary muscle action?
    A. Breathing
    B. Heartbeat
    C. Peristalsis
    D. Flexion
    E. Pupil dilation

44. The prefixes apo-, de-, and ab- mean
    A. Against
    B. Before
    C. Within
    D. Outside
    E. Away from

45. Food is conveyed from the mouth to stomach by the
    A. Trachea
    B. Esophagus
    C. Salivary glands
    D. Tonsils
    E. Tongue

46. An abnormal lateral curvature of the spine is known as
    A. Kyphosis
    B. Spondylosis
    C. Lordosis
    D. Scoliosis
    E. Ankylosis

47. The beta cells in the pancreas are responsible for the production of
    A. Glucagon
    B. HCl
    C. Insulin
    D. Gastrin
    E. Pepsin

48. The creation of an opening in the abdomen to bring some portion of the colon onto the surface is a
    A. Cholecystectomy
    B. Gastropexy
    C. Gastrostomy

D. Colectomy
E. Colostomy

49. The cranial nerve that is involved in the sense of smell is the
    A. Facial
    B. Oculomotor
    C. Trigeminal
    D. Olfactory
    E. Optic

50. To confirm a fracture of the lower leg, a radiograph should include the
    A. Femur and trochanter
    B. Tibia and fibula
    C. Radius and ulna
    D. Femur and patella
    E. Humerus and scapula

51. Deaths must be reported to a coroner in each of the following situations *except*
    A. Violence
    B. Industrial injuries
    C. Occurring while in custody of the law
    D. Following long-term illnesses
    E. Occurring without medical attendance

52. A complimentary close that is appropriate for a business letter is
    A. As ever
    B. Regards
    C. Respectfully
    D. Medically yours
    E. Sincerely yours

53. A physician performed a breast augmentation on a patient and later published an article with photos of the patient in a medical journal. The patient did not give permission to publish the pictures. This constitutes
    A. Negligence
    B. Fraud
    C. Assault
    D. Invasion of privacy
    E. Battery

54. Which is *not* an example of anxiety?
    A. Not hearing instructions
    B. Asking relevant questions
    C. Frequent use of the bathroom
    D. Moist hands
    E. Frequently moistening the lips

55. Which is *not* a criterion for establishing negligence?
    A. Duty owed
    B. Dereliction of duty

C. Direct cause
D. Damages
E. Informed consent

56. The initial report for a workers' compensation claim should be filed
    A. After a diagnosis is established
    B. After the patient requests
    C. Immediately after the initial visit
    D. After the patient is discharged
    E. After the insurance company requests it

57. When a physician accepts a patient for treatment, the physician has a duty to
    A. Be free from errors in judgment
    B. Guarantee a successful surgical outcome
    C. Use care, diligence, and skill in treatment
    D. Restore the patient to better condition than before treatment began
    E. Make sure the patient has insurance coverage

58. Which of the following patients would require a legal agent to consent to surgery?
    A. A six-year-old child
    B. A 21-year-old woman for elective plastic surgery
    C. A 90-year-old mentally competent woman
    D. A 19-year-old married woman
    E. A 22-year-old man with diabetes

59. Under "Respondent Superior," the physician may be held liable for which of the following?
    A. The pharmacist who fills the prescription incorrectly
    B. The hospital lab tech who performs a lab test incorrectly
    C. An intern at the hospital who injures a patient
    D. A medical assistant who administers an incorrect medicine
    E. The insurance company

60. Patients are most likely to remember instructions when
    A. The most important information is given first
    B. The instructions are given verbally
    C. Medical terms are used
    D. The instructions are detailed
    E. Instructions are given hurriedly

61. When communicating with a hearing-impaired person,
    A. Speak loudly
    B. Speak naturally
    C. Use medical terms
    D. Speak quickly
    E. Do not maintain eye contact

62. When a physician treats a Medicaid patient, the physician agrees
    A. To accept payment in full from the patient
    B. To accept the fee approved by Medicaid as payment in full
    C. To accept Medicaid payment and bill patient for balance
    D. To submit the claim to Medicaid
    E. To charge the patient a copayment

63. Which of the following is subjective information?
    A. Lab reports
    B. Treatment modalities
    C. EKG reports
    D. Past surgical history
    E. Diagnosis

64. When the release of medical records is authorized, the medical assistant should
    A. Give the patient the original record
    B. Notify the insurance company
    C. Have the physician sign a release form
    D. Give the patient a copy of the original records
    E. All of the above

65. Which is *not* an element of the communication process?
    A. Channel
    B. Source
    C. Message
    D. Receiver
    E. Noise

66. Elisabeth Kubler-Ross established
    A. The five stages of dying
    B. Nursing care practices
    C. The hierarchy of needs
    D. A communication process
    E. The AAMA

67. All of the following are considered a tort except
    A. Abandonment
    B. Assault and battery
    C. Breach of contract
    D. Defamation of character
    E. Invasion of privacy

68. Which of the following is a mandatory form of credential?
    A. Regulation
    B. Licensure
    C. Certification
    D. Registration
    E. Accreditation

69. The opposite of lateral is
    A. Proximal
    B. Anterior

C. Medial
D. Distal
E. Posterior

70. Communication can best be defined as
   A. The process of sharing meaning
   B. The process of talking
   C. The process of explaining
   D. The process of nonverbal actions
   E. The process of analyzing meaning

71. Which of the following documentation situations could create a liability?
   A. Altering a document
   B. Failing to document a procedure
   C. Recording incorrect information
   D. Scribbling out an error
   E. All of the above

72. The basic structural and functional unit of the body is the
   A. Cell
   B. Tissues
   C. Organs
   D. Organ system
   E. Nucleus

73. A group of similar cells make up
   A. Organs
   B. Organ systems
   C. Organelles
   D. Tissue
   E. Glands

74. The outer membrane of a bone is the
   A. Diaphysis
   B. Epiphysis
   C. Endosteum
   D. Periosteum
   E. Marrow

75. Types of muscle tissue include
   A. Smooth muscle
   B. Cardiac muscle
   C. Skeletal muscle
   D. A and C
   E. A, B, and C

76. The heart muscle is the
   A. Pericardium
   B. Myocardium
   C. Endocardium
   D. Ventricle
   E. Epicardium

77. Another name for the voice box is the
   A. Pharynx
   B. Larynx

C. Trachea
D. Paranasal sinus
E. Vocal cords

78. The primary site of absorption of nutrients is the
   A. Mouth
   B. Stomach
   C. Small intestines
   D. Large intestine
   E. Liver

79. Which is *not* a function of the urinary system?
   A. Eliminate waste
   B. Regulate salt levels
   C. Balance water gain and loss
   D. Production of insulin
   E. Regulate pH balance

80. The region between the vaginal opening and the rectum is the
   A. Peritoneum
   B. Perineum
   C. Hymen
   D. Fimbriae
   E. Labia majora

81. Male sterilization is performed on the
   A. Epididymis
   B. Fallopian tubes
   C. Vas deferens
   D. Seminal vesicles
   E. Prostate gland

82. The central nervous system is made up of
   A. Peripheral nerves
   B. Neurons
   C. Brain and spinal cord
   D. Brain
   E. Spinal cord

83. The brainstem is made up of the
   A. Midbrain
   B. Pons
   C. Medulla oblongata
   D. None of the above
   E. All of the above

84. Olfactory receptors are located in the
   A. Mouth
   B. Nose
   C. Ear
   D. Eye
   E. Skin

85. The ''master gland'' is the
   A. Brain
   B. Hypothalamus

C. Pituitary gland
D. Thyroid gland
E. Pancreas

86. One who specializes in the study of cells is
    A. Cytology
    B. Cytologist
    C. Histology
    D. Histologist
    E. Pathologist

87. The abbreviation meaning "four times a day" is
    A. bid
    B. tid
    C. qid
    D. qod
    E. q4h

88. Which is not a common reaction to illness?
    A. Fear
    B. Depression
    C. Anxiety
    D. Euphoria
    E. Stress

89. The prefix "hypo-" means
    A. Above
    B. Below
    C. Excessive
    D. Skin
    E. Before

90. An oncologist
    A. Diagnoses and treats female reproductive disorders
    B. Delivers babies
    C. Cares for infants and children
    D. Diagnoses and treats cancers
    E. Administers anesthesia

91. Rendering care to a patient without consent could result in a charge of
    A. Rape
    B. Battery
    C. Slander
    D. Libel
    E. Abuse

92. A commitment or obligation to act in certain way(s) is a(n)
    A. Duty
    B. Beneficence
    C. Ethic
    D. Veracity
    E. Right

93. The medical assistant's signature on an informed consent form means that the medical assistant
    A. Prepared the form
    B. Explained the procedure to the patient
    C. Witnessed the discussion of the procedure between the physician and patient
    D. Verified the patient's signature
    E. Verified the physician's signature

94. Poor eye contact is an example of
    A. Therapeutic communication
    B. Verbal communication
    C. Nontherapeutic communication
    D. Nonverbal communication
    E. Silence

95. A person's failure to act in a prudent and reasonable manner is known as
    A. Negligence
    B. Malpractice
    C. Dereliction of duty
    D. Assault
    E. Intent

96. Athlete's foot is also called
    A. Pediculosis
    B. Moniliasis
    C. Tinea pedis
    D. Tinea cruris
    E. An abrasion

97. Small, purple hemorrhagic spots on the skin are called
    A. Bruises
    B. Petechiae
    C. Ecchymosis
    D. Thrombosis
    E. Acupuncture

98. Suppuration means
    A. Blood formation
    B. Dryness
    C. Mucus formation
    D. Pus formation
    E. Urine formation

99. Which is *not* a disease process of the skin
    A. Dermatitis
    B. Urticaria
    C. Eclampsia
    D. Impetigo
    E. Psoriasis

100. Coryza is associated with
    A. The common cold
    B. Pinkeye
    C. Rash

D. Indigestion

E. Fainting

101. The matrix of a schedule is the
    A. Hospital calls
    B. Times available
    C. Times not available
    D. Facilities available
    E. Staff available

102. Scheduling patients with the same medical complaints on the same day is
    A. Wave scheduling
    B. Modified wave scheduling
    C. Open hours
    D. Grouping scheduling
    E. Double booking

103. A major advantage of using a computer for word processing is
    A. Extensive editing capability
    B. Speed of processing
    C. Spell-check
    D. Column layout
    E. Storage capacity

104. Which is *not* true of certified mail?
    A. Insurance coverage is available
    B. Receipt of delivery can be obtained for a fee
    C. Only first-class mail can be certified
    D. Record of delivery is kept by the Post Office
    E. Restricted delivery can be obtained for a fee

105. Which of the following must be sent by first-class mail?
    A. Magazines
    B. Books
    C. Printed materials
    D. Personal letters and postcards
    E. Equipment catalogues

106. A Medicare claim for a deceased beneficiary may be paid directly to the physician if
    A. The physician accepts assignment
    B. The spouse assigns benefits to the physician
    C. Social Security verifies Medicare coverage
    D. Charges are paid by the intermediary
    E. The estate is billed

107. All checks received as payment for charges should be endorsed
    A. Immediately
    B. At the end of the day
    C. When they are deposited
    D. After they are posted
    E. Monthly

108. In an alphabetic file, which is filed first?
    A. A. R. Stephenson
    B. John Stephenson
    C. George Stephens
    D. Ann Stephenson-Bailey
    E. Andrew Stephen

109. A superbill
    A. Is given to a patient who has been seen by two or more physicians within a clinic
    B. Is a form designed to help in filing insurance claims
    C. Is a combined bill from the physician and the hospital
    D. Is a complete accounting system
    E. Lists all accounts receivable

110. Which is correct for an inside address?
    A. Dr. David Roberts
    B. Dr. David Roberts, M.D.
    C. Mr. David Roberts, M.D.
    D. Roberts, David, M.D.
    E. David Roberts, M.D.

111. Which is *not* true about a postage meter?
    A. It prints its own postage
    B. Some can seal the envelope
    C. It locks when the postage is used up
    D. The mailer leases the machine and purchases the postage
    E. A license must be obtained from the Post Office

112. The two-letter abbreviation for Nebraska is
    A. NB
    B. NE
    C. NA
    D. NR
    E. NK

113. Which letter style requires the complimentary closing and typed signature be placed in line with the left margin of the body of the letter?
    A. Block style
    B. Semiblock style
    C. Full block style
    D. Indented style
    E. Semi-indented style

114. Which of the following is *not* included in a memorandum?
    A. Date
    B. Subject
    C. Complimentary close
    D. Writer's name
    E. Reference initials

115. The second page of a two-page letter contains
which of the following in the heading?
- **A.** Name and date
- **B.** Name and page number
- **C.** Name, page number, and date
- **D.** Name, page number, date, and subject
- **E.** Name, writer's name, subject, and date

116. The complimentary close of a letter is typed how
many lines below the last line of the body?
- **A.** Two
- **B.** Three
- **C.** Four
- **D.** Five
- **E.** Ten

117. A computer program is
- **A.** Hardware
- **B.** Software
- **C.** Network
- **D.** Server
- **E.** Input device

118. A fee profile is derived from
- **A.** Insurance payments
- **B.** Patient's payments
- **C.** Government payments
- **D.** Physician charges
- **E.** Insurance charges

119. Which of the following is demographic informa-
tion included in a medical record?
- **A.** Present illness
- **B.** Date of birth
- **C.** Lab reports
- **D.** X-ray findings
- **E.** Complete physical exam

120. ICD-9-CM coding applies to
- **A.** Proctoscopy
- **B.** Pap smear
- **C.** Appendectomy
- **D.** Irritable bowel syndrome
- **E.** Mastectomy

121. When it is 4:00 P.M. in New York City, what time
is it in Seattle, WA?
- **A.** 12:00 P.M.
- **B.** 1:00 P.M.
- **C.** 2:00 P.M.
- **D.** 3:00 P.M.
- **E.** 4:00 P.M.

122. Which of the following is available to depen-
dents of active-duty military personnel?
- **A.** CHAMPVA
- **B.** Workers' compensation

- **C.** PPO
- **D.** Medicaid
- **E.** CHAMPUS

123. Ideally, a phone should be answered before the
- **A.** Second ring
- **B.** Third ring
- **C.** Fourth ring
- **D.** Fifth ring
- **E.** The other line picks up the call

124. An E code in the ICD-9-CM coding system
- **A.** Refers to external causes
- **B.** Refers to hypertension
- **C.** Refers to neoplasms
- **D.** Refers to suicide attempt
- **E.** Refers to disease

125. The universal claim form developed by HCFA is
- **A.** Form 1904
- **B.** ICD-9
- **C.** Form 1040
- **D.** HCFA-1500
- **E.** HCFA-1999

126. Patients who are always late or who habitually
cancel appointments should be scheduled
- **A.** First in the morning
- **B.** Right before lunch
- **C.** Midafternoon
- **D.** At the end of the day
- **E.** On Fridays

127. In which of the following do physicians provide
services on a discounted fee-for-service basis?
- **A.** A PPO
- **B.** An HMO
- **C.** Medicare
- **D.** Workers' compensation
- **E.** Private insurance carrier

128. An error was made in charting the patient's rec-
ord. The method used to correct the error is to
- **A.** Erase the error and write in the correction
- **B.** Re-enter the notation on the next line
- **C.** Draw a single line through the error, write
the word "error," make the correction, date
and initial the entry
- **D.** Cross out the error and make the correction
in the margin
- **E.** Cross out the entry and correct it.

129. SOAP is an acronym for
- **A.** Child protection services
- **B.** A medical assistant society
- **C.** Source-oriented medical records

D. Problem-oriented progress notes

E. Traditional medical records

130. A patient refuses to follow medical advice and the physician decides to terminate the relationship. The letter to the patient should state all of the following *except*

A. A referral to another physician

B. An offer to make records available

C. That the physician withdraws from the case

D. A future date after which the physician is not available

E. That the patient still needs medical care

131. When the medical office works on a fixed appointment schedule and a patient arrives without an appointment requesting to see the physician, the patient

A. Should be sent away

B. Should be referred to another physician

C. Should be called as soon as there is a cancellation

D. Should be told to come back tomorrow

E. Should be squeezed in for a brief visit so the physician can decide what the next treatment step should be

132. If a patient calls to cancel his or her appointment

A. Express regret

B. Immediately offer a new appointment time

C. Have the patient speak to the office manager

D. Discourage cancellations sternly

E. All of the above

133. A good telephone technique is a

A. High-pitched voice

B. Low-pitched and expressive voice

C. Monotone voice

D. Breathless and excited voice

E. Soft-spoken voice

134. A pegboard system is often referred to as

A. A trial-balance system

B. A basic system

C. A daily accounting system

D. A write-it-once system

E. A write-it-twice system

135. The process of recording transactions to an account

A. Journalizing

B. Posting

C. Debiting

D. Crediting

E. Editing

136. If a patient's account has been turned over to a collection agency and the patient calls about the bill, the patient should be told

A. To remit payment to the physician's office

B. To deal with the collection agency

C. To talk with the office manager

D. To disregard further statements

E. To find another physician

137. Preparing the magnetic surface of a blank disk to accept data is done by

A. Blocking

B. Formatting

C. Revealing

D. RAM

E. Merging

138. The entry, editing, manipulation, and storage of text using the computer is

A. Telecommunications

B. Documentation

C. Interfacing

D. Word processing

E. Formatting

139. When a shipment of supplies is received, the supplies should be checked against the

A. Advertised prices

B. Enclosed packing slip

C. Invoice

D. Requisition slip

E. Inventory

140. A credit balance on an account occurs when

A. The patient's check was returned for insufficient funds

B. The insurance company disallows the claim

C. The patient pays in advance

D. A discount is given

E. The patient is sent to collection

141. An endorsement that contains a signature and a "for deposit only" statement is known as

A. Blank

B. Restrictive

C. Special

D. Third-party

E. Certified

142. Which of the following abbreviations is not correct?

A. Feb.

B. T_4

C. Rh

D. mm Hg

E. bl pr

143. For payment purposes, Medicare is primary to
    A. Medicaid
    B. Disability insurance
    C. Workers' compensation
    D. HMO
    E. PPO

144. A procedure was charted but not performed. The entry in the medical record should
    A. Be erased
    B. Be crossed out
    C. Have a single line drawn through it and marked "error"
    D. Have a single line drawn through it and marked "not done"
    E. Be left alone

145. A signature stamp may be used for
    A. "Return to school" forms
    B. Workers' compensation claims
    C. Transcribed operative notes
    D. Disability reports
    E. Dictated discharge summaries

146. The complimentary close may be omitted in which letter style?
    A. Block
    B. Semiblock
    C. Modified block
    D. Simplified
    E. Open punctuation

147. Failure to assign insurance benefits results in
    A. Payments made to the patient
    B. Claim rejection
    C. A write-off
    D. Less-than-usual payment amounts
    E. Collection proceedings

148. For an ICD-9 code to be valid, the maximum number of code digits is
    A. Six
    B. Five
    C. Four
    D. Three
    E. Ten or more

149. Which is true of the medical record?
    A. If it is not recorded, it was not done
    B. The patient owns the information
    C. The physician owns the record
    D. A signed release is waived if the record is subpoenaed
    E. All of the above

150. The portion of a fee that the patient with insurance must pay is called the
    A. Cost of coverage
    B. Premium
    C. Copayment
    D. Coordination of benefits
    E. Claim

151. The fastest type of U.S. mail service is
    A. Certified
    B. First class
    C. Second class
    D. Fourth class
    E. Express

152. Which of the following steps in the filing process checks for and repairs damaged documents?
    A. Storing
    B. Inspecting
    C. Conditioning
    D. Indexing
    E. Releasing

153. The insurance company that sells and administers a policy is called the
    A. Carrier
    B. Policy holder
    C. Provider
    D. Beneficiary
    E. Vendor

154. A check may be dishonored for which of the following reasons?
    A. Overdraft
    B. Postdated
    C. NSF
    D. All of the above
    E. None of the above

155. Which is *not* considered to be a closing of a letter?
    A. Salutation
    B. Complimentary closing
    C. Signature line
    D. Enclosure notation
    E. Reference notation

156. Which is *not* recorded when taking a telephone message?
    A. Date of call
    B. Time of call
    C. Message
    D. Person called
    E. Caller's Social Security number

157. The most common color-coding system color codes the
    A. Physician's name
    B. Patient's given name
    C. Patient's surname

D. Patient's demographic data
E. Patient's Social Security number

158. A physician must accept assignment on all of the following patients *except*
    A. Medicaid
    B. Independent commercial carriers
    C. Title 19
    D. CHAMPUS
    E. Workers' compensation

159. "Dear Mrs. McEvoy:" is an example of the
    A. Signature line
    B. Complimentary close
    C. Inside address
    D. Salutation
    E. Certified mail

160. A patient calls to cancel an appointment. This should be noted by
    A. Writing the date and "canceled" in the chart
    B. Writing "canceled" in the appointment book
    C. Sending a letter and confirming the cancellation
    D. Both A and B
    E. All of the above

161. A disadvantage of alphabetic filing is
    A. Difficulty in classifying
    B. Misfiling common names
    C. Difficulty in retrieving
    D. Difficulty in indexing
    E. Incompatibility with color-coding

162. Which of the following must always match the deposits for the month?
    A. Accounts receivable
    B. Received on account
    C. Total of ledger cards
    D. Patient charges
    E. Accounts payable

163. The reason for clearly marking an allergy in a patient's chart is
    A. It is unpredictable
    B. It is dangerous to the providers
    C. It is closely related to drug therapies
    D. It is infectious
    E. It is long-lasting

164. Which of the following telephone calls from a patient should not be charted?
    A. A request for a change in appointment time
    B. A request for a prescription renewal
    C. A request for a referral to a specialist

D. Patient report that symptoms have disappeared
E. A pharmacist's request for a prescription renewal

165. A patient may base his or her perception of the medical office on
    A. Previous experiences at this office
    B. Previous medical care experiences
    C. The attitude and appearance of the receptionist
    D. Fear
    E. Charges of care

166. Who is the "responsible person" on the new patient information form?
    A. The patient
    B. The parent
    C. The insurance company
    D. The person who will pay the bill
    E. The referring physician

167. What information is needed to properly matrix the appointment book?
    A. Hours of hospital rounds
    B. Times to schedule routine physical exams
    C. Hours for walk-ins
    D. Patient preferences for appointment times
    E. Times for immunization clinics

168. Which of the following dates is correctly written for the heading of a business letter?
    A. 12/30/00
    B. Dec. 30th, 2000
    C. December 30, 2000
    D. December 30, '00
    E. 30/12/00

169. Why should all documents be proofread, even if spell-check is used?
    A. Correctly spelled words may be used incorrectly
    B. Sometimes errors are missed
    C. There is no spell-check for medical terms
    D. Spell-check is expensive to use
    E. All of the above

170. The purpose of OUT guides is to ensure
    A. That folders do not slide under the others
    B. That temporary folders can be easily identified
    C. Files are easy to find in the drawer
    D. The place to replace a file
    E. Help with correct alphabetical order

171. If a patient's insurance has a $15.00 copay for an office visit, who pays the copay?
    A. The insurance company
    B. The patient

C. The patient's employer
D. Copays cannot be collected
E. Supplemental insurance

172. If a required preauthorization is not obtained for a procedure, who is responsible for the charges?
A. The referring physician
B. The physician performing the procedure
C. The patient
D. The insurance company
E. The patient's employer

173. Which is *not* considered to be an input device?
A. Keyboard
B. Light pen
C. Mouse
D. Printer
E. Joystick

174. Which of the following is objective information?
A. Health habits
B. High blood pressure
C. Previous illnesses
D. Medical insurance
E. Family history

175. Accounts receivable include
A. Petty cash
B. Listing of patient account cards
C. Summary of amount owed physician by patients
D. Summary of charges over a period of time
E. Record of daily office financial activity

176. A key element in standard precautions is
A. Handling all blood and body fluids as if they are infected
B. Wearing gloves when handling specimens
C. Washing hands before handling specimens
D. Handling body secretions with care
E. Handling blood-stained items with care

177. The most important function of handwashing is to
A. Remove infectious microorganisms
B. Sterilize the hands
C. Clean the hands
D. Kill infectious microorganisms
E. Keep healthcare workers free from Hepatitis B

178. Used disposable syringes and needles must be disposed of in
A. The nearest trash can
B. A sharps container
C. A biohazard box

D. A biohazard bag
E. A waste container with a lid

179. The normal pulse rate for an adult is
A. 60-80 beats per minute
B. 80-90 beats per minute
C. 80-120 beats per minute
D. 110-130 beats per minute
E. 130-160 beats per minute

180. The pulse rate is
A. Usually higher in adults than children
B. Usually higher in children than adults
C. The same for adults and children
D. Usually lower in children than adults
E. Usually higher in adults than infants

181. On an initial exam for a new patient, the blood pressure should be taken on
A. The left arm of a right-handed patient
B. The right arm of a left-handed patient
C. The right arm
D. The left arm
E. Both arms

182. Pulse rate can be increased by
A. Hypothyroidism
B. Fear
C. Fever
D. Physical activity
E. B, C, and D

183. A rectal temperature registers approximately how many degrees higher than an oral temperature?
A. 1 degree C
B. 2 degrees C
C. 3 degrees F
D. 2 degrees F
E. 1 degree F

184. The carotid artery is located
A. At the temple
B. On the upper surface of the foot
C. At the right and left sides of the neck
D. At the back of the knee
E. In the groin

185. A patient who weighs 150 pounds also weighs
A. 52.12 kg
B. 58.91 kg
C. 67.5 kg
D. 68.18 kg
E. 88.45 kg

186. A patient who is 65 inches tall is
A. 5 feet, 3 inches
B. 5 feet, 5 inches

    C. 5 feet, 6 inches
    D. 6 feet
    E. 6 feet, 2 inches

187. The probable outcome of a disease process in a patient is the
    A. Prodrome
    B. Diagnosis
    C. Syndrome
    D. Prognosis
    E. Cure

188. A stethoscope is used during
    A. Auscultation
    B. Palpation
    C. Mensuration
    D. Percussion
    E. Inspection

189. Additional tests that may be performed as part of a complete physical exam would be
    A. EEG
    B. BUN
    C. O&P
    D. CBC
    E. IVP

190. A Pap smear can detect
    A. Unusual cell growth on the cervix
    B. Unusual cell growth on the rectum
    C. Unusual cell growth in the colon
    D. Unusual cell growth in the bladder
    E. STDs

191. Patients should be instructed not to douche, use creams, or foams, or have intercourse for how long before a Pap smear?
    A. No restrictions
    B. 8–12 hours
    C. 12–18 hours
    D. 18–22 hours
    E. 24–48 hours

192. How many feet away from the Snellen Chart should the patient stand or sit?
    A. 10
    B. 20
    C. 30
    D. 40
    E. 50

193. A patient lying on the back with feet placed in stirrups is in the
    A. Lithotomy position
    B. Jackknife position
    C. Knee-chest position
    D. Trendelenburg position
    E. Fowler's position

194. An audiometer is used to measure
    A. Vision
    B. Pupil reaction to light
    C. Hearing
    D. Deep reflexes
    E. Color vision

195. For a sigmoidoscopy, a patient should be placed in which of the following positions?
    A. Sims'
    B. Lithotomy
    C. Prone
    D. Trendelenburg
    E. Supine

196. If a patient's vision is recorded as OS 20/40, this would mean that the patient can read with
    A. Both eyes at 20 feet what a normal eye can read at 40 feet
    B. The right eye at 40 feet what a normal eye can read at 20 feet
    C. The right eye at 20 feet what a normal eye can read at 40 feet
    D. The left eye at 20 feet what a normal eye can read at 40 feet
    E. The left eye at 40 feet what a normal eye can read at 20 feet

197. Routine blood tests that may be performed at an initial obstetrical exam include
    A. CBC, VDRL, glucose, and blood chemistries
    B. CBC and glucose
    C. CBC, glucose, blood type and Rh
    D. CBC, blood type and Rh, VDRL, HIV, and rubella titer
    E. CBC, cholesterol, glucose, and HIV

198. A substance that is capable of inhibiting the growth of microorganisms and is safe for use on body tissues is a(n)
    A. Germicide
    B. Antibiotic
    C. Antiseptic
    D. Disinfectant
    E. Soap

199. The most common temperature and pressure used to sterilize in an autoclave are
    A. Temp: 350° F; pressure: 20 lb
    B. Temp: 250° F; pressure: 15 lb
    C. Temp: 250° F; pressure: 20 lb
    D. Temp: 150° F; pressure: 15 lb
    E. Temp: 150° F; pressure: 20 lb

200. The complete destruction of all forms of microbial life is
   A. Medical asepsis
   B. Sanitization
   C. Disinfection
   D. Sterilization
   E. Germicide

201. Instruments that are sterilized should be used
   A. Immediately
   B. Within 24 hours
   C. Within 1 week
   D. Within 1 month
   E. Before they cool down

202. The type of immunity that develops when an antigen is introduced into the body is
   A. Passive
   B. Active
   C. Natural
   D. Maternal
   E. Unnatural

203. The type of immunity that results from an immunization is called
   A. Passive
   B. Artificial passive
   C. Natural active
   D. Artificial active
   E. Congenital

204. Of the following group, the thickest suture material is
   A. 10-0
   B. 4-0
   C. 000
   D. 00
   E. 0

205. Transfer forceps are removed from the container with the prongs
   A. Separated and facing upward
   B. Separated and facing downward
   C. Together and facing upward
   D. Together and facing downward
   E. Touching the side of the container to remove excess fluid

206. Betadine (providone-iodine) may be used for
   A. Cleaning the sterile field
   B. Handwashing before a medical procedure
   C. Disinfecting the skin at the surgical site
   D. Disinfecting instruments
   E. Marking the surgical site

207. Incision into, and removal of, a part of a lesion is a(n)
   A. Aspiration biopsy
   B. Incisional biopsy
   C. Excisional biopsy
   D. Punch biopsy
   E. Needle biopsy

208. The angle for the insertion of the needle for an IM injection is
   A. 10-15 degrees
   B. 30 degrees
   C. 45 degrees
   D. 90 degrees
   E. Not important

209. A needle for a subcutaneous injection is inserted at which angle?
   A. 15 degrees
   B. 30 degrees
   C. 45 degrees
   D. 90 degrees
   E. 60 degrees

210. A topical medication
   A. Is injected
   B. Is applied to the skin
   C. Is placed under the tongue
   D. Is placed between the cheek and gum
   E. Is swallowed

211. The size and gauge of the needle for a subcutaneous injection are
   A. 1½ inch, 21 gauge
   B. 1 inch, 25 gauge
   C. ¼ inch, 21 gauge
   D. ⅝ inch, 22 gauge
   E. ⅝ inch, 25 gauge

212. A drug that is used to relieve pain is an
   A. Antidote
   B. Antidepressant
   C. Anesthetic
   D. Analgesic
   E. Antiemetic

213. The physician orders 500 mg Amoxil to be given to the patient. The stock on hand is 250 mg per capsule. How many capsules would be given to the patient?
   A. ½ capsule
   B. 2 capsules
   C. 3 capsules
   D. 1 capsule
   E. 5 capsules

214. When a lab report is received in the office, it should be
    A. Filed in the patient's chart
    B. Filed in the patient's chart only if normal
    C. Filed in the patient's chart only if abnormal
    D. Given to the physician to review
    E. Given to the physician to review only if abnormal

215. A stool specimen is tarry and black. This may indicate
    A. Ulcerative colitis
    B. Biliary obstruction
    C. UTI
    D. Upper gastrointestinal bleeding
    E. Lower gastrointestinal bleeding

216. A medication that may interfere with accurate Hemoccult results is
    A. Antibiotics
    B. Vasodilators
    C. Aspirin
    D. Diuretic
    E. Vitamin E

217. Pyuria is
    A. Blood in stool
    B. Pus in sputum
    C. Pus in urine
    D. Blood in urine
    E. Blood in sputum

218. An important symptom of diabetes mellitus is
    A. Oliguria
    B. Glycosuria
    C. Anuria
    D. Proteinuria
    E. Hematuria

219. The most common sites used for venipuncture are the
    A. Superior and inferior vena cavae
    B. Great saphenous veins
    C. Cephalic and basilic veins
    D. Femoral and cephalic veins
    E. Brachial and basilic veins

220. Blood collected in a tube with EDTA added would be used for
    A. Blood alcohol levels
    B. Hematology studies
    C. Blood chemistries
    D. Coagulation studies
    E. Total cholesterol panel

221. An effective X-ray exam used for detecting early breast cancer is
    A. Thermography
    B. CAT scan
    C. Tomography
    D. Xeroradiography
    E. Mammography

222. The therapeutic use of cold is referred to as
    A. Diathermy
    B. Cryotherapy
    C. Thermotherapy
    D. Electrotherapy
    E. Hydrotherapy

223. Another term for rapid heart beat is
    A. Tachycardia
    B. Bradycardia
    C. Myocardial infarction
    D. Fibrillation
    E. Defibrillation

224. This wave on an EKG represents the contraction of the ventricles
    A. P
    B. QRS
    C. T
    D. U
    E. R

225. Each cardiac cycle takes approximately
    A. 0.1 second
    B. 0.8 second
    C. 1 second
    D. 1 minute
    E. 80 seconds

226. For the universally accepted standardization of the EKG, the stylus should deflect
    A. 5 mm
    B. 10 mm
    C. 15 mm
    D. 20 mm
    E. 25 mm

227. It is best to use which of the following in a steam autoclave
    A. Tap water
    B. Tap water and baking soda
    C. Tap water and vinegar
    D. Distilled water
    E. Saline solution

228. The timing of an autoclave load begins when
    A. The door is secured
    B. The pressure begins to rise
    C. The desired temperature is reached
    D. The chamber is preheated
    E. Steam flows from the exhaust vent

229. A common lab test that may be ordered for a patient who is on Lasix (furosemide) is
A. WBC count
B. Hemoglobin determination
C. Sed rate
D. Cholesterol level
E. Potassium determination

230. A dressing that adheres to a wound may be soaked off with
A. Alcohol
B. Benzoin
C. Hydrogen peroxide
D. Betadine
E. Sterile saline

231. The artery that is used most often to take a blood pressure is the
A. Temporal
B. Femoral
C. Dorsalis pedis
D. Radial
E. Brachial

232. Hematocrit is the
A. Coagulation of blood
B. Concentration of hemoglobin
C. Volume of packed cells
D. Number of red blood cells in a sample
E. Number of white blood cells in a sample

233. For proper insertion of a needle for venipuncture, the needle should be inserted
A. Bevel up, about ½ inch penetration
B. Bevel down, about ½ inch penetration
C. Bevel up, entire length of needle inserted
D. Bevel down, entire length of needle inserted
E. Bevel in any position, ½ inch penetration

234. Which cannot be detected on a urine dipstick?
A. Bilirubin
B. Casts
C. Ketones
D. Blood
E. Glucose

235. The pulse rate taken at the wrist uses which of the following arteries?
A. Femoral
B. Brachial
C. Radial
D. Temporal
E. Carotid

236. The best urine sample to use for a pregnancy test is a
A. 24-hour specimen
B. Random sample
C. 2-hour post-prandial
D. Second-voided specimen
E. First morning specimen

237. A lens on the microscope is 100x. The ocular is 10x. Total magnification would be
A. 10
B. 100
C. 1,000
D. 10,000
E. 100,000

238. Sedimentation rate can be used to screen for
A. Cardiovascular function
B. Liver function
C. Kidney function
D. Blood clotting
E. Inflammation

239. The hematocrit is approximately
A. Three times the hemoglobin
B. Four times the hemoglobin
C. Two times the hemoglobin
D. The same as the hemoglobin
E. Less than the hemoglobin

240. Which urinary constituents are not reported on a urinalysis?
A. Casts
B. RBCs
C. WBCs
D. Artifacts
E. Trichomonas vaginalis

241. According to the food pyramid, which of the following groups of nutrients should be consumed the most?
A. Dairy products
B. Oils and fats
C. Grains
D. Fruits
E. Vegetables

242. Characteristics of the pulse include all of the following *except*
A. Depth
B. Texture of the artery wall
C. Volume
D. Rate
E. Rhythm

243. A sudden loss of blood or body fluids may cause
A. Cardiogenic shock
B. Hypovolemic shock
C. Anaphylactic shock
D. Neurogenic shock
E. Death

244. *Candida albicans* is the most common cause of
  - **A.** The common cold
  - **B.** UTI
  - **C.** URI
  - **D.** Yeast infection
  - **E.** Malaria

245. The position of lead V-1 is the
  - **A.** Third intercostal space left of the sternum
  - **B.** Fourth intercostal space right of the sternum
  - **C.** Third intercostal space right of the sternum
  - **D.** Fourth intercostal space left of the sternum
  - **E.** Left leg

246. The official name of a drug is its
  - **A.** Trade name
  - **B.** Generic name
  - **C.** Common name
  - **D.** Chemical name
  - **E.** Medical name

247. Which of the following needles is the largest?
  - **A.** 19 gauge
  - **B.** 21 gauge
  - **C.** 23 gauge
  - **D.** 25 gauge
  - **E.** 27 gauge

248. The classification of a drug that destroys bacteria is an
  - **A.** Antifungal
  - **B.** Antibiotic
  - **C.** Antitussive
  - **D.** Anti-inflammatory
  - **E.** Antipyretic

249. The rhythm strip on an EKG is the same as
  - **A.** Lead V-1
  - **B.** aVR
  - **C.** Lead I
  - **D.** Lead II
  - **E.** Lead III

250. When a specimen is being prepared for transport to an outside lab, specimen labels should be affixed to the
  - **A.** Requisition form
  - **B.** Container
  - **C.** Lid
  - **D.** All of the above
  - **E.** A and B

251. *Helicobacter pylori* has been discovered to be a possible cause of
  - **A.** Colitis
  - **B.** Food poisoning
  - **C.** Head lice
  - **D.** Ulcers
  - **E.** Cold sores

252. A common medication that is contraindicated for use in children because of the link to Reye's syndrome is
  - **A.** Acetaminophen
  - **B.** Aspirin
  - **C.** Benadryl
  - **D.** Ibuprofen
  - **E.** Penicillin

253. Another term for pain when urinating is
  - **A.** Hematuria
  - **B.** Anuria
  - **C.** Dysuria
  - **D.** Pyuria
  - **E.** Polyuria

254. Which blood element is involved in the coagulation process?
  - **A.** Platelets
  - **B.** WBCs
  - **C.** RBCs
  - **D.** Plasma
  - **E.** Protein

255. A drug that is given parenterally is given
  - **A.** By mouth
  - **B.** By injection
  - **C.** By application to the skin
  - **D.** By a parent
  - **E.** Under the tongue

256. Another name for earwax is
  - **A.** Catharsis
  - **B.** Canthus
  - **C.** Conjunctive
  - **D.** Cerumen
  - **E.** Sebum

257. The normal value range for a hematocrit of a female is
  - **A.** 20–35%
  - **B.** 30–50%
  - **C.** 37–47%
  - **D.** 40–52%
  - **E.** 50–100%

258. Decreased numbers of RBCs are seen in patients with
  - **A.** Polycythemia
  - **B.** Infection
  - **C.** Leukemia
  - **D.** Anemia
  - **E.** Diabetes

259. A barium sulfate mixture is ingested by a patient before a(n)
  A. Upper GI series
  B. Lower GI series
  C. IVP
  D. Cholecystogram
  E. Mammogram

260. The position in which the X-ray beam is directed from front to back is
  A. Oblique
  B. Lateral
  C. Medial
  D. Anteroposterior
  E. Posteroanterior

261. Ultrasound can be used to
  A. Treat acne
  B. Treat psoriasis
  C. Treat muscle strains and sprains
  D. Heal wound infections
  E. Treat cancer

262. All of the following are granulocytes *except*
  A. Monocytes
  B. Basophils
  C. Neutrophils
  D. Bands
  E. Eosinophils

263. Cheyne-Stokes is
  A. A type of stethoscope
  B. A type of respiration
  C. An examination position
  D. A type of pulse
  E. The name of blood pressure equipment

264. The vitamin involved with the coagulation process is
  A. Vitamin A
  B. Vitamin B
  C. Vitamin C
  D. Vitamin D
  E. Vitamin K

265. Which of the following guidelines governs quality control, quality assurance, record keeping, and qualified personnel for the clinical lab?
  A. COLA
  B. CDC
  C. CLIA '88
  D. DEA
  E. OSHA

266. Amoxicillin is a(n)
  A. Diuretic
  B. Antibiotic
  C. Antifungal
  D. Antipyretic
  E. Antianginal

267. Zoloft and Paxil are classified as
  A. Antihistamines
  B. Antidepressants
  C. Antihypertensives
  D. Antibiotics
  E. Diuretics

268. Which of the following are included in the "Seven Rights" of drug administration?
  A. Right patient
  B. Right dose
  C. Right drug
  D. Right documentation
  E. All of the above

269. The part of the eye that enables a person to see color is/are the
  A. Fovea centralis
  B. Cones
  C. Rods
  D. Retina
  E. Macula

270. Dehydration and electrolyte imbalance are of a particular concern in children with
  A. Colic
  B. Influenza
  C. Hepatitis B
  D. Diarrhea
  E. Common cold

271. Which of the following procedures may cause discomfort to the patient?
  A. CT scan
  B. MRI
  C. EEG
  D. Lumbar puncture
  E. EKG

272. Control samples in the lab
  A. Help to standardize the equipment
  B. Determine CLIA'88 compliance
  C. Ensure the accuracy of the test results
  D. Guide the handling of biohazards
  E. Help to create new procedures

273. Which is *not* correct procedure when performing a capillary puncture?
  A. Wiping away the first drop of blood
  B. Performing the procedure quickly
  C. Warming the finger before the procedure
  D. Cleansing the site with alcohol
  E. Squeezing the finger to encourage blood flow

274. Which of the following can cause a poor EKG tracing?
   A. Loose electrodes
   B. Poor grounding of the machine
   C. Muscle tremors
   D. Electrical interference
   E. All of the above

275. Which of the following is classified as an anticoagulant?
   A. Haldol
   B. Inderal
   C. Elavil
   D. Coumadin
   E. Glucagon

276. Which of the following routes gives the quickest effect?
   A. ID
   B. IM
   C. IV
   D. Subq
   E. PO

277. How many pairs of chromosomes are in the nucleus of a normal cell?
   A. 23
   B. 32
   C. 46
   D. 64
   E. Varies according to cell type

278. The diaphragm separates which two body cavities?
   A. Cranial/spinal
   B. Abdominal/pelvic
   C. Thoracic/abdominal
   D. Thoracic/pelvic
   E. Dorsal/ventral

279. A partial thickness burn that results in blisters and redness is classified as
   A. Fourth degree
   B. Third degree
   C. Second degree
   D. First degree
   E. Excoriation

280. The tough band of tissue that connects bone to bone at a joint is the
   A. Fascia
   B. Articulation
   C. Ligament
   D. Epiphysis
   E. Tendon

281. Paralysis on one side of the body is called
   A. Paresthesia
   B. Paraplegia
   C. Quadriplegia
   D. Biparesis
   E. Hemiplegia

282. The medical term for farsightedness is
   A. Emmetropia
   B. Hyperopia
   C. Myopia
   D. Nystagmus
   E. Astigmatism

283. Which of the following structures creates an opening between the pharynx and the middle ear?
   A. Tympanic membrane
   B. Pinna
   C. Auditory meatus
   D. Eustachian tube
   E. Organ of Corti

284. A freely moving blood clot in the circulation is called a(n)
   A. Embolus
   B. Thrombus
   C. Occlusion
   D. Thrombocyte
   E. Aneurysm

285. The term that means "to control or stop bleeding" is
   A. Hemolysis
   B. Hemostasis
   C. Hematocrit
   D. Hemopoiesis
   E. Hemophilia

286. The medical term for a nosebleed is
   A. Epistaxis
   B. Croup
   C. Dyspnea
   D. Rhinorrhea
   E. Atelectasis

287. An abnormal bubbling or rattling sound heard on auscultation is
   A. Atelectasis
   B. Coryza
   C. Rales
   D. Wheezing
   E. Dyspnea

288. The medical term for a loss of appetite is
   A. Polyphagia
   B. Anorexia
   C. Polyphasia
   D. Bulimia
   E. Ascites

289. All of the following are part of the large intestine *except* the
    A. Appendix
    B. Ascending colon
    C. Rectum
    D. Descending colon
    E. Ileum

290. A condition is characterized by stones in the gallbladder is
    A. Cholecystitis
    B. Cholangitis
    C. Choledochiasis
    D. Cholelithiasis
    E. Cholecystectomy

291. The structural and functional unit of the kidney is the
    A. Calyx
    B. Nephron
    C. Bowman's capsule
    D. Glomerulus
    E. Loop of Hinle

292. The basic unit of heredity is
    A. An autosome
    B. A gene
    C. DNA
    D. RNA
    E. A gamite

293. The process of cell division is known as
    A. Mitosis
    B. Diffusion
    C. Mutation
    D. Recession
    E. Remission

294. The surgical removal of tubes and ovaries is called a(n)
    A. Panhysterectomy
    B. Hysterectomy
    C. Salpingectomy
    D. Histerosalpingectomy
    E. Salpingo-oophorectomy

295. An unborn child during the first two months of prenatal development is referred to as a(n)
    A. Embryo
    B. Fetus
    C. Neonate
    D. Corpus albicans
    E. Corpus luteum

296. An absence of menstrual flow is called
    A. Oligomenorrhea
    B. Dysmenorrhea
    C. Amenorrhea
    D. Menstruation
    E. Metrorrhagia

297. The smallest of all pathogens are
    A. Fungi
    B. Bacteria
    C. Viruses
    D. Protozoa
    E. Nematodes

298. The first line of defense against invading microorganisms is the
    A. WBCs
    B. Skin
    C. Mucous membranes
    D. Complement
    E. Immunity

299. The superior vena cava returns blood to the
    A. Left atrium
    B. Left ventricle
    C. Right atrium
    D. Right ventricle
    E. None of the above

300. The combining form for "heart" is
    A. Hemo-
    B. Cranio-
    C. Electro-
    D. neuro-
    E. cardio-

Medical Terminology 1

- Language of medicine
- Mostly Latin and Greek origins
- Made up of word parts:
  1. Root word
     - Core of the word
     - Tells the fundamental meaning of the word
     - There may be more than one root word in a medical term
  2. Suffix
     - Word part attached to the end of a root word
     - Changes/modifies its meaning
     - Can be
       - Symptomatic: describes evidence of illness
       - Diagnostic: names a medical condition
       - Operative: describes a surgical treatment
       - General: general applications
  3. Prefix
     - Word part attached to the beginning of a root word
     - Changes/modifies its meaning
  4. Combining vowel/form
     - Used between two root words or between a root word and a suffix to make pronunciation easier
     - Not used between a prefix and the root word
     - Usually an "o"
     - Combining form is a root word with the combining vowel attached

To analyze a medical term:
- Divide the word into word parts
- Divide the word by slashes and label each word part

  Example: leukocytosis

  Leuk/o/cyt/osis

  rw cv rw s

To define a medical term:
- Give each word part a meaning.
- Begin by defining the suffix, then the prefix, then the root word.

To build a medical term, use the same procedure as above.

A. BODY STRUCTURE COMBINING FORMS

1.	blast/o	immature form; developing cell
2.	carcin/o cancer/o	cancer
3.	cyt/o	cell
4.	epitheli/o	epithelium
5.	eti/o	cause
6.	gno/o	knowledge
7.	hist/o	tissue
8.	iatr/o	physician; medicine
9.	kary/o	nucleus
10.	lei/o	smooth
11.	lip/o	fat
12.	my/o	muscle
13.	neur/o	nerve
14.	onc/o	tumor
15.	organ/o	organ
16.	path/o	disease
17.	rhabd/o	rod-shaped
18.	sarc/o	flesh; connective tissue
19.	somat/o	body
20.	system/o	system
21.	viscer/o	internal organs; viscera

B. INTEGUMENTARY SYSTEM COMBINING FORMS

1.	aden/o	gland
2.	aut/o	self
3.	bi/o	life
4.	coni/o	dust
5.	crypt/o	hidden
6.	cutane/o derm/o dermat/o	skin
7.	fibr/o	fibrous tissue; fiber
8.	heter/o	other
9.	hidr/o	sweat
10.	kerat/o	hard; horny tissue
11.	myc/o	fungus
12.	necr/o	death
13.	onych/o ungu/o	nail
14.	pachy/o	thick

27

15. rhytid/o — wrinkle
16. seb/o — sebum (oil)
17. staphyl/o — grapelike clusters
18. strept/o — chainlike
19. trich/o — hair
20. xer/o — dry

C. MUSCULOSKELETAL SYSTEM COMBINING FORMS

1. ankyl/o — stiff
2. aponeur/o — aponeurosis
3. arthr/o — joint
4. burs/o — bursa
5. carp/o — carpals
6. chondr/o — cartilage
7. clavic/o clavicul/o — clavicle
8. cost/o — rib
9. crani/o — skull
10. disk/o — intervertebral disk
11. femor/o — femur
12. fibul/o — fibula
13. humer/o — humerus
14. ili/o — ilium
15. ischi/o — ischium
16. kinesi/o — movement
17. kyph/o — hump
18. lamin/o — thin, flat layer
19. lord/o — bent forward
20. mandibul/o — mandible
21. maxill/o — maxilla
22. menisc/o — meniscus
23. myel/o myelon/o — bone marrow
24. my/o myos/o — muscle
25. oste/o — bone
26. patell/o — patella
27. phalang/o — phalanges
28. pub/o — pubis
29. radi/o — radius
30. scapul/o — scapula
31. scoli/o — bent; curved
32. stern/o — sternum
33. synovi/o — synovial fluid; synovial membrane
34. tars/o — tarsals
35. ten/o tend/o tendin/o — tendon
36. tibi/o — tibia
37. uln/o — ulna
38. vertebr/o rachi/o spondyl/o — vertebrae; vertebral column

D. NERVOUS SYSTEM COMBINING FORMS

1. cerebell/o — cerebellum
2. cerebr/o — cerebrum
3. dur/o — dura mater
4. encephal/o — brain
5. esthesi/o — feeling; sensation; sensitivity
6. gangli/o ganglion/o — ganglion
7. meningi/o mening/o — meninges
8. mon/o — one; single
9. myel/o — spinal cord
10. neur/o — nerve
11. phas/o — speech
12. poli/o — gray; gray matter
13. psych/o ment/o phren/o — mind
14. quadr/i — four

E. CARDIOVASCULAR AND LYMPHATIC SYSTEMS COMBINING FORMS

1. angi/o — vessel
2. aort/o — aorta
3. arteri/o — artery
4. ather/o — fatty deposit
5. bacteri/o — bacteria
6. cardi/o — heart
7. ech/o — sound
8. electr/o — electrical activity; electricity
9. hem/o hemat/o — blood
10. isch/o — blockage; deficiency
11. lymph/o — lymph
12. phleb/o ven/o — vein
13. plasm/o — plasma
14. sphygm/o — pulse
15. splen/o — spleen
16. therm/o — heat
17. thromb/o — clot
18. thym/o — thymus gland
19. valv/o valvul/o — valve
20. ventricul/o — ventricle

F. RESPIRATORY SYSTEM COMBINING FORMS

1. adenoid/o — adenoid
2. alveol/o — alveolus
3. atel/o — incomplete; imperfect
4. bronchi/o bronch/o — bronchus
5. bronchiol/o — bronchiole
6. diaphragmat/o — diaphragm
7. epiglott/o — epiglottis
8. laryng/o — larynx
9. lob/o — lobe
10. muc/o — mucus
11. nas/o rhin/o — nose

12. orth/o — straight
13. ox/o — oxygen
    ox/i
14. pharyng/o — pharynx
15. pleur/o — pleura
16. pneum/o — lung; air
    pneumat/o
    pneumon/o
17. pulmon/o — lung
18. py/o — pus
19. sinus/o — sinus
20. sept/o — septum; wall off
21. spir/o — breathe; breathing
22. thorac/o — thorax; chest
23. tonsill/o — tonsil
24. trache/o — trachea

G. DIGESTIVE SYSTEM COMBINING FORMS

1. an/o — anus
2. appendic/o — appendix
3. cec/o — cecum
4. duoden/o — duodenum
5. chol/e — bile; gall
6. cholecyst/o — gallbladder
7. cholangi/o — bile duct
8. choledoch/o — common bile duct
9. col/o — colon
10. dent/i — tooth
11. diverticul/o — diverticulum; blind pouch extending from an organ
12. duoden/o — duodenum
13. enter/o — small intestines
14. esophag/o — esophagus
15. gastr/o — stomach
16. gingiv/o — gum
17. gloss/o — tongue
    lingu/o
18. hepat/o — liver
19. herni/o — hernia
20. ile/o — ileum
21. jejun/o — jejunum
22. lapar/o — abdomen
    abdomin/o
    celi/o
23. palat/o — palate
24. pancreat/o — pancreas
25. peritone/o — peritoneum
26. proct/o — rectum
    rect/o
27. polyp/o — polyp; small growth on a stalk
28. pylor/o — pylorus; pyloric sphincter
29. sial/o — saliva
30. sigmoid/o — sigmoid colon
31. stomat/o — mouth
    or/o
32. uvul/o — uvula

H. URINARY SYSTEM COMBINING FORMS

1. albumin/o — albumin
2. azot/o — urea; nitrogen
3. cyst/o — bladder; sac
    vesic/o
4. glomerul/o — glomerulus
5. glyc/o — sugar
    glycos/o
6. hydr/o — water
7. lith/o — stone; calculus
8. meat/o — meatus; opening
9. nephr/o — kidney
    ren/o
10. noct/i — night
11. olig/o — scanty; few
12. pyel/o — renal pelvis
13. son/o — sound
14. ureter/o — ureter
15. urethr/o — urethra
16. urin/o — urine; urinary tract
    ur/o

I. ENDOCRINE SYSTEM COMBINING FORMS

1. acr/o — extremities
2. adeno/o — gland
3. adren/o — adrenal glands
    adrenal/o
4. calc/i — calcium
5. cortic/o — cortex
6. dips/o — thirst
7. endocrin/o — endocrine
8. hormon/o — hormone
9. kal/i — potassium
10. natr/o — sodium
11. parathyroid/o — parathyroid glands
12. thyroid/o — thyroid gland
    thyr/o
13. toxic/o — poison

J. MALE REPRODUCTIVE SYSTEM COMBINING FORMS

1. andr/o — male; man
2. balan/o — glans penis
3. epididym/o — epididymis
4. prostat/o — prostate gland
5. vas/o — vessel; duct
6. vesicul/o — seminal vesicles
7. orchid/o — testicle; testes
    orchi/o
    orch/o
8. sperm/o — sperm
    spermat/o
9. test/o — testicle; testes

K. FEMALE REPRODUCTIVE SYSTEM COMBINING FORMS

1. arche/o — beginning; first
2. cervic/o — cervix

3. colp/o   vagina
   vagin/o
4. gynec/o   female; woman
   gyn/o
5. hymen/o   hymen
6. hyster/o   uterus
   metr/o
   metri/o
   uter/o
7. lact/o   milk
8. mamm/o   breast
   mast/o
9. men/o   menstruation
10. oophor/o   ovary
11. ov/o   egg; ovum
    ov/i
12. perine/o   perineum
13. salping/o   fallopian tubes
14. vulv/o   vulva
    episi/o

L. COMBINING FORMS INDICATING COLORS
1. albin/o   white
   leuk/o
2. chlor/o   green
3. cyan/o   blue
4. erythr/o   red
5. melan/o   black
6. xanth/o   yellow

M. SUFFIXES USED TO INDICATE PATHOLOGICAL CONDITIONS
1. -algia   pain
   -dynia
2. -cele   hernia
3. -ectasis   dilation; swelling
4. -edema   swelling
5. -emesis   vomiting
6. -emia   blood condition
7. -ia   state of; condition
8. -iasis   abnormal condition
9. -itis   inflammation
10. -lith   stone; calculus
11. -lysis   destruction; separation; breakdown
12. -malacia   softening
13. -megaly   enlargement
14. -oma   tumor; mass
15. -osis   abnormal increase; abnormal condition
16. -pathy   disease process
17. -penia   decrease; deficiency
18. -phobia   irrational fear
19. -plegia   paralysis
20. -ptosis   drooping; sagging; prolapse
21. -ptysis   spitting
22. -rrhage   bursting forth
    -rrhagia
23. -rrhea   flow; discharge
24. -rrhexis   rupture
25. -sclerosis   hardening
26. -spasm   involuntary contraction
27. -stenosis   narrowing
28. -y   process; state; condition

N. SUFFIXES USED TO INDICATE DIAGNOSTIC AND SURGICAL PROCEDURES
1. -centesis   surgical puncture to remove fluid
2. -desis   surgical binding; surgical fusion
3. -ectomy   excision; surgical removal
4. -gram   record; writing
5. -graph   instrument used to record
6. -graphy   process of recording; producing images
7. -meter   instrument used to measure
8. -metry   to measure; measurement
9. -opsy   to view
10. -pexy   surgical fixation
11. -plasty   surgical repair; surgical reconstruction
12. -rrhaphy   suture; sew
13. -scope   instrument used to visually examine
14. -scopy   process of visually examining
15. -stasis   stoppage; stopping; controlling
16. -stomy   new opening
17. -tome   instrument used to cut
18. -tomy   process of cutting; incision into
19. -tripsy   surgical crushing

O. GENERAL SUFFIXES
1. -ase   enzyme
2. -blast   immature form
3. -cyte   cell
4. -er   specialist; one who specializes
   -or
   -ician
   -logist
   -ist
5. -ion   process
6. -ium   membrane
7. -logy   study of
8. -ose   sugar
9. -phagia   to eat; swallow
10. -phasia   speech
11. -plasia   formation; development
12. -pnea   breathing
13. -poiesis   production; formation
14. -trophy   development; growth
15. -uria   urine

P. SUFFIXES USED TO CREATE ADJECTIVE FORMS

1. -ac   pertaining to
   -al
   -ar
   -ary
   -eal
   -ic
   -ine
   -ior
   -ose
   -ous
   -tic
2. -genous   produced by; producing
   -genic
3. -oid   like; resembling
4. -ole   small
   -ule

Q. PREFIXES USED TO INDICATE DIRECTION AND POSITION

1. ab-   away from
2. ad-   toward
3. ante-   before
4. circum-   around
5. dia-   complete; through
6. ecto-   outside
7. endo-   within
8. e-   out; outward; outside
   ex-
   exo-
   extra-
9. epi-   upon; on; above
10. eso-   inward; within
11. hyper-   above; excessive
12. hypo-   below; under; deficient
13. in-   in; into
14. infra-   below; beneath
15. inter-   between
16. intra-   within
17. meta-   beyond; change
18. para-   beside; near
19. per-   through
20. peri-   around
21. post-   after
22. pre-   before; in front of
23. pro-   before
24. retro-   back; behind
25. sub-   under; below
26. supra-   above
27. trans-   across

R. PREFIXES REFERRING TO NUMBER OR MEASUREMENT

1. bi-   two
   di-
2. hemi-   half
   semi-
3. mono-   one
   uni-
4. multi-   many
   poly-
5. nulli-   none
6. primi-   first
7. quadri-   four
8. tri-   three

S. MISCELLANEOUS PREFIXES

1. a-   no; not; lack of
   an-
2. ana-   apart
3. anti-   against
4. auto-   self
5. brady-   slow
6. contra-   against
7. dys-   bad; abnormal; difficult; painful
8. in-   not
   ir-
   im-
9. macro-   large
10. mal-   bad
11. micro-   small
12. neo-   new
13. pan-   all
14. syn-   together; joined; with
    sym-
15. tachy-   fast; rapid

T. PLURALS

■ To form a plural, change the:

a as in burs**a**	→	**ae** as in burs**ae**
ax as in thor**ax**	→	**aces** as in thor**aces**
en as in foram**en**	→	**ina** as in foram**ina**
is as in cris**is**	→	**es** as in cris**es**
is as in ir**is**	→	**ides** as in ir**ides**
is as in femor**is**	→	**a** as in femor**a**
ix as in append**ix**	→	**ices** as in append**ices**
nx as in phala**nx**	→	**ges** an in phalan**ges**
on as in spermato-zo**on**	→	**a** as in spermatozo**a**
um as in ov**um**	→	**a** as in ov**a**
us as in nucle**us**	→	**i** as in nucle**i**
y as in arter**y**	→	**ies** as in arter**ies**

Abbreviations

A. CHARTING TERMS

abd	abdomen
ADL	activities of daily living
approx	approximately
ASAP	as soon as possible
ax	axillary
BE	barium enema
BM	bowel movement
BMR	basal metabolic rate
BP, B/P	blood pressure
bx	biopsy

cath	catheterization; catheter
CC	chief complaint
chemo	chemotherapy
c/o	complains of
CSF	cerebrospinal fluid
D&C	dilatation (dilation) and currettage
Disc, d/c, dc	discontinue
DOB	date of birth
Dr.	doctor
drsg	dressing
dx	diagnosis
EDC	estimated date of confinement
EEG	electroencephalogram
EKG, ECG	electrocardiogram
ETOH	ethyl alcohol
FH	family history
FU	follow up
fx	fracture
GI	gastrointestinal
GP	general practitioner
grav, gravida	pregnancy
GYN	gynecology
H&P	history and physical
HEENT	head, eye, ear, nose, throat
hr	hour
hs	hour of sleep; bedtime
ht	height
hx	history
I&D	incision and drainage
ID	intradermal
IM	intramuscular
IV	intravenous
KUB	kidney, ureter, bladder
Ⓛ	left
LLQ	left lower quadrant
LMP	last menstrual period
LUQ	left upper quadrant
med(s)	medication(s)
mets	metastasis
N&V	nausea and vomiting
NPO	nothing by mouth
NVD	nausea, vomiting, diarrhea
OB	obstetrics
OC	oral contraceptives
OR	operating room
os	opening
P	pulse
para	live birth
PE, px	physical exam
PEARL	pupils equal and reactive to light
peds	pediatrics
PH	patient (past) history
pt	patient

QNS	quantity not sufficient
R	respiration
®	right
RLQ	right lower quadrant
r/o	rule out
ROM	range of motion
RUQ	right upper quadrant
Rx	prescription
SQ, subQ, SC	subcutaneous
stat	immediately
sx	symptoms
T	temperature
T&A	tonsilloadenoidectomy (tonsils and adenoids)
TLC	tender loving care
tx	treatment, therapy
UCHD	usual childhood diseases
vo	verbal order
VS	vital signs
WDWN	well-developed, well-nourished
WNL	within normal limits
wt	weight

B. DIAGNOSTIC TERMS

AIDS	acquired immune deficiency syndrome
ASHD	arteriosclerotic heart disease
CA	cancer
CHF	congestive heart failure
COPD	chronic obstructive pulmonary disease
CVA	cerebral vascular accident
HIV	human immunodeficiency virus
IDDM	insulin-dependent diabetes mellitus
MI	myocardial infarction
NIDDM	non-insulin-dependent diabetes mellitus
PMS	premenstrual syndrome
SIDS	sudden infant death syndrome
SOB	shortness of breath
STD	sexually transmitted disease
TB	tuberculosis
URI	upper respiratory infection
UTI	urinary tract infection

C. PRESCRIPTION TERMS

aa	of each
ac	before meals
AD	right ear
ad lib	as desired
AM	morning
amt	amount

AS	left ear
AU	both ears
bid	twice daily, two times a day
$\bar{c}$	with
et	and
noct	night
OD	right eye
OS	left eye
OU	both eyes
$\bar{p}$	after
pc	after meals
po	by mouth
PM	afternoon
prn	as needed
$\bar{q}$	every
qd	every day
qh	every hour
qid	four times daily, four times a day
qod	every other day
qoh	every other day
$\bar{s}$	without
$\overline{ss}$	half
tab	tablet
tid	three times daily, three times a day

D. LABORATORY TERMS

ABO	main blood grouping system
AP	anterior/posterior (X-ray)
BUN	blood urea nitrogen
CBC	complete blood count
diff, dif	differential white blood cell count
ESR	erythrocyte sedimentation rate, sed rate
FBS	fasting blood sugar
H&H	hemoglobin and hematocrit
hct	hematocrit
hgb	hemoglobin
HCG	human chorionic gonadotropin
GTT	glucose tolerance test
lat	lateral (X-ray)
O&P	ova and parasites
obl	oblique (X-ray)
Pap	Pap smear
pH	degree of acidity or alkalinity
PKU	phenylketonuria
RBC	red blood cell
UA	urinalysis
WBC	white blood cell

E. MEASURES

C	centigrade
cc	cubic centimeter
cm	centimeter
dr	dram
F	Fahrenheit
gm	gram
gr	grain
gtt(s)	drop(s)
kg	kilogram
L	liter
lb, #	pound
mcg, μ	microgram
mg	milligram
ml	milliliter
mn	minum
oz	ounce
pt	pint
qt	quart
tbsp, T	tablespoon
tsp, t	teaspoon
U	unit

F. COMPOUNDS/CHEMICALS

Ca	calcium
Cl	chloride
CO_2	carbon dioxide
Fe	iron
H	hydrogen
H_2O	water
Hg	mercury
K	potassium
Na	sodium
NaCl	sodium chloride
O_2	oxygen

G. SYMBOLS

♂	male
♀	female
>	greater than
<	less than
↑	increase, above
↓	decrease, below
×	times (multiply by)
%	percent
=	equal
+	plus
−	minus
:	ratio
::	proportion
⊕	positive
⊖	negative
⦵	standing
⌐	sitting
○—	lying down

Anatomy and Physiology

I. Introduction to the Body

A. GENERAL
- Anatomy
  - Study of body structures
- Physiology
  - Study of body functions

B. LEVELS OF ORGANIZATION
— Arranged from smallest to largest
- Chemical
  - Includes atoms and molecules
- Cell
  - Basic unit of all life
- Tissue
  - Group of cells with similar structure and function
- Organ
  - Group of tissues that work together and perform a function
- System
  - Group of organs working together to accomplish a set of functions
- Organism
  - Made up of systems that work together to maintain life

C. ORGAN SYSTEMS
— Each has a specific function, but all systems work together
- Integumentary system
  - Made up of skin and accessory organs
  - Provides protection, temperature regulation, chemical synthesis, water balance, and sense reception
- Skeletal system
  - Made up of bones, joints, tendons, and ligaments
  - Provides protection, provides a framework for the body, assists with movement, stores minerals, hemopoiesis
- Muscular system
  - Made up of muscles
  - Provides movement, body heat, and storage of energy

- Nervous system
  - Made up of brain, spinal cord, and nerves
  - Coordinates all body activities and detects changes in the outside environment
- Endocrine system
  - Made up of glands that secrete chemical messengers (hormones)
  - Coordinates and balances body activities and regulates reproductive systems
- Cardiovascular system
  - Made up of heart and blood vessels
  - Transports substances to the tissues and removes waste products from tissues
- Lymphatic system
  - Made up of lymph, lymph vessels, lymph nodes, and lymphoid organs
  - Removes excess fluid and helps to protect the body against disease
- Digestive system
  - Made up of mouth, esophagus, stomach, intestines, rectum, liver, gallbladder, and pancreas
  - Takes in food and processes it into molecules that can be used by the body; eliminates solid waste products
- Urinary system
  - Made up of kidneys, ureters, bladder, and urethra
  - Removes liquid nitrogenous waste products and helps to regulate water balance
- Respiratory system
  - Made up of nose, pharynx, larynx, trachea, bronchi, and lungs
  - Brings O_2 into the lungs and removes CO_2 from the body
- Reproductive system
  - Made up of gonads (ovaries and testes) duct systems, accessory glands, and support structures
  - Produces new individuals

D. LIFE PROCESSES
- Characteristics that distinguish a living organism from a nonliving organism

■ Organization
  • Each part has a function and cooperates with all other parts
■ Metabolism
  • All chemical reactions in the body
■ Responsiveness
  • Ability to detect changes in the internal and external environment and respond to them
■ Movement
  • All activities accomplished by the muscular system
■ Reproduction
  • Formation of new cells; formation of a new individual
■ Growth
  • Increase in size by an increase in the number of cells
■ Respiration
  • Exchange of O_2 and CO_2
■ Digestion
  • Ability to break down complex foodstuffs into simpler molecules that the body can use
■ Excretion
  • Process of removing waste products from the body
■ Maintaining boundaries
  • Keeping the inside environment separate from the outside

E. SURVIVAL NEEDS
■ Requirements of an organism to sustain life
■ Physical factors that come from the environment
■ Water
  • Probably more necessary than food
  • Provides a medium for all chemical reactions
  • Provides a fluid base for body secretions and excretions
  • Makes up about 60% of body weight
■ Oxygen
  • Necessary for metabolic reactions
■ Nutrients
  • Taken in from diet
  • Provide raw materials necessary for growth, replacement, and repair
  • Provide energy for body processes
■ Temperature
  • Necessary for chemical reactions to occur
  • Optimum is 98.6 degrees Fahrenheit
■ Pressure
  • Application of a force
  • Necessary for breathing and blood pressure

F. HOMEOSTASIS
■ Body's ability to maintain a constant internal environment regardless of the external environment
■ When the body is healthy, the internal environment remains stable within limited normal ranges
■ Lack of homeostasis can lead to illness and eventually death

G. ANATOMICAL TERMS
■ Universal language
■ Used to describe directions and regions of the body
■ Anatomical position
  • Beginning position for point of reference
  • Body is standing erect, face forward, arms at sides with palms facing forward, toes pointing forward
■ Directions in the body (see Figure 2-1)
  1. Superior
    • Part above another part; toward the head
  2. Inferior
    • Part below another part; toward the feet
  3. Anterior (ventral)
    • Toward the front
  4. Posterior (dorsal)
    • Toward the back
  5. Medial
    • Toward or near the midline of the body
  6. Lateral
    • Toward or near the side of the body; away from the midline
  7. Proximal
    • Closer to the point of attachment
  8. Distal
    • Farther away from the point of attachment
  9. Superficial
    • On or near the surface
  10. Deep
    • Away from the surface
■ Planes and sections of the body (see Figure 2-1)
  1. Used to visualize spatial relationships of body parts
  2. Sagittal plane
    • Divides the body into left and right parts
  3. Midsagittal plane
    • Divides the body into equal right and left halves
  4. Transverse plane
    • Divides the body into upper and lower parts; cross section
  5. Frontal (coronal) plane
    • Divides the body into front and back parts
■ Body cavities (see Figure 2-2)
  • Hollow body spaces that contain internal organs
  1. Dorsal cavity
    • Made up of two cavities along the back of the body
    a) Cranial cavity
      ■ Contains the brain

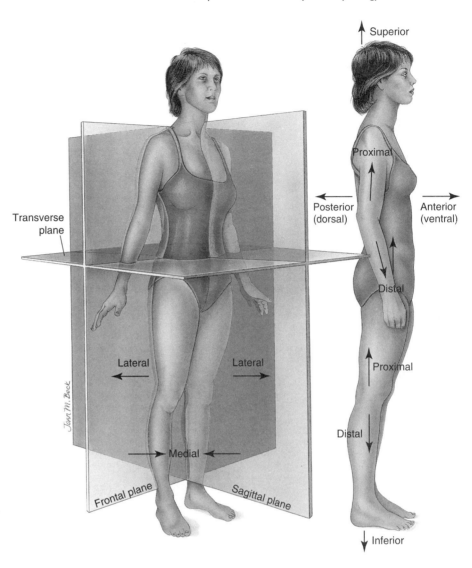

FIGURE 2-1 Directions and planes of the body. (From Patton KT, Thibodeau G: The Human Body in Health and Disease, ed 2, St. Louis, 1997, Mosby, p. 4.)

b) Spinal cavity
  ■ Contains the spinal cord
2. Ventral cavity
  • Made up of two cavities along the front of the body
  a) Thoracic cavity
    ■ Contains heart, lungs, esophagus, and trachea
  b) Abdominopelvic cavity
    ■ Contains organs below the diaphragm
  c) Diaphragm
    ■ Separates the thoracic and abdominopelvic cavities
■ Abdominal regions (see Figure 2-3)
  • Used to describe locations of body organs or pain
  • Two methods
1. Quadrants
  • Divides abdomen into four regions
    ■ Right upper quadrant (RUQ)
    ■ Left upper quadrant (LUQ)

■ Right lower quadrant (RLQ)
    ■ Left lower quadrant (LLQ)
2. Nine regions
  • More specific
    ■ Epigastric
    ■ Umbilical
    ■ Hypogastric
    ■ Right and left hypochondriac
    ■ Right and left lumbar
    ■ Right and left iliac
■ Body areas
  • Abdominal: portion of trunk below diaphragm; between thorax and pelvis
  • Antebrachial: forearm; region between elbow and wrist
  • Antecubital: space in front of elbow
  • Axillary: armpit area
  • Brachial: arm; region between elbow and shoulder
  • Buccal: cheek area
  • Carpal: wrist area

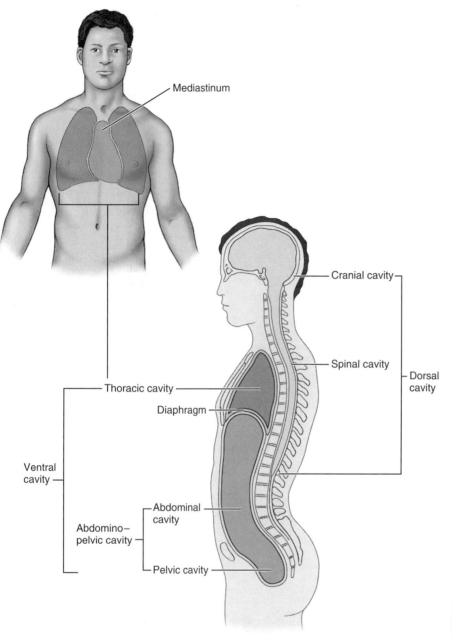

FIGURE 2-2   Major body cavities. (From Herlihy B, Maebius N: The Human Body in Health and Illness, Philadelphia, 1999, Saunders, p. 14.)

- Celiac: abdomen
- Cephalic: head
- Cervical: neck area; cervix
- Costal: ribs
- Cranial: skull
- Cutaneous: skin
- Femoral: thigh area; region between the hip and knee
- Frontal: forehead
- Gluteal: buttock area
- Inguinal: groin
- Lumbar: lower back area between ribs and pelvis
- Mammary: breast

- Occipital: lower portion of back of head
- Ophthalmic: eyes
- Oral: mouth
- Otic: ears
- Palmar: palm of the hand
- Pectoral: chest area
- Pedal: foot
- Pelvic: inferior region of abdominal cavity
- Perineal: region between the anus and pubic symphysis; includes region of external reproductive organs
- Plantar: sole of the foot
- Popliteal: area behind the knee
- Sacral: posterior region between hipbones

Chapter 2 ■ Anatomy and Physiology   **39**

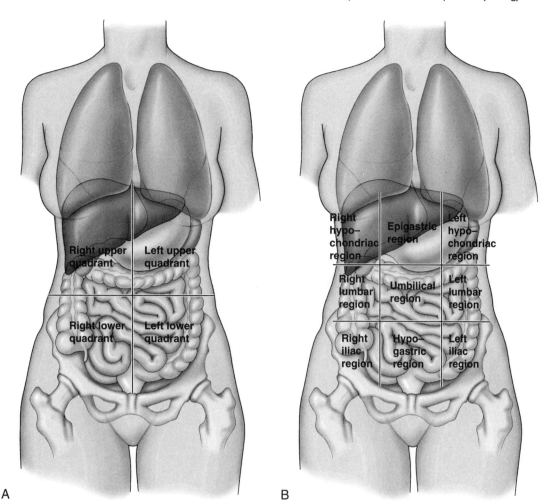

A   B

FIGURE 2-3 Areas of the abdomen. A, Four quadrants. B, Nine regions. (From Herlihy B, Maebius N: The Human Body in Health and Illness, Philadelphia, 1999, Saunders, p. 15.)

- Sternal: anterior midline of thorax
- Tarsal: ankle area
- Thoracic: chest
- Umbilical: navel
- Vertebral: backbone

II. Cell

A. GENERAL
- ■ Basic structural and functional unit of the body
- ■ Vary in size, shape, and function
- ■ Very well organized in structure

B. STRUCTURE (see Figure 2-4)
1. Cell membrane
   - Thin, flexible, outermost barrier of the cell
   - Made up of a double layer of phospholipids
   - Allows water and chemicals to pass in and out
   - Permeable and selective
2. Cytoplasm
   - Cytosol

- Thick, semisolid substance that contains mostly water
   - Site of cellular activity
   - Holds organelles in place
3. Nuclear membrane
   - Encloses the nucleus
4. Nucleus
   - Control center of the cell
   - Contains genetic material (DNA)
5. Nucleolus
   - Small, dense structure located in the nucleus
   - Important in the synthesis of ribosomes
6. Centrioles
   - Hollow, rod-shaped structures found in the cytoplasm near the nucleus
   - Play an important role in cell division
7. Endoplasmic reticulum
   - Complex network of tubular channels
   - "Transportation system" of the cell
   - Allows molecules to move from one part of the cell to the other

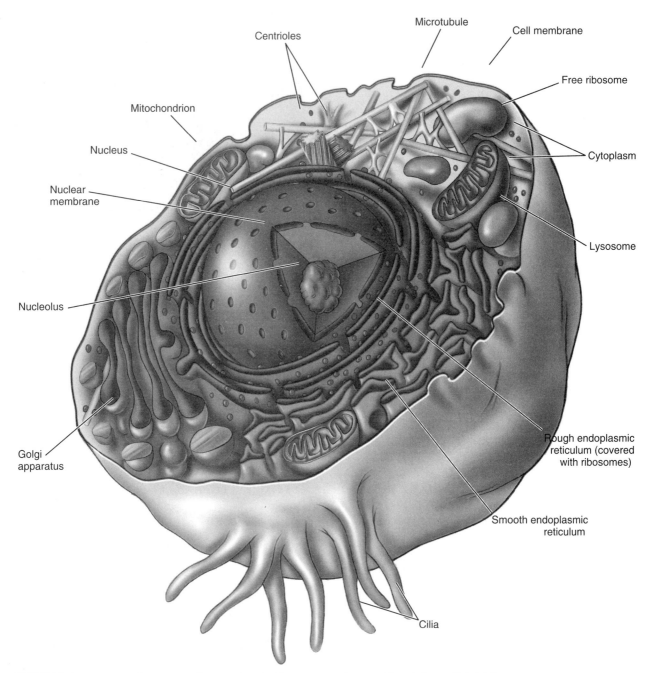

FIGURE 2-4 A typical cell. (From Herlihy B, Maebius N: The Human Body in Health and Illness, Philadelphia, 1999, Saunders, p. 38.)

- Two types
  a) Rough: ribosomes attached; transports proteins
  b) Smooth: without ribosomes; manufactures lipids and hormones
8. Golgi apparatus
  - Stack of flattened sacs
  - Located near the nucleus
  - Processes and packages proteins
9. Lysosomes
  - Sacs of various sizes and shapes

- Contain strong chemicals that digest various substances that enter the cytoplasm
10. Mitochondria
  - Sausage-shaped sacs
  - Inner layer arranged in folds
  - "Powerhouse" of the cell
  - Source of energy for cells and tissues
11. Microtubules
  - Extremely small, hollow tubes
  - Criss-cross cytoplasm to form a "skeleton"
  - Give cells strength and shape

12. Peroxisomes
    - Membranous sacs that resemble lysosomes
    - Contain enzymes that detoxify harmful substances
13. Ribsomes
    - Composed of ribonucleic acid (RNA) and protein
    - Form amino acids into new protein molecules
    - Some are free floating in the cytoplasm; some are attached to endoplasmic reticulum
14. Vacuoles
    - Membrane-bound sacs that appear in the cytoplasm when the cell membrane folds inward on itself
    - Contain fluid or solid substances
    - Lysosomes can empty their enzymes into the sac
    - Aid in metabolic activity of the cell
15. Microvilli
    - Tiny fingerlike extensions that project from the surface of certain cells
    - Increase absorptive surface of cell
16. Cilia
    - Hairlike projections on the surface of the cell
    - Move substances along the cell surface
17. Flagella
    - Hairlike projection from surface of the cell
    - Provides movement

C. TYPES OF MOVEMENT ACROSS THE CELL MEMBRANE
    - Ability of the cell to carry out its function depends on movement or exchange of fluids, particles, and molecules
    - Movement controlled and facilitated by cell membrane
    1. Diffusion
        - Movement of solids from an area of higher concentration to an area of lower concentration
        - Does not require cellular energy
    2. Filtration
        - Movement of a fluid by hydrostatic pressure
        - Does not require cellular energy
    3. Osmosis
        - Movement of water from an area of higher concentration to an area of lower concentration
        - Does not require cellular energy
    4. Phagocytosis
        - ''cell eating''; cell engulfs particle
        - Requires cellular energy
    5. Pinocytosis
        - ''cell drinking''; cells engulfs fluid
        - Requires cellular energy

6. Active transport
    - Movement of substances from an area of lower concentration to an area of higher concentration
    - Requires cellular energy

D. CELL DIVISION
    - Mitosis
    - Results in two identical daughter cells
    - Consists of two separate operations:
      1. Division of the nucleus (karyokinesis)
      2. Division of cytoplasm (cytokinesis)
    - Entire process has several phases:
      1. Interphase: chromosomes double
      2. Prophase: centrioles move to opposite ends of the cell, trailing a thin, threadlike substance that forms a structure resembling a spindle
      3. Metaphase: chromosomes line up across the spindles and begin to move toward the opposite ends of the cell
      4. Telophase: nuclear area becomes pinched in the middle until two regions have formed; similar change happens in the cell membrane; the cell eventually splits in two

III. Tissues and Membranes

A. GENERAL
    - Group of cells similar in structure and function
    - Organized into four general types

B. TYPES OF TISSUES
    1. Connective tissue
        - Variety of forms throughout the body
        - Serves as a framework for other tissues
        - Combines to form more complex tissues (organs)
        - Provides support and protection
        - Serves as storage sites
        - Fills in spaces between body structures
        - Types include:
          a) Loose (areolar)
            - Attaches skin to underlying tissues
            - Surrounds blood and lymph vessels
            - Fills spaces around muscles and other organs
          b) Dense
            - Provides great strength
            - Makes up tendons and ligaments
          c) Elastic
            - Capable of stretching
          d) Adipose
            - Stores fat
            - Serves to insulate body and as an energy reserve
          e) Reticular
            - Associated with the formation of blood

f) Cartilage
  ▪ Rigid connective tissue
  ▪ Forms sliding surface for joints
  ▪ Contains no blood vessels
  ▪ Three types:
    1) Hyaline cartilage
    2) Elastic cartilage
    3) Fibrocartilage
g) Bone (osseous)
  ▪ Compact and rigid
  ▪ Calcium deposits in fibers give it hardness and strength
  2. Epithelial tissue
  • Epithelium
  • Provides covering and lining for surfaces
  • Classified according to number of cells, arrangement of cells, location of tissue, and shape of cells at the surface of the tissue
  3. Muscle tissue
  • Makes up muscles
  • Has ability to contract (shorten)
  • Basis of and provides for movement
  • Three kinds:
    a) Skeletal muscle tissue
      ▪ Attaches to bone and produces movement
      ▪ Voluntary (under conscious control)
    b) Smooth muscle
      ▪ Found in internal organs
      ▪ Involuntary (not under conscious control)
    c) Cardiac muscle tissue
      ▪ Found in the heart
      ▪ Complex network of cells
      ▪ Involuntary
  4. Nervous tissue
  • Composed of cells that can respond to surroundings
  • Cells called neurons: supported and nourished by neuroglial cells
  • Regulates all activities and functions of the body

C. MEMBRANES (see Figure 2-5)
  ■ Thin sheet of tissue
  ■ Can cover a surface, serve as a partition, line organs and cavities, or anchor an organ
  1. Serous membrane
  • Serosa
  • Lines walls of body cavities that do not open to the outside
  • Has two layers:
    a) Parietal layer: layer attached to the wall of the cavity or sac
    b) Visceral layer: layer attached to the internal organ

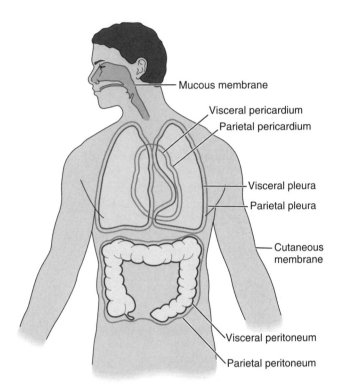

FIGURE 2-5   Epithelial membranes: cutaneous membrane (skin), mucous membranes, and serous membranes (pleura, pericardium, and peritoneum). (From Herlihy B, Maebius N: The Human Body in Health and Illness, Philadelphia, 1999, Saunders, p. 88.)

  • Three main serous membranes
    a) Pleura: lines thoracic cavity and covers the lungs
    b) Pericardium: sac that encloses the heart
    c) Peritoneum: largest serous membrane; lines the wall of the abdominal cavity and covers the abdominal organs
  2. Mucous membrane
  • Mucosa
  • Lines the walls of body cavities that open to the outside
  • Produces a thick, sticky substance (mucus)
  3. Cutaneous membrane
  • The skin
  4. Synovial membrane
  • Lines joint cavities
  • Secretes a lubricating fluid that reduces friction

IV. Integumentary System

A. GENERAL
  ■ Considered to be the largest system and organ of the body
  ■ Made up of skin and its appendages (hair, glands, nails)
  ■ Forms outer boundary of the body

B. FUNCTIONS
1. Protection from radiation, water loss, drying, and invasion of microorganisms
2. Control of body temperature
3. Detection of sensation
4. Secretion of waste products
5. Production of vitamin D

C. STRUCTURE (see Figure 2-6)
■ Two main layers:
1. Epidermis
   • Outer layer
   • Made up of 4 to 5 sublayers (strata)
   • Innermost layer continuously supplies cells that move up to the next strata
   • Cells continue to pick up keratin as they pass through the strata
   • Outermost layer contains lifeless, keratin-filled cells that continually slough off
   • Contains melanocytes that produce pigment (melanin), which gives skin color
   • Contains no blood supply
2. Dermis
   • Corium; "true skin"
   • Innermost layer
   • Contains nerve and blood supply
   • Also contains appendages of the skin
   • Provides strength to the skin
   • Stores water and electrolytes

■ Appendages
   • Special structures that perform a variety of functions
1. Sudoriferous glands
   • Sweat glands
   • Coiled, tubelike structures in the dermis
   • Produce and transport sweat to the skin surface
   • Sweat then evaporates and cools the body
2. Ceruminous glands
   • Modified sweat glands found in the ear
   • Secrete cerumen (earwax)
3. Sebaceous glands
   • Oil glands
   • Connected to hair follicle
   • Secrete sebum that oils the hair and lubricates the skin
4. Hair
   • Covers most of the body
   • Made up of dead, keratinized tissue
   • Connected to small muscles (erector pili)
5. Nails
   • Hard, keratinized structures found on the fingertips and tips of toes
   • Protective function
■ Subcutaneous tissue
   • Layer of tissue below the dermis
   • Connects dermis to the surface of muscles
   • Made up of adipose tissue, elastic fibers, and fibers
   • Injection site

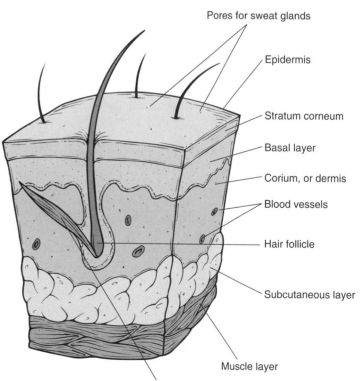

FIGURE 2-6   Normal skin. (From Frazier MS, Drzymkowski JW: Essentials of Human Diseases and Conditions, ed 2, Philadelphia, 2000, Saunders, p. 149.)

Pores for sweat glands
Epidermis
Stratum corneum
Basal layer
Corium, or dermis
Blood vessels
Hair follicle
Subcutaneous layer
Muscle layer
Sebaceous gland duct

D. DISEASES AND DISORDERS

1. Abrasion: scrape
2. Acne vulgaris: inflammation of a sebaceous gland; characterized by papules, pustules, and comedos
3. Albinism: whiteness of skin due to lack of melanin
4. Alopecia: baldness
5. Avulsion: torn-away tissue
6. Bulla: large vesicle
7. Burn: tissue injury resulting from thermal, chemical, electrical, or radioactive agents
   - First-degree: superficial involvement of epidermis; characterized by erythema, tenderness, and pain
   - Second-degree: involves epidermis and dermis; characterized by vesicles
   - Third-degree: involves epidermis, dermis, and injury to underlying tissues; characterized by charring, tissue damage, and loss of fluid
   - Rule of Nines: method of determining percentage of body surface area affected:
     - Head and neck = 9%
     - Torso = 36%
     - Arms = 18%
     - Legs = 36%
     - Genitals = 1%
8. Callus: thickened area of epidermis due to pressure or friction
9. Carcinoma: skin cancer: caused by exposure to UV rays and radiation; types include
   - basal cell: malignant tumor of the basal cell layer of epidermis
   - squamous cell: malignant tumor of the squamous epithelial cells of the epidermis
   - malignant melanoma: cancerous growth of melanocytes
10. Comedo: papule having a small, dark central region (blackhead) or pale region (whitehead)
11. Cyanosis: blue coloration of the skin due to lack of oxygen
12. Cyst: raised or flat fluid-filled or solid-filled sac
13. Decubitus ulcer: bedsore; open lesion caused by poor or no circulation to the area resulting from pressure against the tissue
14. Dermatitis: inflammation of the skin; characterized by pruritis, various lesions, erythema
    - Seborrheic dermatitis: chronic dermatitis; caused by an increase in sebaceous secretions; characterized by greasy scales, pruritis, dandruff
    - Atopic dermatitis: inflammation with rash
    - Eczema: dry, leathery vesicles in adults; characteristic pattern on face, neck, elbows, and knees
    - Contact dermatitis: inflammation caused by irritant
15. Dermatophytosis: superficial fungal infection; caused by *Tinea* species: lesions are round, scaly, and/or ring-shaped
    - Tinea corporis: ringworm; involves exposed skin
    - Tinea unguium: involves toenail
    - Tinea pedis: athlete's foot
    - Tinea cruris: jock itch
16. Erythema: redness due to local inflammation or irritation
17. Eschar: scab or crust
18. Excoriation: scratch
19. Fissure: crack, groove, or crevice
20. Furuncle: boil
21. Hematoma: bruise; caused by collection of blood under the tissue from a blood vessel injury
22. Herpes simplex: cold sore/fever blister; small painful vesicles that erupt around the mouth, lips, nose, or mucous membranes; caused by herpes simplex type I virus
23. Herpes zoster: shingles; acute inflammatory eruption of painful vesicles along the course of a peripheral nerve; caused by herpes zoster virus
24. Impetigo: infectious bacterial infection caused by *staphylococci* or *streptococci;* vesicles dry to form crusts especially around the mouth and nose
25. Jaundice: yellowing of the skin; can be caused by liver, blood, or gallbladder disorders
26. Keloid: abnormal scar formation
27. Lesion: any injury, wound, or area of disease
28. Macule: flat lesion (freckle)
29. Nevus: mole
30. Nodule: raised lesion made of a solid tissue mass
31. Papule: firm, raised lesion (pimple)
32. Pediculosis: infection by lice (genus: *Pediculus*)
    - Pediculosis capitas: head lice
    - Pediculosis corporis: body lice
    - Pediculosis palpebrarus: infestation of eyebrows and lashes
    - Pediculosis pubis: "crabs": genital lice
33. Polyp: cyst on a stalk
34. Pruritis: itching
35. Psoriasis: chronic disease characterized by red lesions and silvery scales; may be autoimmune
36. Pustule: pus-filled vesicle
37. Scleroderma: thick, dense, fibrous skin
38. Ulcer: open sore

39. Urticaria: hives; usually due to allergic reaction
40. Verruca(e): warts; caused by papilloma virus
41. Vesicle: fluid-filled lesion (blister)
42. Vitiligo: white patches on skin due to lack of melanin production
43. Wheal: circular, raised lesion having central pallor and circumscribed redness

V. Skeletal System

A. GENERAL (see Figure 2-7)
■ Composed of bones, cartilage, and ligaments
■ Adult skeleton composed of 206 bones

B. FUNCTIONS
1. Provides a framework for the body: shape and support for other structures
2. Provides for movement: places for muscles to attach
3. Provides protection: surrounds body cavities
4. Provides hematopoiesis: blood cell formation in marrow
5. Provides storage: inorganic minerals (Ca, D, Mg, K, Na) stored in matrix and released into circulation as needed

C. ANATOMY OF LONG BONE
1. Diaphysis: shaft of the long bone; made up of compact and cancellous bone
2. Epiphysis: ends of the long bone
3. Epiphyseal cartilage (plate): "growth plate"; layer of cartilage between the diaphysis and epiphysis where the growth in length occurs
4. Articular cartilage: thin sheet of cartilage that covers the end of the epiphysis; provides a cushion and lubrication for joint
5. Periosteum: tough, vascular covering of the bone; made up of fibrous connective tissue; does not cover the epiphysis
6. Endosteum: lining of the medullary cavity
7. Medullary cavity: cavity in the center of long bones; contains marrow
   • Red marrow: produces red blood cells
   • Yellow marrow: made up of fat

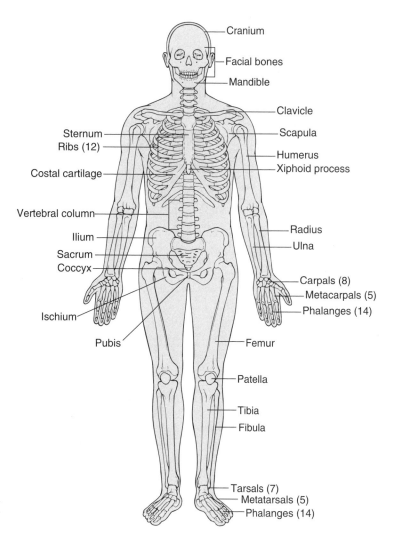

FIGURE 2-7 Normal skeletal system, anterior view. (From Frazier MS, Drzymkowski JW: Essentials of Human Diseases and Conditions, ed 2, Philadelphia, 2000, Saunders, p. 183.)

8. Process: bony projection on the surface of a bone
9. Foramen: an opening in a bone
10. Sinus: bony cavity in a bone

D. BONE CLASSIFICATIONS
 1. Long: length exceeds width
 2. Short: smaller than long bone with expanded ends
 3. Flat: thin, sheetlike
 4. Sesamoid: rounded bones embedded in tendons; round bones
 5. Irregular: various shapes

E. ORGANIZATION OF THE SKELETON
 1. Axial skeleton: consists of bones of the skull, spine, and chest (see Figure 2-8)
  a) Cranium: bones enclose the brain
   1) Frontal: forms forehead
   2) Parietal: forms sides and top
   3) Temporal: forms lower sides and floor; contains ossicles (bones of middle ear): malleus, incus, and stapes; external auditory meatus (opening into middle ear)
   4) Mastoid process: projection located on temporal bone
   5) Styloid process: sharp projection inferior to external auditory meatus
   6) Zygomatic process: projects anteriorly to form prominence of cheek
   7) Occipital: single bone forming post of cranium; contains foramen magnum where spinal cord exits skull
   8) Sphenoid: butterfly-shaped bone that bridges the temporals to form the floor of the cranium; contains sella turcica where the pituitary gland sits
   9) Ethmoid: single bone that forms most of bony area between the nasal cavity and orbits
  b) Facial: forms the basic framework for the face
   1) Nasal: two bones forming the bridge of the nose
   2) Vomer: thin bone that forms the inferior nasal septum
   3) Lacrimal: located in the medial walls of the orbits; contains the lacrimal glands
   4) Zygomatic: forms the arch of the cheekbone
   5) Palatine: forms the post-portion of the hard palate
   6) Mandible: lower jawbone (only movable bone in the face)
   7) Hyoid: U-shaped bone that supports the tongue; only bone that does not articulate with another

  c) Spinal column: composed of 26 vertebrae separated by pads of cartilage (intervertebral disks); houses the spinal cord; 4 distinct curves; common structural pattern (see Figure 2-9)
   1) Cervical vertebrae: first 7, C-1 through C-7; forms the neck
    C-1: atlas; supports the skull
    C-2: axis; allows for rotation of skull
   2) Thoracic vertebrae: next 12, T-1 through T-12; articulate with the ribs
   3) Lumbar vertebrae: next 5, L-1 through L-5; forms the small of the back
   4) Sacrum: triangular-shaped bone; forms the posterior wall of the pelvic cavity
   5) Coccyx: tailbone
  d) Thorax: thoracic cage; protects heart, lungs, and great vessels (see Figure 2-10)
   1) Sternum: breastbone; 3 parts
    • Manubrium: superior, triangular part
    • Body: middle, slender part
    • Xiphoid process: projection at end of body; landmark for CPR
   2) Ribs
    • Curved, flat bones that form the lateral sides of thorax
    • 12 pairs
     (a) True ribs; first 7 pairs; articulate with the sternum by means of costal cartilage
     (b) False ribs: next 3 pairs; articulate with the seventh rib by means of costal cartilage
     (c) Floating ribs: last 2 pairs; do not articulate with the sternum
 2. Appendicular skeleton: made up of bones of upper and lower extremities and girdles that are anchored to the axial skeleton (see Figure 2-11)
  a) Shoulder girdle
   1) Clavicle: collarbone (2); forms a bridge between shoulder blades and breastbone
   2) Scapula: (2) shoulder blade
   3) Humerus: bone of the upper arm
   4) Radius: lateral bone of the forearm (thumb side)
   5) Ulna: medial bone of the forearm (little finger side)
   6) Carpals: 2 rows of 4 bones tightly bound by ligaments; make up the wrist
   7) Metacarpals: 5 bones that make up the hand
   8) Phalanges
    • 3 bones in each finger (proximal, medial, and distal)

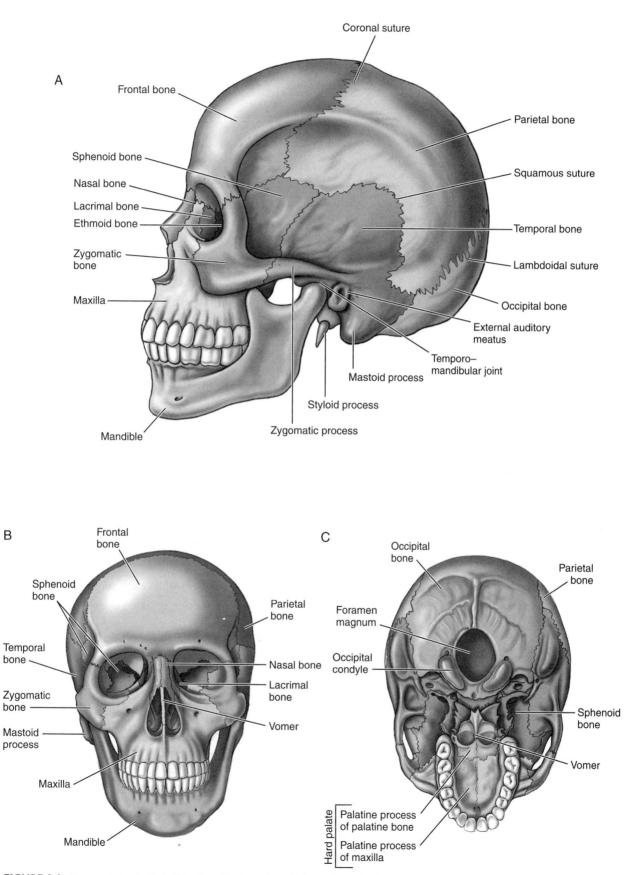

FIGURE 2-8 Bones of the skull. *A,* Side view. *B,* Front view. *C,* Base of the skull. (From Herlihy B, Maebius N: The Human Body in Health and Illness, Philadelphia, 1999, Saunders, p. 118.)

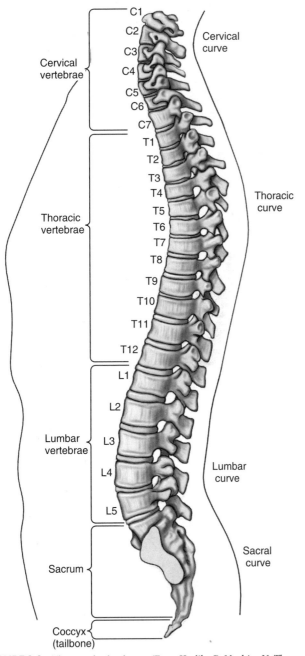

FIGURE 2-9 The vertebral column. (From Herlihy B, Maebius N: The Human Body in Health and Illness, Philadelphia, 1999, Saunders, p. 121.)

- 2 bones in each thumb (proximal and distal)

b) Pelvic girdle: attaches lower extremities to axial skeleton (see Figure 2-12)

  1) Pelvis: os coxae basin-shaped bones on floor of trunk; 3 parts

    • Ilium: superior, wing-shaped bones of hips

    • Ischium: inferior portion; "sit-down" bone

    • Pubis: anterior portion; right and left sides join at symphysis pubis (pad of cartilage)

  2) Femur: thighbone; largest, longest, and strongest bone in the body

  3) Patella: kneecap; triangular-shaped, enclosed in tendon

  4) Tibia: shinbone

    • Lateral malleolus: bulge on outside of ankle

    • Medial malleolus: bulge on inside of ankle

  5) Fibula: smaller leg bone lateral to the tibia

  6) Tarsals: 7 bones that make up the ankle; largest is calcaneous (heel bone)

  7) Metatarsals: 5 bones that make up the instep of the foot

  8) Phalanges: 14 bones that make up the toe

    • 3 in each toe (proximal, medial, and distal)

    • 2 in each great toe (proximal and distal)

c) Articulations: joints; where two bones come together; classified by the amount of movement allowed (see Figure 2-13)

  1) Synarthroses: immovable joints (example: sutures in skull)

  2) Amphiarthroses: slightly movable joints; bones are connected by cartilage (example: symphysis pubis)

  3) Diarthroses: freely movable joints; ends covered with cartilage; separated by a space containing synovial fluid for lubrication (example: elbow)

F. DISEASES AND DISORDERS

  1. Abnormal spinal curvatures

    a) Scoliosis: abnormal lateral curvature of the spine

    b) Kyphosis: humpback; abnormal outward curvature of the spine

    c) Lordosis: swayback; abnormal inward curvature of the spine

  2. Arthritis: inflammation of the joints

    a) Osteoarthritis

      ■ Chronic inflammation of joint

      ■ Results in degeneration of cartilage, which causes hypertrophy of bone

    b) Rheumatoid

      ■ Chronic, systemic inflammatory disease of joint

      ■ Causes erosion of cartilage

    c) Ankylosing spondylitis

      ■ Rheumatoid arthritis of the spine

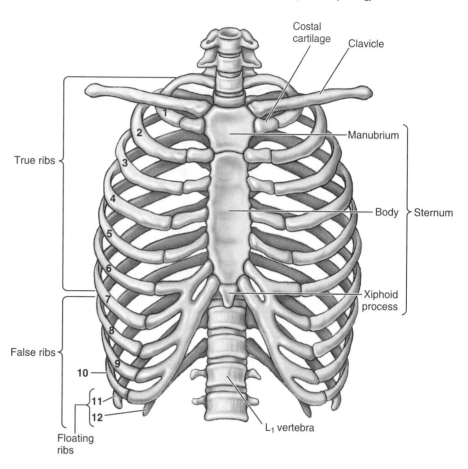

FIGURE 2-10 The thoracic cage. (From Herlihy B, Maebius N: The Human Body in Health and Illness, Philadelphia, 1999, Saunders, p. 124.)

d) Gout
 ■ Arthritis caused by deposit of uric acid in joint
3. Bursitis: inflammation of the bursa (thin sac that helps tendons and muscles move over bones)
4. Fractures: crack or break in a bone
 a) Simple (closed): fracture with no external wound
 b) Compound (open): fracture with external break in the skin
 c) Greenstick: incomplete break
 d) Comminuted: shattering of the bone (bone fragments)
 e) Impacted: one broken end is forced into the other
5. Neoplasms
 a) Osteosarcoma: malignant tumor of connective tissue arising from the bone
 b) Osteochondroma: tumor of bone and cartilage
 c) Chondrosarcoma: tumor of cartilage
6. Osteomalacia: condition of softening of bones; due to low level of vitamin D
7. Osteomyelitis: inflammation of bone, usually following compound fracture or symptoms

8. Osteoporosis: condition of porous, brittle bones, especially in menopausal women; due to low levels of calcium and potassium
9. Paget's disease: osteitis deformans; chronic metabolic disease causing bones to thicken and soften
10. Pott's disease: tuberculosis of the vertebrae
11. Spina bifida: congenital abnormality characterized by failure of vertebrae to close around the spinal cord
12. Sprain: acute partial tear of a muscle, tendon, or ligament
13. Strain: result of overuse, overstretching, or excessive forcible stretching of a muscle
14. Talipes: club foot

VI. Muscular System

A. GENERAL
 ■ Approximately 650 muscles in the body
 ■ Makes up approximately 40% of body weight

B. FUNCTIONS
1. Movement: contractions (shortening) allows movement of bone
2. Protection: sheets of muscle protect internal organs

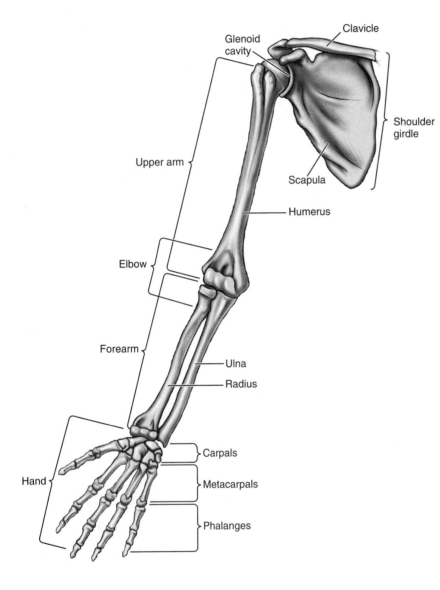

FIGURE 2-11   Bones of the upper limb. (From Herlihy B, Maebius N: The Human Body in Health and Illness, Philadelphia, 1999, Saunders, p. 125.)

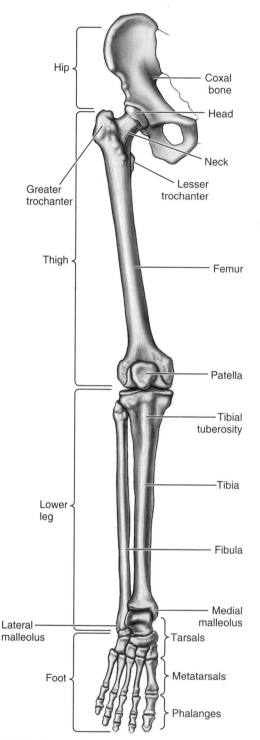

2. Smooth: involuntary muscles (operate automatically); appears nonstriated; helps with metabolic functions
3. Cardiac: found only in the heart; involuntary; causes contraction of heart muscle to maintain blood flow

D. CHARACTERISTICS OF MUSCLE
  1. Excitability: ability to receive and respond to a stimulus
  2. Contractility: ability to shorten (contract)
  3. Extensibility: ability to stretch
  4. Elasticity: ability to return to original shape and length

E. SKELETAL MUSCLE STRUCTURE: Composed of bundles of fibers held together by fibrous connective tissue
  1. Fiber: skeletal muscle cell
  2. Endomysium: connective tissue membrane that covers a muscle fiber
  3. Fasciculus: bundle of muscle fibers
  4. Perimysium: connective tissue membrane that surrounds the fasciculus
  5. Epimysium: tough tissue membrane that covers the entire muscle
  6. Fascia: connective tissue outside of the epimysium; surrounds and separates the muscles
  7. Tendon: strong, cordlike structure that attaches muscles to bones
  8. Aponeurosis: sheetlike tendon that attaches muscle to muscle

F. NAMING OF MUSCLES: May be named according to the following
  1. Size: maximus, medius, longus
  2. Shape: deltoid, latus
  3. Fiber direction: rectus, oblique
  4. Points of attachment:
    a) Origin: point of attachment that does not move on contraction
    b) Insertion: point of attachment that moves on contraction
  5. Number of attachments: biceps, quadriceps
  6. Action of muscle: adductor, flexor, levator

G. MUSCLE ACTIONS
  1. Prime mover: provides movement
  2. Antagonist: opposes prime mover; can cause opposite movement or provide more control and precision to prime mover
  3. Synergist: helps prime mover to work more efficiently and effectively
  4. Fixator: stabilizes the origin of the prime mover

H. MOVEMENT
  ■ Caused by contraction (shortening) of muscle
  ■ Complex series of events based on chemical reactions at cellular level
  ■ Begins with stimulation by nerve cell and ends when the muscle is relaxed
  ■ Requires ATP for energy source

FIGURE 2-12 Bones of the lower limb. (From Herlihy B, Maebius N: The Human Body in Health and Illness, Philadelphia, 1999, Saunders, p. 128.)

3. Posture: provides position and alignment of body parts
4. Heat production: movement produces heat
5. Shape: muscles + bones give the body shape

C. TYPES OF MUSCLE TISSUE (see Figure 2-14)
  1. Skeletal: under conscious control (voluntary); appears striated (striped); provides movement of body

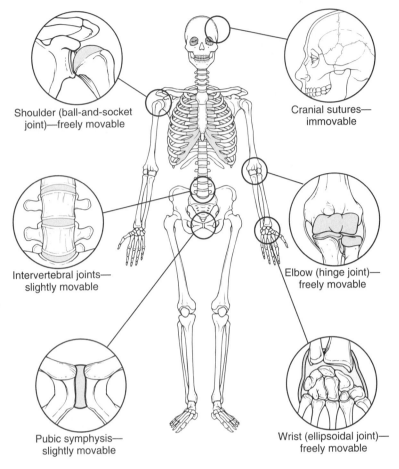

Shoulder (ball-and-socket joint)—freely movable

Cranial sutures—immovable

Intervertebral joints—slightly movable

Elbow (hinge joint)—freely movable

Pubic symphysis—slightly movable

Wrist (ellipsoidal joint)—freely movable

FIGURE 2-13 Examples of types of joints. (From Frazier MS, Drzymkowski JW: Essentials of Human Diseases and Conditions, ed 2, Philadelphia, 2000, Saunders, p. 184.)

I. TYPES OF MOVEMENTS (see Figure 2-15)
1. Flexion: to bend; brings 2 bones closer together and decreases the angle between them
2. Extension: to straighten; opposite of flexion; increases the angle between bones
3. Hyperextension: extension beyond the anatomical position; joint angle in excess of 180 degrees
4. Abduction: to take away; movement of a bone or limb away from the midline of the body
5. Adduction: to bring together; opposite of abduction; movement of a bone or limb toward the midline of the body
6. Circumduction: circular motion of a body part or segment; the proximal end is stationary while the distal end outlines a large circle
7. Rotation: movement of a bone around its own axis
8. Inversion: turning a body part inward
9. Eversion: opposite of inversion; turning a body part outward
10. Supination: movement of a body part to face upward
11. Pronation: opposite of supination; movement of a body part to face downward

J. MAJOR SKELETAL MUSCLES (see Figures 2-16, 2-17)
1. Muscles of facial expression
a) Frontalis: over the frontal bone; raises eyebrows and wrinkles forehead
b) Orbicularis oris: circular muscle that surrounds mouth; closes mouth, forms words, puckers lips
c) Orbicularis oculi: circular muscle that surrounds the eye; helps in winking, blinking, and squinting
d) Buccinator: principle muscle of the cheek; helps in whistling, sucking, and blowing out air
e) Zygomaticus: extends from the zygomatic arch to corner of mouth; raises the corners of the mouth when smiling
2. Muscles of mastication (chewing)
a) Temporalis: largest; inserts in mandible; responsible for chewing
b) Masseter: inserts in mandible; used for chewing
3. Neck muscles
a) Sternocleidomastoid: runs across front of neck from the sternum to clavicle to mastoid process; flexes neck
b) Trapezius: extends from occipital bone to end of thoracic vertebrae; extends head

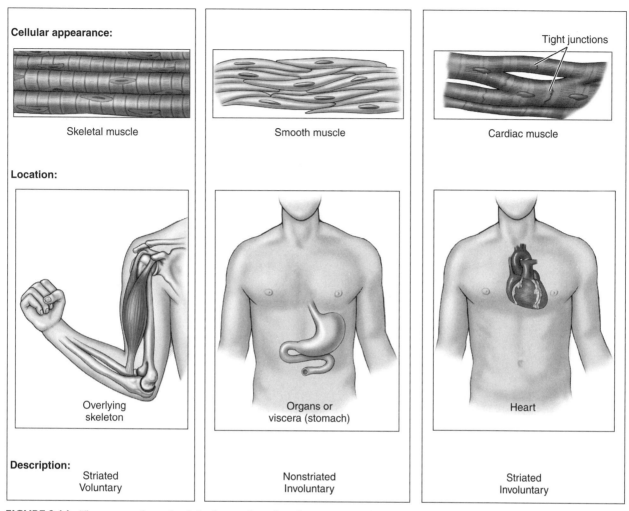

Cellular appearance:

Skeletal muscle

Smooth muscle

Cardiac muscle

Tight junctions

Location:

Overlying skeleton

Organs or viscera (stomach)

Heart

Description:

Striated
Voluntary

Nonstriated
Involuntary

Striated
Involuntary

FIGURE 2-14 Three types of muscle: skeletal, smooth, and cardiac. (From Herlihy B, Maebius N: The Human Body in Health and Illness, Philadelphia, 1999, Saunders, p. 140.)

4. Vertebral column muscles
   a) Erector spinae: group of muscles on each side of vertebral column from sacrum to skull; keeps vertebral column erect
   b) Quadratus lumborum (deep back muscles): short muscles between vertebrae; responsible for movement of vertebral column
5. Thoracic wall muscles
   a) Intercostal muscles (internal and external): located between ribs; helps with breathing
   b) Diaphragm: dome-shaped muscle located between thorax and abdomen; muscle of respiration
6. Abdominal wall muscles
   a) External oblique: fibers run medially and inferiorly
   b) Internal oblique: fibers run opposite of external obliques
   c) Transversus abdominus: fibers run horizontally
   d) Rectus abdominus: fibers run vertically

7. Muscles that move the shoulder and arm
   a) Trapezius: large, triangular muscle of the back; used to shrug shoulders
   b) Serratus anterior: located on side of chest; used in pushing
   c) Pectoralis major: superficial muscle on anterior chest; adductor; moves arm medially across chest
   d) Latissimus dorsi: large superficial muscle of lower back
   e) Deltoid: large triangular muscle that covers the shoulder; used to abduct arm; injection site
   f) Rotator cuff muscles: infraspinatus, supraspinatus, subscapularis, teres minor; assists with movement of the humerus; form cuff over proximal humerus
8. Muscles that move the forearm and hand
   a) Triceps brachii: posterior of arm; extends the forearm
   b) Biceps brachii: flexes the forearm

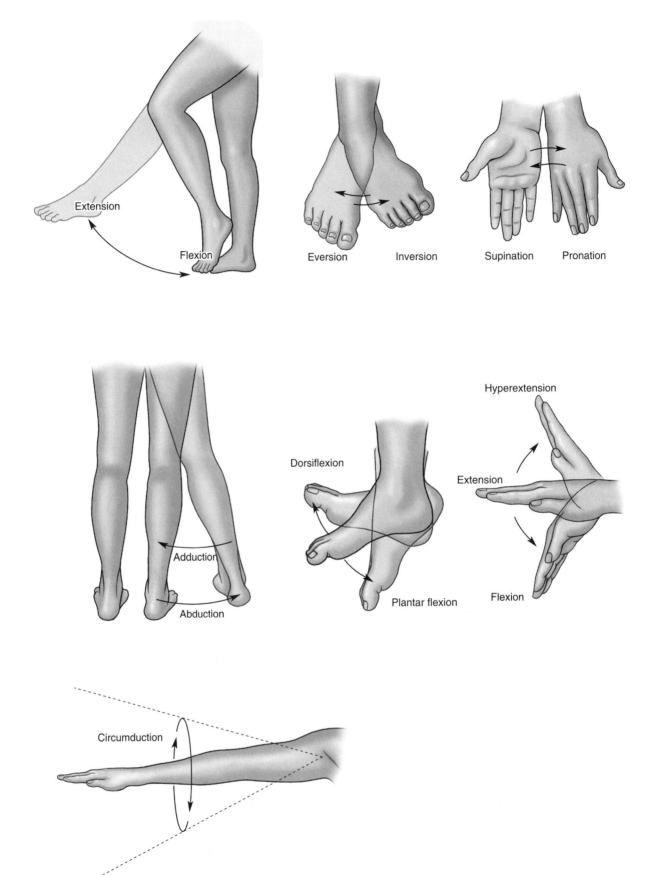

FIGURE 2-15 Types of movements at joints. (From Herlihy B, Maebius N: The Human Body in Health and Illness, Philadelphia, 1999, Saunders, p. 134.)

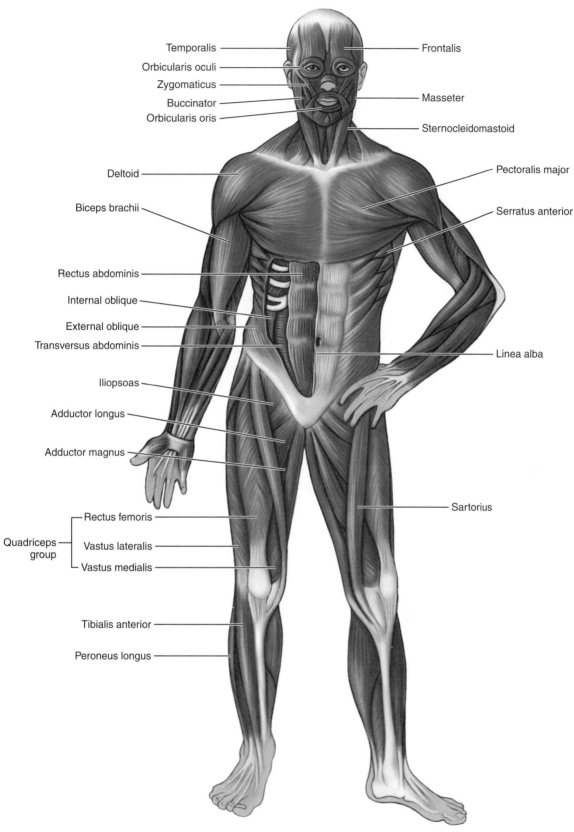

FIGURE 2-16 Major muscles of the body, anterior view. (From Herlihy B, Maebius N: The Human Body in Health and Illness, Philadelphia, 1999, Saunders, p. 150.)

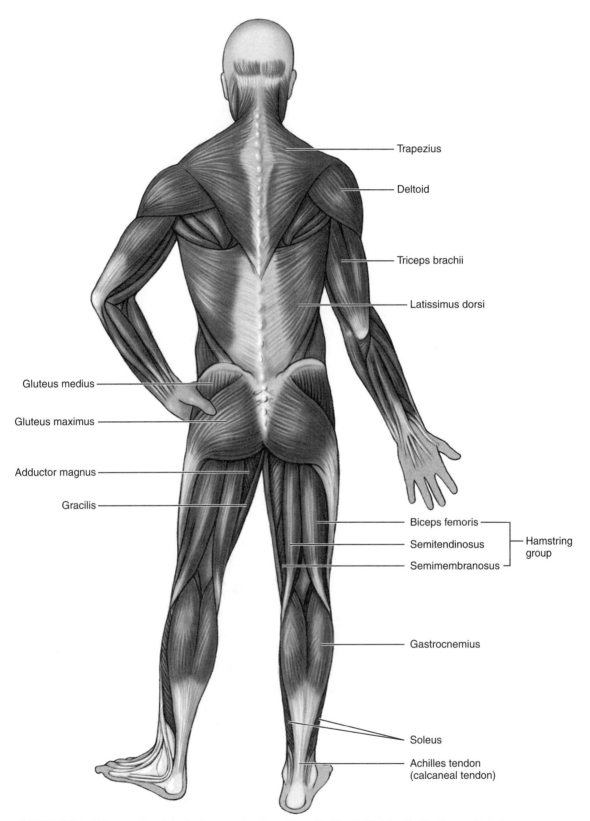

FIGURE 2-17   Major muscles of the body, posterior view. (From Herlihy B, Maebius N: The Human Body in Health and Illness, Philadelphia, 1999, Saunders, p. 151.)

c) Brachialis: flexes the forearm

d) Brachioradialis: lateral side of forearm; flexes the forearm

9. Muscles that move the thigh

   a) Gluteus maximus: forms the buttocks; extends and straightens the thigh at the hip

   b) Gluteus medius: deep to the gluteus maximus; common injection site; abducts the thigh

   c) Gluteus minimus: deepest of gluteal group; abducts the thigh

   d) Iliopsoas: anterior muscle; flexes the thigh

   e) Adductor longus: medial muscle; adduct the thigh

   f) Adductor brevis: medial muscle; adduct the thigh

   g) Adductor magnus: medial muscle; adduct the thigh

   h) Gracilis: medial muscle; adducts the thigh

10. Muscles that move the leg

   a) Quadriceps femoris: group of muscles located on anterior and lateral sides of thigh; extend the leg and straighten the leg at the knee

     1) Vastus lateralis: injection site for infants and children; extends leg and supports knee joint

     2) Vastus intermedius: extends leg

     3) Vastus medialis: extends leg

     4) Rectus femoris: extends leg

   b) Sartorious: longest muscle in the body; runs obliquely over the quad group; flexes and medially rotates the legs (to sit cross-legged)

   c) Hamstrings: posterior to the thigh; flexes the leg at the knee; strong tendons; includes

     1) Biceps femoris

     2) Semi tendinosus

     3) Semi membranosus

11. Muscles that move the ankle and foot

   a) Tibialis anterior: primary muscle of anterior group; dorsiflexion of foot

   b) Peroneus longus: lateral to the leg; everts the foot

   c) Gastrocnemius: posterior to leg (calf); plantar flexion (''toe-dancer's'' muscles)

   d) Soleus: posterior to the leg (calf)

   e) Achilles tendon: common tendon for gastrocnemius and soleus; connects muscles to calcaneus; largest tendon in body

K. DISEASES AND DISORDERS

1. Muscular dystrophy: congenital disorder; characterized by progressive wasting of muscle tissue

2. Myasthenia gravis: chronic, progressive neuromuscular disease; may be autoimmune; characterized by muscle weakness, dysphagia and blepharoptosis

3. Tendinitis (sometimes spelled *tendonitis*): inflammation of tendon

VII. Nervous System

A. GENERAL

■ Major controlling, regulating, and communicating system of the body

■ Works with the endocrine system to regulate and maintain homeostasis

B. FUNCTIONS

1. Control: regulates internal body functions and processes

2. Communication: directs processes among body systems

3. Mental processes: generates thoughts, feelings, perception, sensations, and emotions

C. ORGANIZATION (see Figure 2-18)

1. Central nervous system (CNS): made up of brain and spinal cord

2. Peripheral nervous system (PNS): made up of nerves and ganglia; includes

   a) 12 pairs of cranial nerves originating in the brain

   b) 31 pairs of spinal nerves originating from spinal cord

   c) Afferent (sensory) division: transmits information to brain

   d) Efferent (motor) division: transmits information from brain to organs and body parts

   e) Somatic nervous system: transmits impulses to voluntary muscles

   f) Autonomic nervous system: transmits impulses to involuntary muscles and glands

   g) Sympathetic nervous system: prepares the body for stressful conditions

   h) Parasympathetic nervous system: coordinates the normal resting activities

D. ORGANS OF THE NERVOUS SYSTEM (see Figure 2-19)

1. Neuron: nerve cell; structural and functional unit of nerve tissue; highly specialized; if destroyed, cannot be replaced (does not go through mitosis)

   a) Cell body: contains nucleus and organelles

   b) Dendrites: one or more branching extensions; receives signals from other neurons and brings them to the cell body

   c) Axon: single extension from the cell body; carries impulses away from the cell body

   d) Myelin sheath: white, segmented, fatty substance that surrounds axons; produced by

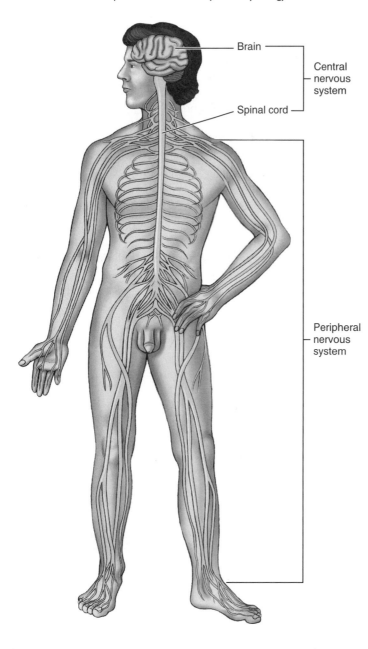

FIGURE 2-18   Divisions of the nervous system: central and peripheral. (From Herlihy B, Maebius N: The Human Body in Health and Illness, Philadelphia, 1999, Saunders, p. 165.)

Schwann cells that cover the axons; serves as an insulator and to speed the conduction of nerve impulses; gives white appearance to fibers (white matter)
- e) Neurilemma: outer membrane of axon
- f) Nodes of Ranvier: gaps in myelin sheath
- g) Neurotransmitter: chemical substance that allows neurons to communicate with each other
2. Neuroglia: "nerve glue"; nonconductive cells of nerve tissue; provides support system (nourishment and protection) for neurons; more numerous than neurons; different types with specialized functions; capable of mitosis
3. Nerves: collection of nerve fibers held together by layers of connective tissue
   a) Afferent (sensory): carry impulses from PNS to CNS

   b) Efferent (motor): carry impulses from CNS to PNS
4. Brain (see Figure 2-20)
   a) Cerebrum: largest superior portion; consists of thin layer of gray matter (cerebral cortex) and white matter (bulk of cerebrum)
      1) Cortex: makes us "human"; concerned with memory, language, reasoning, intelligence, personality, and other factors associated with human life
      2) Divided into two halves (hemispheres) by longitudinal fissure
         (a) Right hemisphere: controls the left side of the body
            • Responsible for auditory perception, tactile perception, and interpretation of spatial relationships

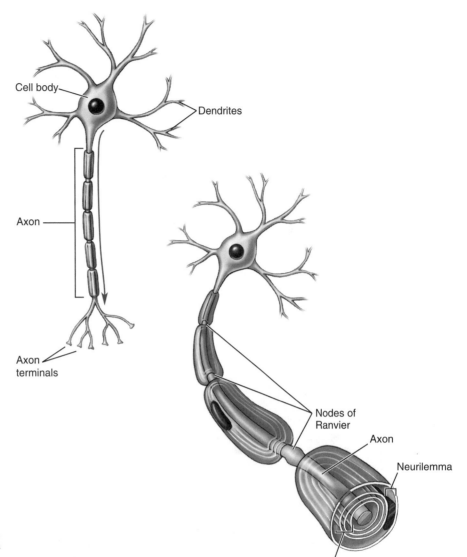

Cell body

Dendrites

Axon

Axon
terminals

Nodes of
Ranvier

Axon

Neurilemma

Myelin sheath

FIGURE 2-19 Structure of a neuron. (From Herlihy B, Maebius N: The Human Body in Health and Illness, Philadelphia, 1999, Saunders, p. 167.)

(b) Left hemisphere: controls the right side of the body
- Responsible for language and hand movements
- Hemispheres divided into 5 lobes

3) Each hemisphere is divided into 5 lobes named for bones that cover them (except for the insula)
   (a) Frontal lobe: controls voluntary muscle movements and speech
   (b) Parietal lobe: receives and integrates sensory output
   (c) Temporal lobe: interprets sound; involved with personality, emotion, memory, and behavior
   (d) Occipital lobe: interprets sight
   (e) Insula: visceral effects

4) Ventricles: cavities within each hemisphere that make and store CSF

b) Diencephalon: centrally located; surrounded by cerebral hemispheres
   1) Thalamus: relay station for all sensory input; associated with pain, temperature, and touch sensations; located between cerebrum and midbrain
   2) Hypothalamus: located below thalamus; important role in regulating heart rate, blood pressure, body temperature, water balance, hunger, sleep, and wakefulness

c) Brain stem
   1) Medulla oblongata: lowest portion of brain, connects to spinal cord; contains vital centers for control of heartbeat, respiration, and blood pressure

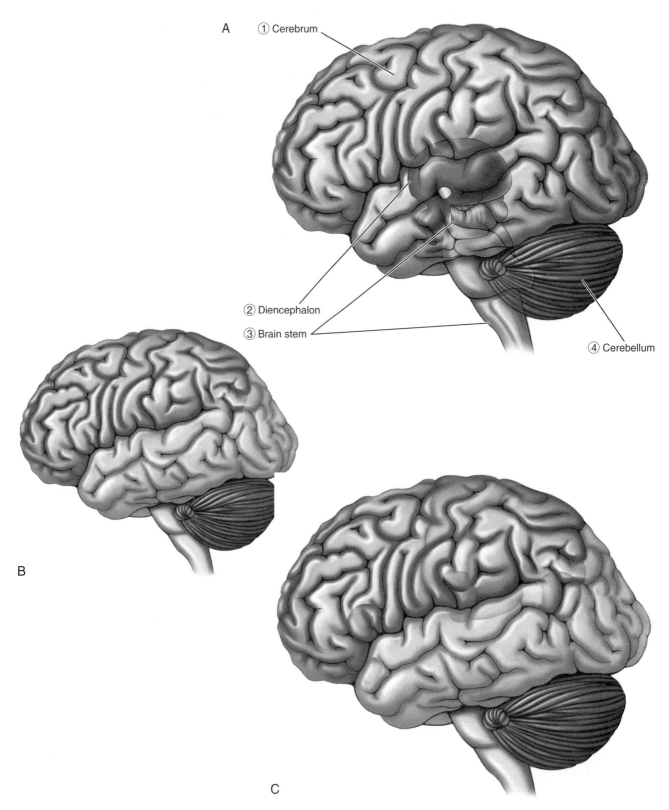

A

① Cerebrum

② Diencephalon

③ Brain stem

④ Cerebellum

B

C

FIGURE 2-20 A, The brain's four major areas. B, The lobes of the cerebrum. C, The functional areas of the cerebrum. (From Herlihy B, Maebius N: The Human Body in Health and Illness, Philadelphia, 1999, Saunders, p. 175.)

2) Pons: bulge at the base of the brain; links the cerebellum to the rest of the nervous system; nerve fibers cross here; one side of the brain controls the other side of the body

3) Midbrain: upper portion of the brain stem; correlates information about muscle tone and posture; relay center for certain eye and ear reflexes

d) Cerebellum: second largest portion of the brain, located below the cerebrum; responsible for coordination of voluntary movement, posture, and balance

e) Spinal cord: extends from the brain stem through the foramen magnum into the vertebral column to the second lumbar vertebra; approximately 17" long; conducts nerve impulses to and from brain; center for spinal reflexes; 31 pairs of spinal nerves connected to cord

f) Meninges: protective membrane covering brain and spinal cord; 3 layers

1) Dura mater: strong, fibrous outer layer

2) Arachnoid: middle, delicate weblike layer that allows for movement of CSF

3) Pia mater: thin inner layer; contains blood vessels to supply the brain

g) Meningeal spaces

1) Epidural space: located between dura mater and bone (skull or vertebra); acts as a cushion

2) Subdural space: located between dura mater and arachnoid; contains serous fluid for lubrication

3) Subarachnoid space: located between arachnoid and pia mater; contains CSF

h) Cerebral spinal fluid (CSF): clear, colorless, watery fluid found in subarachnoid space and in the ventricles of the brain; is constantly circulating; provides protective cushion for the brain; can detect physiological changes in the body

E. DISEASES AND DISORDERS OF THE BRAIN

1. Alzheimer's disease: senile dementia; chronic organic brain syndrome; characterized by degeneration of nervous tissue resulting in lowered intellectual functioning and untimely death

2. Amyotrophic lateral sclerosis (ALS); also known as Lou Gehrig's disease; affects motor neurons; characterized by muscle atrophy and weakness

3. Cerebral palsy: due to congenital brain defects or injury at birth; characterized by loss of sensation and/or control of muscle movements

4. Encephalitis: inflammation of the brain

5. Epilepsy: abnormal electrical activity of the brain; characterized by random, intense electrical discharges that result in seizure activity

6. Guillain-Barré syndrome: acute rapidly progressive disease of the spinal nerves

7. Hydrocephalus: excessive amount of CFS causing macroencephaly

8. Meningitis: inflammation of meninges; can be caused by virus or bacteria

9. Migraine: periodic severe headaches; accompanied by nausea and vomiting, auras, and throbbing pain

10. Multiple sclerosis (MS): chronic inflammation of CNS; attacks myelin sheath causing sensory and motor abnormalities

11. Neuritis: inflammation of peripheral nerves

12. Paralysis: loss of voluntary muscular control and sensation to a body part or organ

a) Hemiplegia: paralysis of one side of body, often due to stroke (CVA)

b) Paraplegia: paralysis of trunk and lower extremities, due to spinal cord injury; the area below the injury is paralyzed

c) Quadriplegia: paralysis of all four extremities

d) Bell's palsy: paralysis of muscles on one side of face

13. Parkinson's disease: chronic disease; characterized by tremors and muscle rigidity

14. Stroke: cerebrovascular accident (CVA); ''brain attack''; caused by occlusion or hemorrhage of blood vessels supplying the brain; results in impairment and paralysis of the affected side

15. Transient ischemic attack (TIA): ''mini'' stroke; temporary, recurrent episodes of impaired neurological activity; due to lack of blood flow to the brain

VIII. Special Senses

A. GENERAL

■ Variety of receptors located in various structures

■ Stimulation of a receptor by an appropriate stimulus results in an impulse, which is sent to the CNS, where it is processed

■ Allows the human to be aware of the world around him/her

■ Depends on sensory receptors classified as
  • General (widely distributed)
  • Special (localized in a specific area)

B. GENERAL SENSES: somatic senses; found throughout the body (see Figure 2-21)

1. Touch and pressure

a) Mechanoreceptor (responds to a bending, or a change in the shape of a cell)

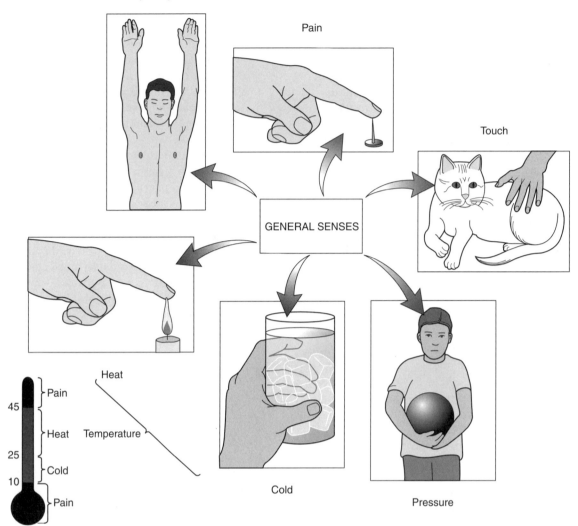

FIGURE 2-21   The general senses. (From Herlihy B, Maebius N: The Human Body in Health and Illness, Philadelphia, 1999, Saunders, p. 217.)

b) Widely distributed in skin
c) Includes free nerve endings, Meissner's corpuscles (touch), Pacinian corpuscles (pressure)
2. Position and orientation: proprioceptors
3. Temperature
a) Thermoreceptor (detects change in temperature)
b) Found immediately under the skin
c) Ten times more cold receptors than heat receptors
4. Pain
a) Nociceptors (responds to tissue damage)
b) Widely distributed in skin and tissues of internal organs
c) Protective function
C. SPECIAL SENSES: located within special organs
1. Gustatory sense
a) Sense of taste
b) Organs of taste (taste buds) localized on the surface of tongue

c) Chemoreceptors (sensitive to chemicals in food)
d) Includes receptors for sensations of salty, sweet, sour, and bitter
2. Olfactory sense
a) Sense of smell
b) Receptors found in upper nose
c) Chemoreceptors
d) Closely related to sense of taste
3. Visual sense: (see Figure 2-22)
a) receptors located in the eye
b) Photoreceptors (detects light)
1) Eye
(a) Found in protective bony socket (orbit)
(b) Three layers (tunics)
(1) Sclera
• Outer layer; white of the eye
• Made of tough fibrous tissue

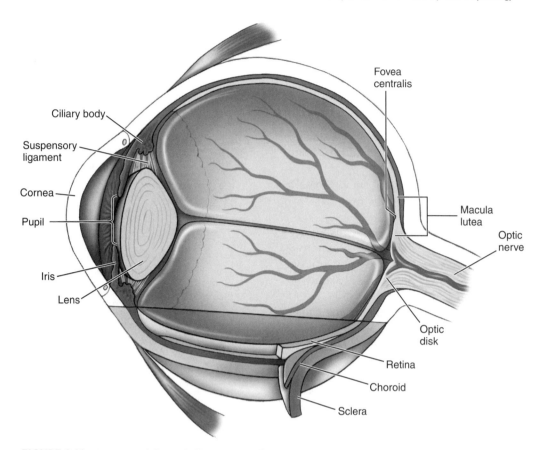

FIGURE 2-22   Structure of the eyeball. (From Herlihy B, Maebius N: The Human Body in Health and Illness, Philadelphia, 1999, Saunders, p. 222.)

- Anterior portion covered by cornea which focuses light rays
(2) Choroid
  - Middle layer
  - Highly vascular
  - Ciliary body; changes shape of the lens
  - Suspensory ligament: connects the ciliary body to lens
  - Iris: colored portion of the eye
    —Doughnut-shaped muscle with hole in the middle (pupil)
    —Continually contracts and relaxes to regulate the amount of light entering the eye
(3) Retina
  - Innermost layer
  - Posterior portion of the eye
  - Contains
    —Rods: receptors sensitive to shades of gray
    —Cones: receptors sensitive to color

- Fovea centralis: area of closely packed cones that function as the area of sharpest vision
  - Optic disk: area on the retina where the optic nerve exits the eye; the "blind spot"
2) Cavities
  (a) Anterior cavity: anterior space between the lens and the cornea; filled with aqueous humor (maintains shape and internal pressure)
  (b) Posterior cavity: between lens and the retina; filled with gel-like substance (vitreous humor); keeps retina against the wall of the eye, supports parts of the eye and helps to maintain shape
3) Accessory structures
  (a) Eyebrows and eyelashes: protects against foreign objects
  (b) Eyelids: opens and closes eye to keep foreign objects out and to keep eye moist
  (c) Lacrimal apparatus: lacrimal glands make tears to lubricate,

moisten, and cleanse the eye; nasolacrimal duct drains tears into the nasal cavity

(d) Conjunctiva: mucous membrane that lines the inner eyelids and anterior eyeball

4) Muscles of the eye

(a) Extrinsic muscles: skeletal muscles attached to the orbital bones and outer eye

(b) Intrinsic muscles: smooth muscles located in the eye

5) Visual pathway

light ray → cornea → aqueous humor → pupil → lens → vitreous humor → retina (rods and cones) → optic nerve fibers → optic chiasma → thalamus → cerebral cortex

4. Auditory sense: receptors located in the ears; mechanoreceptors (see Figure 2-23)

a) Ear: found on both sides of the head

1) External ear

(a) Auricle (pinna): fleshy part visible on sides of head; collects sound waves and directs them toward the auditory meatus

(b) External auditory meatus: short tube that extends from the auricle to the tympanic membrane;

lined with glands that produce cerumen (earwax) to protect and lubricate

2) Middle ear: found in the temporal bone

(a) Tympanic membrane: eardrum

(b) Auditory tube: eustachian tube; extends from the middle ear to the throat; equalizes pressure between the outside air and the middle ear cavity

(c) Ossicles: 3 tiny bones of the middle ear

• Malleus: attached to the tympanic membrane

• Incus: connects the malleus to the stapes

• Stapes: attached to the incus and oval window

(d) Oval window: membrane covering the opening into the vestibule

3) Inner ear

(a) Bony labyrinth

• Series of interconnecting chambers in the temporal bone

• Contains membranous labyrinth filled with fluid (endolymph)

• Space between the bony and membranous labyrinth is filled with fluid (perilymph)

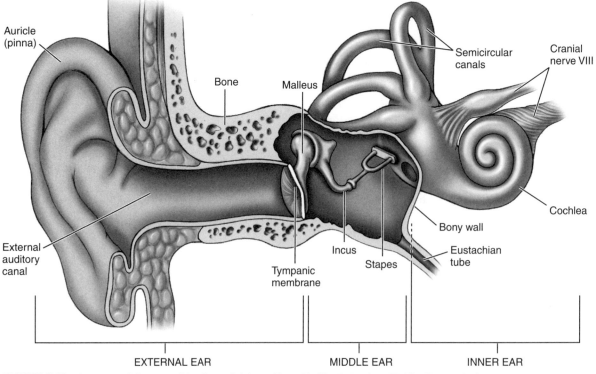

FIGURE 2-23   Structure of the ear and its three divisions. (From Herlihy B, Maebius N: The Human Body in Health and Illness, Philadelphia, 1999, Saunders, p. 229.)

• Divided into 3 sections:
—Vestibule: involved with balance
—Semicircular canals: involved with equilibrium
—Cochlea: snail-shaped structure involved with hearing; contains the organ of Corti which contains receptors for sound

b) Auditory pathway
sound wave → pinna → external auditory meatus → tympanic membrane → malleus → incus → stapes → oval window → cochlea → perilymph → auditory nerve fibers → cerebral cortex

D. DISEASES AND DISORDERS
1. Astigmatism: irregular focusing of light rays due to a nonspheroid cornea
2. Blepharitis: inflammation of the eyelids
3. Cataract: opaqueness, cloudiness of the lens of the eye
4. Conjunctivitis: "pinkeye"; inflammation of the conjunctiva
5. Deafness: inability to hear
6. Diplopia: double vision
7. Glaucoma: accumulation of fluid in the eye: increases pressure that can cause damage to the retina and the optic nerve
8. Hordeolum: "stye"; infection of the sebaceous gland of eye
9. Hyperopia: farsightedness; ability to clearly see far objects but not near objects
10. Impacted cerumen: solidified earwax compacted within the ear canal
11. Keratitis: inflammation of the eyelids
12. Macular degeneration: degenerative disease in the center of the field of vision (macular lutea); affects central vision, not peripheral
13. Ménière's disease: chronic disease of the inner ear; characterized by vertigo, tinnitus, progressive hearing loss, and sensation of fullness, pressure, in the ear
14. Myopia: nearsightedness; ability to clearly see near objects but not far objects
15. Nystagmus: repetitive involuntary movement of the eye
16. Otitis media: inflammation of the middle ear
17. Otosclerosis: bone formation around the oval window and stapes; causes partial to complete deafness
18. Presbyopia: inability to focus quickly; due to loss of lens elasticity due to aging
19. Retinal detachment: partial/complete separation of the retina from the choroid; results in blindness
20. Ruptured tympanic membrane: an opening in the eardrum due to middle ear inflammation caused by sharp objects in the canal or a blow to the ear; major risk is infection developing in the middle ear
21. Strabismus: "lazy eye"; inability of both eyes to focus on the same thing
22. Tinnitus: ringing in ears
23. Vertigo: dizziness

IX. Blood

A. GENERAL
■ Primary transport medium of the body
■ Pumped by the heart through a closed system of vessels
■ Classified as connective tissue (cells and matrix)
■ About 5 liters in adult
■ 8% of body weight

B. FUNCTIONS
1. Transportation
   a) Carries oxygen and nutrients to cells
   b) Carries carbon dioxide and wastes from the tissues to the lungs and kidneys for removal
   c) Carries hormones from the endocrine glands to other parts of the body
2. Regulation
   a) Regulates body temperature by removing heat from active areas and transporting that heat to skin for dissipation
   b) Helps regulate fluid and electrolyte balance
   c) Regulates pH through buffers
3. Protection
   a) Provides clotting mechanism to prevent fluid loss when vessels are damaged
   b) White blood cells engulf and destroy invading microorganisms
   c) Antibodies react with the offending agents

C. COMPOSITION OF BLOOD (see Figure 2-24)
1. Plasma
   a) Liquid portion of circulating blood
   b) 55% of total blood volume
   c) 90% water
   d) Continuously changing due to dissolved solutes
   e) Contains plasma proteins
      1) Albumin: maintains osmotic pressure
      2) Globulin: functions in lipid transport and immune reaction
      3) Fibrinogen: formation of blood clots
   f) Also contains amino acids, urea, uric acids, nutrients, hormones, oxygen, carbon dioxide, antibodies, and electrolytes

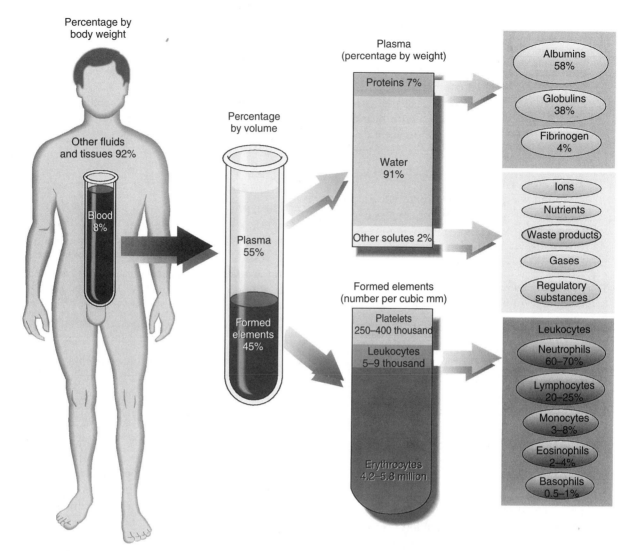

FIGURE 2-24 Components of blood. (From Patton KT, Thibodeau G: The Human Body in Health and Disease, ed 2, St. Louis, 1997, Mosby, p. 294.)

2. Formed elements: produced by hemopoiesis (red blood cells in red bone marrow; white blood cells in lymphoid tissue); all types develop from stem cell (hematocytoblast)
   a) Erythrocytes (red blood cells; RBCs)
      1) Most numerous of formed elements
      2) Normal range: 4.5 to 6 million per cubic millimeter of blood
      3) Biconcave disks (thin in the middle and thick around the edge)
      4) Mature cells have no nucleus
      5) Primary function: to carry oxygen to all body cells; oxygen combines with hemoglobin and is transported
      6) Formation regulated by hormone erythropoietin
      7) Iron, vitamin B-12, and folic acid are essential to RBC production
      8) Live about 120 days; are then destroyed by spleen and liver
   b) Leukocytes (white blood cells; WBCs)
      1) Larger in size than RBCs, but fewer in number
      2) Normal range: 5,000 to 10,000 per/cubic millimeter of blood
      3) Each contains a nucleus
      4) Able to move through capillary walls into tissue
      5) Primary function: to provide defense against invading microorganisms; promote or inhibit inflammatory response
      6) Types:
         (a) Granulocytes: contains granules in cytoplasm
            • Neutrophil: most common; have multilobed nucleus; responds first to tissue damage;

number increases in acute infection
- Eosinophil: two-lobed nucleus; large granules in cytoplasm; neutralize histamine; numbers increase during allergic reaction and parasitic infections
- Basophil: least numerous of WBCs; has large U-shaped nucleus; can leave blood and enter tissue, where they release histamine and heparin

(b) Agranylocytes: granules absent in cytoplasm
- Lymphocytes: large round nucleus surrounded by small amount of cytoplasm; role in body's defense system
  —T-lymphocytes: directly attacks microorganisms
  —B-lymphocytes: produce antibodies

- Monocytes: largest in size of all WBCs; can enter the tissue (macrophage); finish the cleanup process of the neutrophils

c) Thrombocytes (platelets)
1) Small fragments of very large cells (megakaryocytes)
2) Normal range: 250,000 to 500,000 per cubic millimeter of blood
3) Initiates formation of blood clots

D. HEMOSTASIS: stoppage of bleeding; includes three processes (see Figure 2-25)
1. Vascular constriction: reduces flow of blood through torn vessel
2. Platelet plug formation: platelets become sticky and adhere to each other
3. Coagulation: complex series of steps that results in clot formation; requires calcium and vitamin K

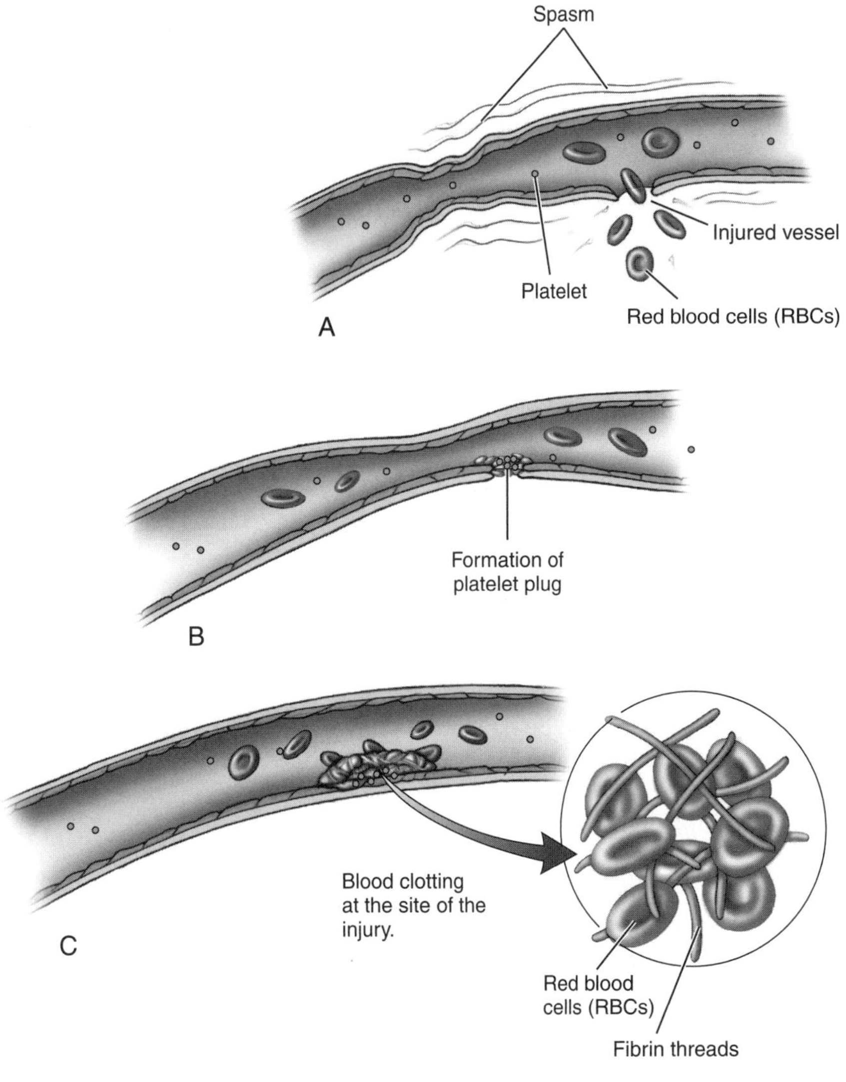

FIGURE 2-25 The steps of hemostasis: *A,* Vascular constriction. *B,* Formation of the platelet plug. *C,* Blood clotting (coagulation). (From Herlihy B, Maebius N: The Human Body in Health and Illness, Philadelphia, 1999, Saunders, p. 273.)

E. BLOOD TYPING
1. Based on specific antigens and antibodies related to RBCs; blood type antigens are found on RBC's; antibodies in plasma
2. Main blood groups ABO blood groups; blood types MUST match in transfusions:
   a) Type A: has A antigens on RBCs; has anti-B antibodies
   b) Type B: has B antigens on RBCs; has anti-A antibodies
   c) Type AB: has A and B antigens on RBCs; has no antibodies
   d) Type O: has neither A or B antigens on RBCs; has both anti-A and anti-B antibodies
3. Rh factor: Rh+ has Rh antigen on RBCs; Rh− has no antigens; neither has anti-Rh in plasma; hemolytic disease of the newborn may develop when Rh− mother has Rh+ fetus

F. DISEASES AND DISORDERS
1. Anemia: abnormal decrease in hemoglobin, RBC count or hematocrit
2. Leukemia: malignant neoplasm of blood-forming organs; usually involves one specific type of blood cell
3. Polycythemia: abnormal increase in hemoglobin, RBC count, or hematocrit
4. Thrombocytopenia: decrease in thrombocytes; results in decrease in clotting capabilities

X. Lymphatic System

A. GENERAL
■ Part of the circulatory system
■ Transports a fluid (lymph) through lymphatic vessels and empties it into venous blood
■ Major role in the body's defense system

B. FUNCTIONS
1. Returns excess interstitial fluid to blood
2. Absorbs fats and fat-soluble vitamins from the digestive system
3. Provides defense against disease

C. ORGANS OF THE LYMPHATIC SYSTEM (see Figure 2-26)
1. Lymph
   a) Similar in composition to blood plasma
   b) Picked up from interstitial fluid and returned to blood plasma
2. Lymphatic vessels
   a) Found in tissue spaces
   b) Carry fluid away from the tissues
   c) Vessels empty into the lymphatic ducts:
      1) Right lymphatic duct: drains lymph from upper right quadrant of the body
      2) Thoracic duct: drains the remainder of the body

3. Lymphatic organs
   a) Lymph nodes
      1) Located along the lymphatic vessels
      2) Superficial nodes found in the groin, axilla, and neck
      3) Filter and cleanse the lymph before it enters the blood
   b) Tonsils
      1) provide protection against pathogens that may enter through the mouth or nose
      2) 3 groups
         (a) pharyngeal tonsils: located near the opening of the nose into the pharynx; adenoids
         (b) palatine tonsils: "the tonsils"; located near the opening of the oral cavity into the pharynx
         (c) lingual tonsils: posterior surface of the tongue
4. Spleen: located in the upper left abdomen beneath the diaphragm, posterior to the stomach; filters blood; acts as a reservoir for the blood
5. Thymus: located posterior to the sternum; large in infants, it atrophies after puberty; produces thymosin (stimulates the maturation of lymphocytes in the lymphatic organs)

D. RESISTANCE TO DISEASE
■ Resistance is the body's ability to counteract pathogens
■ Susceptibility is the lack of resistance
■ Resistance is accomplished through defense mechanisms:
1. Nonspecific defense mechanisms: directed against all pathogens and foreign substances; provides first line of defense against invasion (see Figure 2-27)
   a) Barriers
      ■ Mechanical (e.g., skin)
      ■ Chemical (e.g., hydrochloric acid in stomach)
   b) Chemical action
      ■ Complement: promotes phagocytosis and inflammation
      ■ Interferon: produced by virus-infected cells to provide protection for neighboring cells
   c) Phagocytosis: neutrophils and macrophages
   d) Inflammation: characterized by redness, warmth, swelling, and pain
2. Specific defense mechanisms: programmed to be selective (specificity); ability to remember invading agent (memory); invading agent called antigen; B-lymphorcytes produce anti-

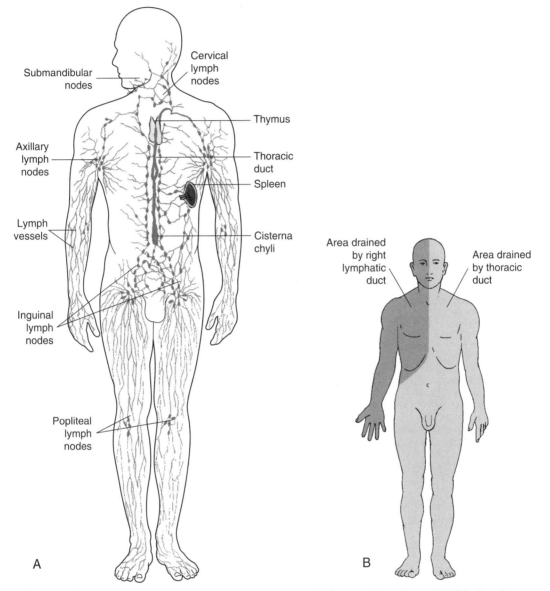

FIGURE 2-26 The lymphatic system. *A,* Principal organs. *B,* Lymph drainage. (From Patton KT, Thibodeau G: The Human Body in Health and Disease, ed 2, St. Louis, 1997, Mosby, p. 356.)

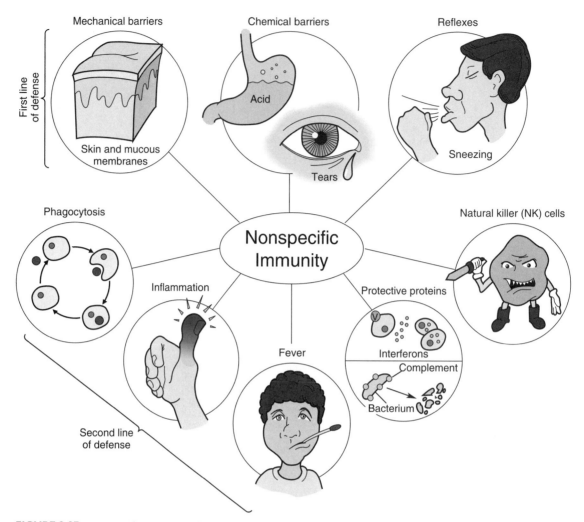

FIGURE 2-27   Nonspecific immunity. The first line of defense includes mechanical barriers, chemical barriers, and reflexes. Processes involved in the second line of defense are phagocytosis, inflammation, fever, protective proteins (complement proteins and interferons) and natural killer cells. (From Herlihy B, Maebius N: The Human Body in Health and Illness, Philadelphia, 1999, Saunders, p. 346.)

bodies that react with the antigen (see Figure 2-28)

   a) Acquired Immunity

      1) Active natural immunity: results when a person has disease

      2) Active artificial immunity: results when a specific antigen is deliberately introduced into a person (immunization)

      3) Passive natural immunity: results when antibodies are transferred from one person to another (as mother to child)

      4) Passive artificial immunity: results when antibodies that developed in another person or animal are injected into a person

   b) Natural immunity: acquired through normal activities

E. DISEASES AND DISORDERS OF THE LYMPHATIC SYSTEM

   1. Acquired immunodeficiency syndrome (AIDS): suppression or deficiency of immune system caused by HIV (human immunodeficiency virus)

   2. Hodgkin's disease: malignant condition of lymphatic tissue in spleen and nodes

   3. Lymphedema: abnormal accumulation of lymph due to obstruction of vessels; occurs in the extremities

   4. Mononucleosis: acute infectious disease caused by Epstein-Barr virus by direct oral contact

   5. Non-Hodgkin's lymphoma: malignant disease of lymphatic system

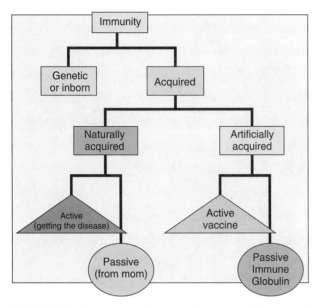

FIGURE 2-28 Immunity is either genetic or acquired. Immunity is acquired either naturally or artificially. Naturally acquired immunity can be either active (triangles) or passive (circles). (From Herlihy B, Maebius N: The Human Body in Health and Illness, Philadelphia, 1999, Saunders, p. 354.)

XI. Cardiovascular System

A. GENERAL
- Closed, sterile system
- Consists of heart and blood vessels

B. FUNCTIONS
1. Transportation: carries important elements throughout the body
2. Temperature regulation: helps with the regulation of body temperature through dilation and constriction of blood vessels
3. Waste removal: assists the lungs, kidneys, and liver
4. Fluid balance: maintains balance between fluid loss and fluid retention

C. ORGANS
1. Heart (see Figure 2-29)
    - Hollow, muscular, cone-shaped organ about the size of a fist; located slightly to the left of midline in the mediastinum; protected by the sternum and ribs; upper end is base; lower end is pointed and is the apex (apical pulse)
    - Made up of 3 layers
      a) Epicardium: outer layer
      b) Myocardium: thick, middle muscular layer
      c) Endocardium: inner layer
    - Covered by pericardium (double-layered sac that decreases friction and protects the heart)
    - Contains 4 chambers
      a) Atria: (singular: "atrium"); 2 upper chambers; receive blood from veins
      b) Ventricles: 2 lower chambers; receive blood from atria and pump it into the body
      c) Septum: divides chambers into right and left
      d) Valves: structures that allow one-way flow of blood throughout the heart
        1) Tricuspid valve: permits blood to flow from right atrium to right ventricle; composed of 3 flaps of tissue
        2) Bicuspid valve: (mitral valve); made up of 2 flaps of tissue; permits blood to flow from left atrium to left ventricle
        3) Pulmonary valve: located at the entrance of the pulmonary artery; prevents backflow of blood into the right ventricle; semilunar (half-mooned shape)
        4) Aortic valve: located at the entrance of the aorta; prevents backflow of blood into the left ventricle; semilunar
          blood enters right atrium → right ventricle → pulmonary artery → pulmonary capillaries (exchange of gases) → pulmonary vein → left atrium → left ventricle → aorta → capillaries in body tissues (exchange in gases) → superior and inferior vena cavae → right atrium
    - Electrical conduction system: initiates and maintains the rhythmic heart contractions (see Figure 2-30)
      a) Sinoatrial node (SA node): pacemaker of the heart; located in the right atrial wall near the superior vena cava; initiates heartbeat and sets its pace
      b) Atrioventricular node (AV node): located in lower right atrial septum; causes the atria to contract
      c) Bundle of His: located in ventricular septum
      d) Bundle branches: two branches extending from bundle of His
      e) Purkinje fibers: extend from the bundle branches; causes ventricles to contract
    - Cardiac cycle: complete heartbeat; consists of contraction (systole) and relaxation (diastole) of both atria and ventricles; complete cycle lasts for 0.8 second (75 bpm); sounds associated with heartbeat described as lubb-dupp
2. Vessels
    a) Artery: vessels that carry blood away from the heart
      - Composed of 3 layers
        1) Tunica adventitia: outermost layer of tough fibrous connective tissue

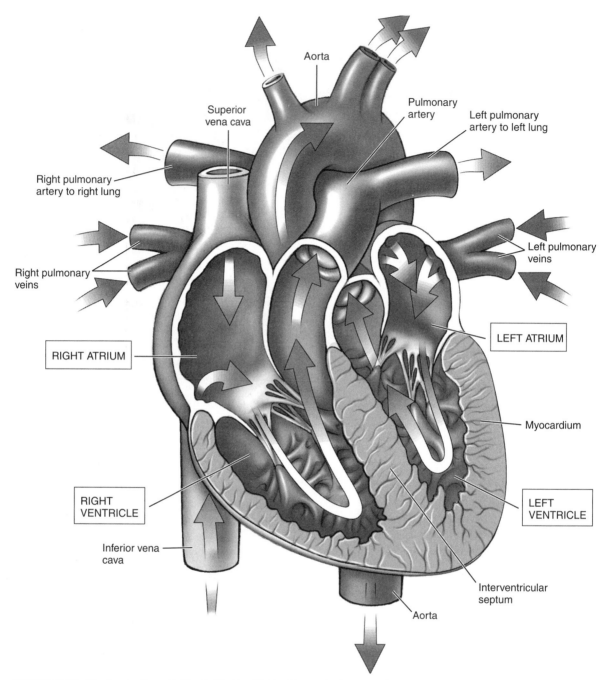

FIGURE 2-29   The heart. (From Herlihy B, Maebius N: The Human Body in Health and Illness, Philadelphia, 1999, Saunders, p. 288.)

2) Tunica media: middle layer of smooth muscle tissue allowing for contraction and dilation

3) Tunica intima: innermost layer
   ■ Arteriole: small arteries

b) Veins: vessels that carry blood toward the heart
   ■ Same layers as arteries, except tunica advinitia is thicker and tunica intima has valves to prevent backflow
   ■ Venules: small veins

c) Capillaries: microscopic vessels, one cell-layer thick
   ■ Connects arterioles and venules
   ■ Exchange of substances takes place here

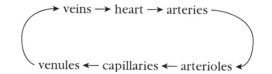

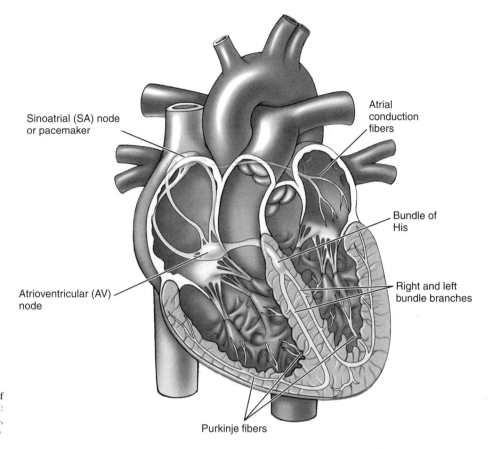

Sinoatrial (SA) node
or pacemaker

Atrial
conduction
fibers

Bundle of
His

Atrioventricular (AV)
node

Right and left
bundle branches

Purkinje fibers

FIGURE 2-30 Conduction system of the heart. (From Herlihy B, Maebius N: The Human Body in Health and Illness, Philadelphia, 1999, Saunders, p. 293.)

3. Major arteries (see Figure 2-31)
   a) Pulmonary: comes from the right ventricle; transports deoxygenated blood to lungs
   b) Aorta: largest artery in the body; comes from the heart; divided into ascending aorta, aortic arch, descending aorta, and abdominal aorta
   c) Coronary: right and left branches off the ascending aorta; supplies the heart with blood
   d) Brachiocephalic: one of 3 major branches off the aortic arch; supplies blood to the neck, head, axilla, and upper arm
   e) Subclavian: supplies arms and vertebrae
      ▪ Left subclavian branches from aortic arch
      ▪ Right subclavian branches from brachiocephalic
   f) Carotid: supplies neck and head
      ▪ Left carotid branches from aortic arch
      ▪ Right carotid branches from brachiocephalic
   g) Facial: branch of carotid; supplies face and cranium
   h) Occipital: branch of carotid; supplies neck and cranium
   i) Axillary: extension of subclavian; supplies the axilla
   j) Brachial: extension of axillary; supplies the upper arm
   k) Radial: branch of brachial; supplies forearm, wrist, and hand
   l) Ulnar: branch of brachial on little finger side; supplies forearm, wrist, and hand
   m) Celiac: branch of abdominal aorta; supplies upper abdomen and organs
   n) Splenic: functions similarly to celiac
   o) Renal: branch of abdominal aorta; supplies kidneys, ureters, and adrenal glands
   p) Mesenteric: branch of abdominal aorta; supplies intestines, colon, and rectum
   q) Iliac: extension of abdominal aorta; branches and supplies abdominal and pelvic regions and lower limbs
   r) Femoral: extension of iliac; supplies abdominal wall, genitalia, and upper leg
   s) Popliteal: extension of femoral; supplies knee and calf
   t) Tibial: extension of popliteal
      ▪ Anterior supplies lower leg, ankle, and foot
      ▪ Posterior supplies lower leg, foot, and heel
   u) Dorsalis pedis: extension of anterior tibial; supplies foot

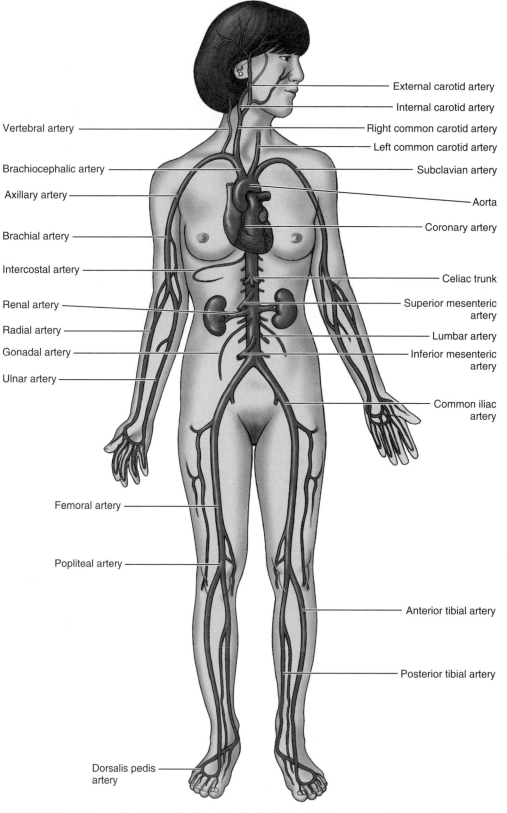

External carotid artery
Internal carotid artery
Right common carotid artery
Left common carotid artery
Subclavian artery
Aorta
Coronary artery
Celiac trunk
Superior mesenteric artery
Lumbar artery
Inferior mesenteric artery
Common iliac artery
Anterior tibial artery
Posterior tibial artery

Vertebral artery
Brachiocephalic artery
Axillary artery
Brachial artery
Intercostal artery
Renal artery
Radial artery
Gonadal artery
Ulnar artery
Femoral artery
Popliteal artery
Dorsalis pedis artery

FIGURE 2-31   Major arteries of the body. (From Herlihy B, Maebius N: The Human Body in Health and Illness, Philadelphia, 1999, Saunders, p. 309.)

4. Major veins (see Figure 2-32)
   a) Pulmonary: transports blood from lungs to left atrium
   b) Coronary: drains blood from the right atrium
   c) Vena cava: largest vein in the body; leads from the body into the right atrium
      ■ Superior vena cava: drains upper body
      ■ Inferior vena cava: drains the lower body
   d) Brachiocephalic: left and right branches go into the superior vena cava; drains the head, neck, and upper extremities
   e) Jugular: branches go into the brachiocephalic; drains the head and neck
   f) Facial: branches go into the jugular; drains the face and cranium
   g) Occipital: branches go into the jugular; drains the cranium
   h) Axillary: branches go into the brachiocephalic; drains the axillary area and the upper arm
   i) Subclavian: branches go into the axillary; drains the upper arm
   j) Cephalic: goes into the axillary; drains the upper and lower arm
   k) Radial: goes into the axillary; drains the thumb side of the forearm and wrist
   l) Basilic: goes into axillary on little finger side; drains the upper and lower arm
   m) Ulnar: goes into the axillary; drains the little finger side of the forearm and wrist
   n) Gastric, cholecystic, and splenic: goes into portal hepatic vein; drains the stomach, gallbladder, and spleen
   o) Mesenteric: goes into the hepatic portal vein; drains the intestines, colon, and rectum
   p) Hepatic: goes into the inferior vena cava; drains the liver
   q) Renal: goes into the Inferior vena cava; drains the kidneys and gonads
   r) Iliac: extension of the inferior vena cava; drains the abdominal, pelvic, and lower limb regions
   s) Femoral: extension of right and left iliac; drains the upper leg
   t) Popliteal: extension of femoral; drains the knee and calf
   u) Saphenous: longest vein in the body:
      ■ Great saphenous goes into femoral; drains the medial leg
      ■ Small saphenous goes into popliteal; drains the lower leg
   v) Tibial: goes into popliteal; drains the lower leg

5. Diseases and Disorders
   1) Angina pectoris: chest pain; usually due to a lack of blood supply to the heart
   2) Aneurysm: abnormal ballooning of a vessel wall
   3) Atherosclerosis: formation of fatty plaques along the vessel walls, causing them to narrow; can be the cause of arteriosclerosis
   4) Arteriosclerosis: hardening of the arteries; walls of vessels become thick and lose elasticity
   5) Bradycardia: abnormally slow heart rate ($<$60 bpm)
   6) Cardiac arrest: unexpected stoppage of the heart function; may follow MI
   7) Congestive heart failure (CHF): characterized by the inability of the heart to keep blood circulating; results in generalized edema
   8) Embolism: a blood clot, air, fat globule, or piece of tissue that has broken loose and entered the circulation
   9) Endocarditis: inflammation of endocardium, including valves
   10) Hypertension (HTN): high blood pressure ($>$140/90)
   11) Mitral stenosis: narrowing of mitral valve that prevents normal flow of blood from the atrium to the ventricle
   12) Myocardial infarction (MI): heart attack; due to occlusion of coronary vessels that decreases the blood supply to the heart; tissue without blood supply necroses
   13) Patent ductus arteriosus: abnormal opening between the aorta and the pulmonary artery
   14) Rheumatic heart disease: can be caused by strep; causes inflammation of the heart and scarring of the valves; can be the result of rheumatic fever or myocardial infarction
   15) Tachycardia: abnormally rapid heart rate ($>$100 bpm)
   16) Tetralogy of Fallot: congenital heart abnormality; characterized by 4 abnormalities
      > Ventricular septal defect
      > Pulmonary stenosis
      > Displacement of the aorta to the right
      > Ventricular enlargement
   17) Thrombophlebitis: inflammation of a vein accompanied by clot formation

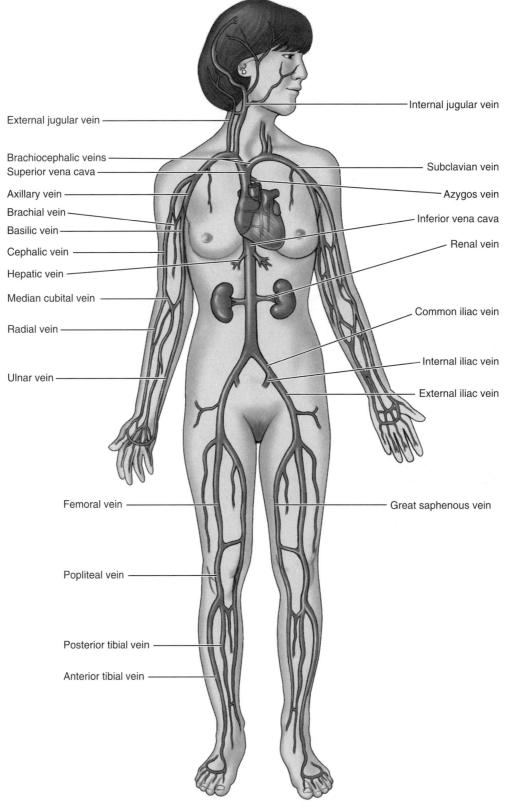

External jugular vein

Brachiocephalic veins
Superior vena cava
Axillary vein
Brachial vein
Basilic vein
Cephalic vein
Hepatic vein
Median cubital vein
Radial vein
Ulnar vein

Femoral vein
Popliteal vein
Posterior tibial vein
Anterior tibial vein

Internal jugular vein
Subclavian vein
Azygos vein
Inferior vena cava
Renal vein
Common iliac vein
Internal iliac vein
External iliac vein
Great saphenous vein

FIGURE 2-32 Major veins of the body. (From Herlihy B, Maebius N: The Human Body in Health and Illness, Philadelphia, 1999, Saunders, p. 311.)

18) Thrombus: blood clot
19) Varicosity (varicose veins): large, twisted, superficial vein; can occur in lower legs, rectum, esophagus

XII. Respiratory System

A. GENERAL
- Supplies continuous supply of oxygen to the body
- Works with the circulatory system to bring oxygen to the entire body and to remove waste products

B. FUNCTIONS
1. Air exchange and distribution: oxygen carried to tissues and carbon dioxide is carried away
2. Filtration: small hairs in nasal cavity trap substances before air enters the trachea
3. Sound production: enhances sounds produced during speech
4. Sense of smell: located in the nose
5. pH regulation: regulates the pH of blood

C. ORGANS: divided into 2 sections (see Figure 2-33):
1. Upper respiratory tract: organs outside of thoracic cavity
    a) Nose
       1) External nose: nasal bones and cartilage; forms nostrils (nares)
       2) Internal nose: nasal cavity; found over roof of mouth; divided into 2 halves by the nasal septum; functions to warm, filter, and humidify air
    b) Pharynx: throat; has 3 divisions
       1) Nasopharynx: nearest to nasal cavity; contains adenoids
       2) Oropharynx: behind the mouth; contains the tonsils
       3) Laryngopharynx: leads to trachea and esophagus
    c) Larynx: voice box; made up of cartilage with ciliated mucous membrane; contains vocal cords; carries air from pharynx to trachea
2. Lower respiratory tract: organs within the thorax
    a) Trachea: windpipe; made up of 16 to 20 C-shaped rings of cartilage that extend from larynx to the bronchi
    b) Bronchi: end of the trachea; divided into right and left bronchi; enters lungs and further divides into secondary bronchi that further branch into bronchioles; branches end in alveolar ducts
    c) Alveoli: air sacs; functional units of respiration; resemble clusters of grapes; these form the terminal end of bronchioles; composed of single layers of epithelium surrounded by capillaries; gases exchanged here
    d) Lungs: cone-shaped organs located in thoracic cavity; each contains approximately 300 million alveoli; responsible for air distribution and exchange; bottom portion (base) rests on diaphragm
       1) Left lung divided into 2 lobes (8 segments)
       2) Right lung divided into 3 lobes (10 segments)
    • Covered by double-layered membrane (pleura); fluid between layers (pleural fluid) lubricates and reduces friction during respiration

D. RESPIRATION
- Controlled by respiratory control center of medulla
- Medulla controls rhythm and depth of inspiration and expiration
- Monitors oxygen, carbon dioxide, and pH of blood, which triggers breathing
- Involves two processes
  1. Pulmonary ventilation: carries out breathing by means of pressure gradient; has 2 phases:
      a) Inspiration: air drawn into lungs by contraction of diaphragm (makes thoracic cavity larger)

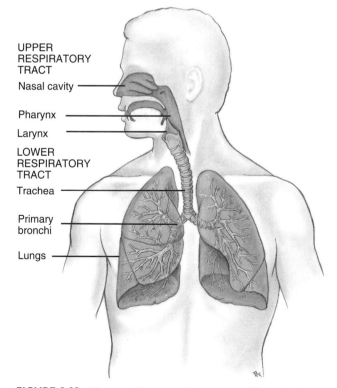

UPPER RESPIRATORY TRACT
Nasal cavity
Pharynx
Larynx
LOWER RESPIRATORY TRACT
Trachea
Primary bronchi
Lungs

FIGURE 2-33 Upper and lower respiratory tract. (From Applegate EJ: The Anatomy and Physiology Learning System, ed 2, Philadelphia, 2000, Saunders, p. 308.)

b) Expiration: air expelled from lungs by relaxation of diaphragm

2. Cellular respiration; has 2 phases
   a) External: exchange of gases between alveoli and capillaries
   b) Internal: exchange of gases between capillaries and body cells

E. DISEASES AND DISORDERS

1. Anoxia: lack of oxygen
2. Apnea: lack of breathing
3. Asphyxia: decrease in oxygen intake
4. Asthma: spasms of bronchus; results in dyspnea and wheezing
5. Atelectasis: partial or complete collapse of alveoli
6. Bronchitis: inflammation of bronchi; may be chronic or acute
7. Carcinoma: malignant tumor of lung and/or respiratory system
8. Cheyne-Stokes respiration: alternating episodes of tachypnea and apnea; usually precedes death
9. Chronic obstructive pulmonary disease (COPD)/chronic obstructive lung disease (COLD): a group of disorders characterized by progressive, irreversible obstruction of airflow; major disorders observed include chronic bronchitis, emphysema, and asthma
10. Croup: acute viral infection characterized by barklike cough
11. Dyspnea: painful or difficult breathing
12. Emphysema: loss of elasticity and enlargement of alveoli
13. Epistaxis: nosebleed
14. Hyperpnea: increase in the volume of breathing
15. Hypoxia: decrease in oxygen
16. Infectious mononucleosis: mono; acute viral infection caused by Epstein-Barr virus; may include upper respiratory symptoms
17. Laryngitis: inflammation of larynx, causes loss of voice
18. Orthopnea: breathing facilitated by an upright position
19. Pertussis: whooping cough; lung disease caused by *Bordella pertussis* bacterium; characterized by "whoop"-sounding cough
20. Pharyngitis: inflammation of throat
21. Pleurisy: inflammation of the pleural membranes
22. Pneumonia: inflammation of bronchioles and alveoli; can be viral or bacterial
23. Pneumothorax: collection of air in the pleural cavity; may cause the lung to collapse
24. Pulmonary edema: accumulation of fluid in lung tissue
25. Pulmonary embolism: clot located in the pulmonary artery or one of its branches; restricts blood flow to the lungs
26. Rales: crackling sounds on inspiration
27. Respiratory acidosis: decreased pH level of body due to inadequate removal of carbon dioxide by the lungs; can progress to tissues outside of the lungs
28. Respiratory alkalosis: increased pH levels due to excessive removal of carbon dioxide by the lungs
29. Sinusitis: inflammation of paranasal sinuses
30. Stridor: high-pitched sounds on inspiration due to obstruction
31. Suffocation: prevention of breathing by external causes
32. Tachypnea: abnormal, rapid breathing
33. Tuberculosis (TB): communicable lung disease caused by *Mycobacterium tuberculosis;* characterized by tubercles in the tissue
34. Upper respiratory infection (URI): acute inflammatory process affecting mucous membranes that line the upper respiratory tract

XIII. Digestive System

A. GENERAL

■ Includes the digestive tract (GI tract, alimentary canal) and accessory organs

■ Digestive tract is a long, continuous tube that starts at the mouth and ends at the anus

■ Processes food into molecules small enough to be utilized by the body

B. FUNCTIONS

1. Digestion: physical and chemical breakdown of complex foodstuffs into simple nutrients
2. Absorption: passage of simple nutrients through the walls of the small intestine into the blood or lymph
3. Elimination: excretion of indigestible waste from the body in the form of feces

C. ORGANS (see Figure 2-34)

1. Mouth (oral cavity)
   • Receives food by ingestion
   • Breaks down food into small particles by mastication (chewing)
   • Mixes food with saliva
   • Lips and cheeks help to hold food in place for chewing
   • Also helps with speech
   a) Palate: separates oral cavity from nasal cavity
      1) Anterior portion (hard palate): supported by bone
      2) Posterior portion (soft palate): made of muscle and connective tissue; ends in fingerlike projection (uvula); uvula and

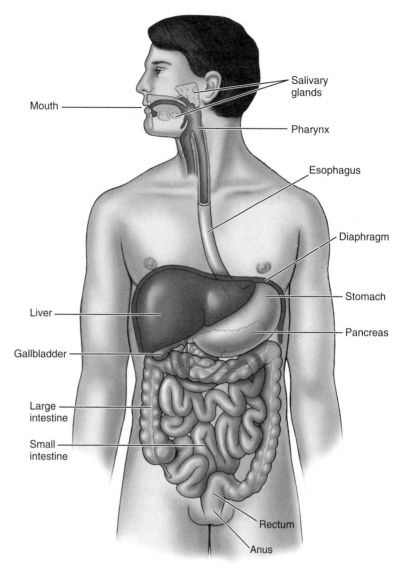

FIGURE 2-34 Major organs of the digestive system. (From Herlihy B, Maebius N: The Human Body in Health and Illness, Philadelphia, 1999, Saunders, p. 389.)

soft palate move upward during swallowing to keep food from entering the nasal cavity
b) Tongue: moves food around in mouth; helps with speech; covered by papillae; papillae provide friction and contain taste buds
c) Teeth: used for mastication
  ■ Two different sets develop
    1) Deciduous ("baby teeth"): first 20 teeth, which eventually fall out
    2) Permanent: set of 32 adult teeth, which replace deciduous teeth
  ■ Shape of tooth corresponds to the way it handles food
    1) Incisors: chisel-shaped and sharp edges for biting foods
    2) Cuspids (canines): conical-shaped with points for grasping and tearing foods

3) Bicuspids: flat surfaces for crushing and grinding
4) Molars: also have flat surfaces for crushing and grinding
  ■ Tooth is divided into
    1) Crown: exposed portion; covered with enamel (hardest surface in the body)
    2) Neck: narrow portion below crown, protected by gums
    3) Root: end portion of neck that fits into socket in mandible and maxilla
    4) Pulp cavity: central core of tooth; contains pulp, which consists of connective tissue, blood vessels, and nerves; surrounded by dentin
d) Salivary glands
  ■ Produce saliva, which contains water, mucus and enzyme amylase; moistens food; begins chemical digestion

■ 3 pairs of exocrine glands secrete saliva into the mouth
1) Parotid: largest pair; located in front of the ears (mumps)
2) Submandibular: located in the floor of the mouth
3) Sublingual: smallest pair; located under the tongue

2. Pharynx (throat): passageway that transports food to esophagus
3. Esophagus: muscular tube that carries food from pharynx to stomach
4. Stomach: located in the left upper quadrant of abdomen
   • Can hold up to 1.5 liters
   • Temporarily stores and partially breaks down food
   • Secretes substances (mucus, HCl, gastrin, pepsinogen) that aid in digestion
   • Destroys bacteria that enters the digestive tract
   • Three regions
     1) Superior region (fundus); opening guarded by the cardiac sphincter
     2) Main portion (body)
     3) Lower portion (pylorus); connects to small intestines; opening to the small intestines guarded by the pyloric sphincter
   • Wall of the stomach has 3 layers made up of smooth muscle; the innermost layer has folds (rugae), which allow for expansion
5. Small intestines
   • Coiled tubular structure about 6 meters in length and about 2.5 centimeters in diameter
   • Fills most of the abdominal cavity
   • Completes chemical digestion
   • Primary site for absorption of nutrients
   • Has 3 divisions:
     1) Duodenum: upper portion
     2) Jejunum: middle portion
     3) Ileum: end portion
   • Suspended from the abdominal wall by a fold of peritoneum (mesentery)
   • Lining contains fingerlike projections (villi); villi contain capillaries and lacteals, which rise off the surface area and absorb nutrients
6. Large intestines
   • Folded tube about 1.5 meters in length and 6 centimeters in diameter
   • Absorbs fluid and electrolytes; eliminates waste products
   • Produces vitamin K (necessary for blood clotting)

• Divided into
  1) Cecum: first division connected to ileum of small intestine; contains ileocecal valve; vermiform appendix attached to cecum
  2) Ascending colon: vertical length of colon that runs along the right side of the abdominal cavity
  3) Transverse colon: horizontal length of colon that runs across the abdominal cavity
  4) Descending colon: vertical length of colon that runs along the left side of the abdominal cavity
  5) Sigmoid colon: S-shaped length of colon that connects to the rectum
  6) Rectum: continues to the anal canal; thick muscular wall
  7) Anal canal: continues from the rectum to outside (anus); guarded by two sphincter muscles

7. Peritoneum
   • Serous membrane that covers most of the abdominal organs and holds them in place
     1) Mesentery: holds intestines in coils
     2) Tansverse mesocolon: binds transverse colon to posterior abdominal wall
     3) Omentum: sheet of serous membrane that contains fat; protects the abdominal organs

8. Accessory organs
   a) Liver
      ■ Accessory organ of digestion
      ■ "Can't Live Without a Liver"
      ■ Largest gland in the body
      ■ Located in the right upper quadrant
      ■ Divided into right and left lobes
      ■ Filters and destroys wastes and toxic substances
      ■ Produces bile, which breaks down (emulsifies) fats
      ■ Stores iron, glycogen, vitamins A, B-12, D, E, and K
      ■ Produces clotting factors
      ■ Recycles iron and hemoglobin from worn-out red blood cells
      ■ Controls carbohydrate and lipid metabolism
   b) Gallbladder
      ■ Pear-shaped sac attached to inferior surface of liver by cystic duct
      ■ Stores, concentrates, and sends bile into the duodenum through the common bile duct (the cystic duct joins the hepatic duct from the liver to form the common bile duct)

c) Pancreas
- Located behind stomach
- Endocrine and exocrine functions
  1) Endocrine: beta cells of the islets of Langerhans secrete insulin (which lowers blood glucose levels); alpha cells of the islets of Langerhans secrete glucagon (which raises blood glucose levels)
  2) Exocrine: acinar cells secrete digestive enzymes (amylase, trypsin, peptidase, and lipase)

D. DIGESTION
- Breakdown of foodstuffs
  - Has 2 processes
1. Mechanical digestion: breaks down food, moves it along the canal, and eliminates the waste from the body
   - Begins with mastication (chewing), which reduces the size of food and mixes the food with saliva to form a bolus
   - Bolus is swallowed (deglutition)
   - Wavelike motion of gastrointestinal tract (peristalsis) moves food along the digestive tract
   - Food is churned in stomach to mix with gastric juices to form chyme
   - Chyme is pushed into the duodenum approximately every 20 seconds until empty
   - Chyme mixes with pancreatic liver and intestinal juices
   - Chyme leaves the jejunum approximately 5 hours after entering the small intestine
   - Residue not absorbed enters the large intestine, where excess water is absorbed and waste (feces) is formed and expelled from the body
2. Chemical digestion: breaks down large complex molecules into smaller molecules for absorption; accomplished by hydrolysis and enzymes
   - Carbohydrates: initially broken down by amylase; final breakdown by sucrase, lactase, and maltase
   - Proteins: broken down into amino acids by proteases: pepsin (stomach), trypsin (pancreas), and peptidase (intestines)
   - Fats: first emulsified by bile in small intestine; finally digested by pancreatic lipase

E. ABSORPTION
- Process of transporting nutrients from small intestinal mucosa to blood or lymph
- Most absorption occurs in small intestine
- Nutrients travel to the liver through portal system

F. ELIMINATION
- Solid waste expelled from body by process of defecation
- Defecation is triggered by stimulation of receptors due to full rectum
- Controlled by internal sphincter (involuntary) and external sphincter (voluntary)

G. DISEASES AND DISORDERS
1. Anorexia: lack of appetite
2. Appendicitis: inflammation of appendix
3. Caries: dental cavities
4. Celiac sprue: malabsorption syndrome; characterized by intolerance to gluten and damage to intestinal mucosa
5. Cholelithiasis: (gallstones); caused by collection of solid cholesterol or calcium in the gallbladder or bile ducts
6. Cirrhosis: degenerative disease of the liver
7. Colitis: inflammation of the colon
8. Constipation: hard stools resulting in difficulty in defecating
9. Crohn's disease: common chronic inflammatory disease of the GI tract; walls of the bowel become edematous and inflamed
10. Diarrhea: loose, watery stools
11. Diverticulitis: inflammation of pouches (diverticula) in the colon
12. Emesis: vomiting
13. Gastritis: inflammation of the stomach
14. Gastroenteritis: inflammation of stomach and intestines
15. Gingivitis: inflammation of the gums
16. Hemorrhoids: inflammation and dilation of surface veins in the rectum and anus
17. Hepatitis: inflammation of the liver; can be acute or chronic
18. Hernia: protrusion of a part of the intestine into an adjacent area or cavity
19. Intussusception: telescoping of one part of the intestine onto another part just below it
20. Irritable bowel syndrome (IBS): collection of symptoms with no organic cause; characterized by abdominal pain, constipation, and diarrhea
21. Malabsorption syndrome: disease process that inhibits absorption of nutrients
22. Mumps: inflammation of parotid salivary glands
23. Pancreatitis: inflammation of the pancreas
24. Stomatitis: inflammation of mouth
25. Thrush: yeast infection of the mouth; caused by *Candida albicans*
26. Ulcer: lesion in the mucosa of the stomach or intestine
27. Vincent's angina: (trench mouth); ulcerations of the mucosa of the mouth

XIV. Urinary System

A. GENERAL
- Produces and excretes urine from the body
- Kidneys clean blood of waste products
- Plays vital role in electrolyte, water, and acid-base balance

B. FUNCTIONS
1. Waste elimination: excretes nitrogen-containing liquid waste (urine) from the body
2. Regulation of blood volume: balances water loss and gain
3. Regulation of pH: balances gain and loss of bicarbonate and hydrogen ions
4. Regulations of electrolytes: balances levels through excretion and reabsorption
5. Detoxification: assists liver in neutralizing substances

C. ORGANS (see Figure 2-35)
1. Kidney: 2 bean-shaped organs located retroperitoneal; surrounded by a cushion of fat; 2 layers
   a) Cortex: outer layer
   b) Medulla: inner layer; contains renal pyramids
      1) Triangle-shaped wedges that contain the nephron
      2) Points of pyramids come together into a cuplike structure (calyx [singular])
      3) Calyces (plural) join together to form renal pelvis where urine is collected
      4) Nephron: microscopic functional unit of kidneys; filters blood and produces urine; made up of
         (a) Bowman's capsule: cup-shaped structure in renal cortex; holds the glomerulus
         (b) Glomerulus: ball-shaped cluster of capillaries that sits in Bowman's capsule; Bowman's capsule and glomerulus make up the renal corpuscle
         (c) Proximal convoluted tubule: extension of Bowman's capsule; makes up first part of the renal tubule
         (d) Loop of Henle: extends from proximal convoluted tubule
         (e) Distal convoluted tubule: extends from the loop of Henle
         (f) Collecting tubule: tubule formed by union of distal convoluted tubules; convoluted tubules join to form one renal pyramid; pyramids join to form calyx
2. Ureter
   a) Tube that runs from kidneys into urinary bladder

b) Renal pelvis narrows as it leaves kidney to form ureter
3. Urinary bladder
   a) Muscular sac located behind symphysis pubis
   b) Capable of great expansion due to folds (rugae) in its inner lining
   c) Serves as temporary storage place for urine
4. Urethra
   a) Tube that carries urine from the bladder to the outside of the body
   b) Opening to outside is urinary meatus

D. BLOOD FLOW TO KIDNEYS
1. Renal artery: enters kidney at hilum
2. Afferent arteriole: enters Bowman's capsule
3. Glomerulus: network of capillaries
4. Efferent arteriole: comes from glomerulus and exits Bowman's capsule
5. Peritubular capillaries: extend from efferent arteriole; surrounds renal tubule
6. Renal venule: extends from peritubular capillaries
7. Renal vein: extends from renal venule; exits kidney at hilum; joins inferior vena cava

E. URINE
1. Formation
   - Series of 3 processes
     a) Filtration: continuous process; glomerular blood pressure causes water and dissolved substances to filter out of the glomeruli and into Bowman's capsule
     b) Reabsorption: movement of substances out of renal tubules into blood in peritubular capillaries; water, nutrients, and electrolytes reabsorbed
     c) Secretion: movement of substances not reabsorbed into urine into collecting tubules
2. Composition
   a) Water: 95% of urine
   b) Nitrogenous waste products: urea, ammonia, uric acid and creatinine (end products of protein metabolism)
   c) Electrolytes: sodium, potassium, phosphate, sulfates, ammonium, bicarbonate, and chloride
   d) Toxins
   e) Pigment: urochrome

F. DISEASES AND DISORDERS
1. Anuria: no urine produced
2. Glycosuria: glucose in the urine
3. Hematuria: blood in the urine
4. Incontinence: voiding urine involuntarily
5. Nephrolithiasis (renal calculi): kidney stones
6. Oliguria: scanty urine output

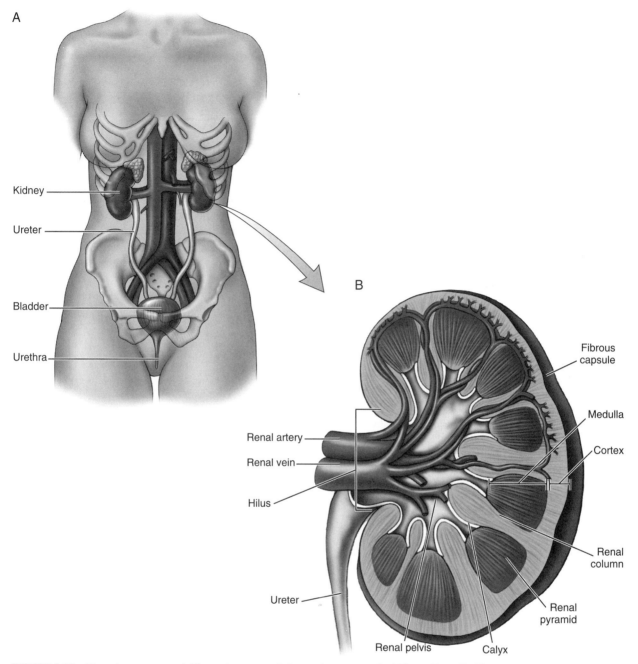

FIGURE 2-35 The urinary system. *A,* The major organs. *B,* Internal structure of a kidney. (From Herlihy B, Maebius N: The Human Body in Health and Illness, Philadelphia, 1999, Saunders, p. 421.)

7. Polycystic kidney disease: collecting tubular disease characterized by swollen, fluid-filled sacs; tubules are unable to empty into the renal pelvis
8. Polyuria: excessive urination
9. Proteinuria: protein in the urine
10. Renal failure: kidneys fail to function; may be chronic or acute
11. Urinary tract infection (UTI): mostly caused by gram-negative bacteria; can occur in any organ in the tract

XV. Endocrine System

A. GENERAL
   ■ Body's slower-acting control system

■ Made up of glands that secrete substances (hormones)

■ Hormones travel through the bloodstream to target organs and cells

B. FUNCTIONS
1. Control: regulates internal body functions and processes
2. Communication: compliments the nervous system; directs communication among the body systems for optimum functioning

C. HORMONES: chemical substances secreted from endocrine glands
1. Tropic hormones: stimulate other endocrine glands to secrete their hormones
2. Sex hormones: stimulate reproductive tissue
3. Anabolic hormones: stimulate cells to grow and repair
4. Prostaglandins: tissue hormones that regulate cellular activity

D. GLANDS (see Figure 2-36)
1. Pituitary gland: master gland; hypophysis
   • Located on inferior surface of the brain
   • Connected to hypothalamus by stalk (infundibulum)
   • Divided into 2 sections
   a) Anterior hypophysis (adenohypophysis) (see Figure 2-37)
      ■ Secretes
        1) Growth hormones (GH): promotes tissue growth; stimulates fat metabolism; helps to maintain blood glucose levels
        2) Prolactin (pRL): promotes development of breast and milk secretion; works with luteinizing hormone during menstrual cycle
        3) Thyroid-stimulating hormone (TSH): stimulates development and hormone production of thyroid gland
        4) Adrenocorticotropic hormone (ACTH): stimulates development and hormone production of adrenal cortex
        5) Follicle-stimulating hormone (FSH)
           > In female: stimulates follicle development and secretion of estrogen
           > In male: stimulates sperm production
        6) Luteinizing hormone (LH)
           > In female: stimulates secretion of estrogen and progesterone
           > In male: stimulates secretion of testosterone
        7) Melanocyte-stimulating hormone (MSH): regulates normal color of skin; helps regulate adrenal gland's response to ACTH

   b) Posterior pituitary (neurohypophysis):
      ■ Does not manufacture hormones
      ■ Stores and releases hormones made in hypothalamus
        1) Antidiuretic hormone (ADH): prevents excessive formation of urine
        2) Oxytocin: stimulates the uterus to contract during childbirth; causes letdown of milk
2. Pineal gland
   • Pine-cone-shaped gland located behind the hypothalamus
   • Produces melatonin that regulates the body's "biological clock"
3. Thyroid gland
   • Butterfly-shaped gland located in the neck, lateral and anterior to the trachea
   • Secretes 2 hormones
     1) Thyroxine (tetraiodothyronine) (T-4) and triiodothyronine (T-3); regulates metabolism of the body; needs iodine for synthesis
     2) Calcitonin: stimulates movement of calcium from the blood to the bone
4. Parathyroid gland
   • Four pea-shaped glands embedded in the thyroid gland
   • Secretes parathormone (PTH), which causes calcium to leave bone and enter the bloodstream
5. Adrenal glands
   • Located on top of each kidney
   • Composed of 2 regions
   a) Adrenal cortex: outer region
      ■ Secretes corticosteroids
        1) Aldosterone: regulates mineral salts
        2) Cortisol: regulates blood pressure
        3) Androgen and estrogen: minor sex hormones
   b) Adrenal medulla: inner region
      ■ Secretes hormones that are important in the sympathetic and parasympathetic nervous system
        1) Epinephrine
        2) Norepinephrine
6. Pancreas
   • Elongated gland that extends posterior to stomach
   • Produces glucagon; from alpha cells; stimulates conversion of glycogen to glucose in liver
   • Produces insulin; from beta cells; decreases glucose levels in blood
   • Produces somatostatin; from delta cells; regulates other pancreatic cells

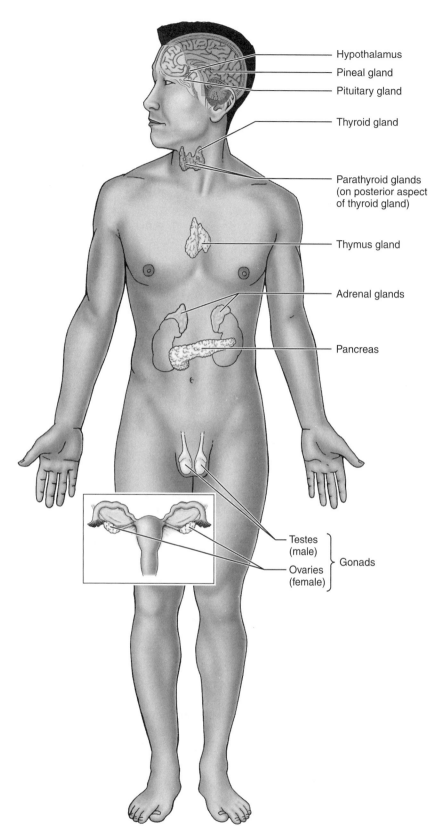

Hypothalamus

Pineal gland

Pituitary gland

Thyroid gland

Parathyroid glands
(on posterior aspect
of thyroid gland)

Thymus gland

Adrenal glands

Pancreas

Testes
(male)

Ovaries
(female)

Gonads

FIGURE 2-36   Major endocrine glands of the body. (From Herlihy B, Maebius N: The Human Body in Health and Illness, Philadelphia, 1999, Saunders, p. 239.)

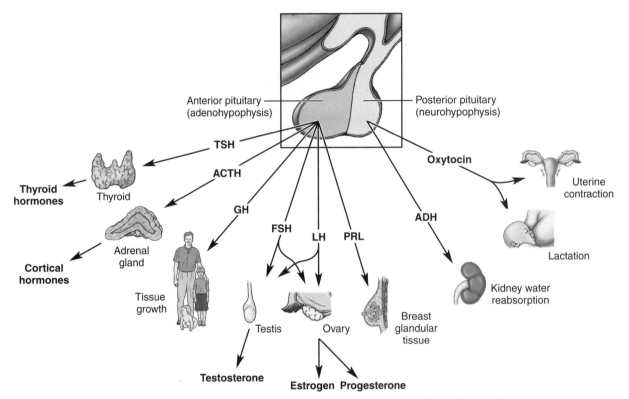

FIGURE 2-37 Hormones secreted by the anterior and posterior pituitary glands. (From Herlihy B, Maebius N: The Human Body in Health and Illness, Philadelphia, 1999, Saunders, p. 246.)

7. Gonads
   • Testes in male
     ▪ Secrete testosterone, which stimulates the development of male sex characteristics
   • Ovaries in female
     ▪ Secrete estrogen: from follicles; stimulates development of female sex characteristics
     ▪ Secrete progesterone: from corpus luteum; maintains a pregnancy
8. Thymus
   • Located in mediastinum below sternum
   • Largest in children; atrophies during adolescence
   • Produces thymosin; stimulates T-lymphocytes for immunity
9. Placenta
   • Produces human chorionic gonadotropin (HCG) during pregnancy

E. DISEASES AND DISORDERS
   1. Acromegaly: hypersecretion of GH after puberty
   2. Addison's disease: hyposecretion of cortisol; characterized by hypotentension and increased skin pigmentation
   3. Cretinism: hypothyroidism due to hyposecretion of thyroxine during infancy; characterized by slow growth, impaired intelligence, and delayed development of secondary sex characteristics
   4. Cushing's syndrome: hypersecretion of cortisol; characterized by "moon face," acne, fatty deposits on upper back
   5. Diabetes insipidus: hyposecretion of ADH; characterized by polyurea and polydipsia
   6. Diabetes mellitus: hyperglycemia; hyposecretion of insulin; characterized by polyurea, polyphagia, and polydipsia
   7. Dwarfism: hyposecretion of GH; characterized by abnormally small size
   8. Giantism: hypersecretion of GH; characterized by abnormally large size
   9. Goiter: enlargement of thyroid gland; due to iodine deficiency
   10. Grave's disease: hyperthyroidism due to hypersecretion of thyroxine; characterized by weight loss, exopthalmia, nervousness, diaphoresis, and heat intolerance
   11. Myxedema: hyposecretion of thyroxine later in life; characterized by fatigue, weight gain, and cold intolerance

XVI. Reproductive System

A. GENERAL: produces offspring for the survival of the species

B. FUNCTIONS
1. Production of egg and sperm cells
2. Nurturing of developing offspring
3. Production of hormones

C. ORGANS/STRUCTURES OF THE MALE SYSTEM
(see Figure 2-38)
1. Testes
   • Essential organs (gonads)
   • Produces sperm (male gamete)
   • Glandular structures located outside of the body in the scrotum
   • Made up of seminiferous tubules (sperm development) and interstitual cells (produces testosterone)
2. Epididymis
   • Continuation of seminiferous tubules
   • Lies on the superior surface of the testes
   • Secretes part of seminal fluid
3. Vas deferens
   • Extension of the epididymis
   • Passes through the inguinal canal into the abdominal cavity; arches over the bladder and joins the seminal vesicles
   • Site of male sterilization (vasectomy)

4. Seminal vesicles
   • Bilateral pouches behind the urinary bladder
   • Secrete a nutrient-rich fluid that nourishes sperm
5. Ejaculatory duct
   • Formed by the union of the vas deferens and seminal vesicles
   • Passes through the prostate gland and enters the urethra
   • Propels sperm and seminal fluid into the urethra during orgasm
6. Prostate gland
   • Doughnut-shaped gland that encircles the base of the urethra on the posterior surface of the bladder
   • Secretes an alkaline fluid that protects the sperm from the acidity of the vagina
7. Bulbourethral gland (Cowper's gland)
   • Pea-shaped glands located on both sides of the urethra
   • Secretes lubrication during intercourse
8. Scrotum
   • Pouch of skin suspended from the perineal area

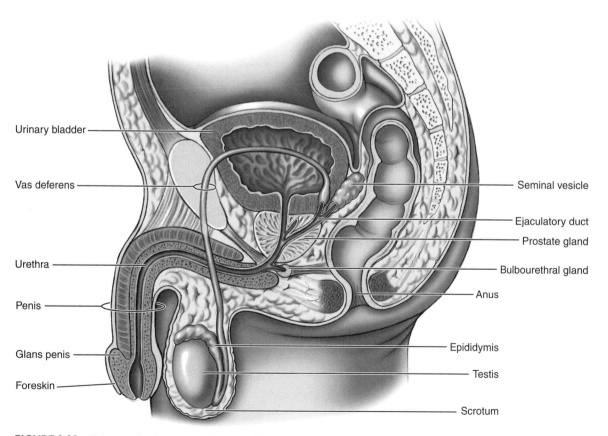

FIGURE 2-38   Male reproductive organs. (From Herlihy B, Maebius N: The Human Body in Health and Illness, Philadelphia, 1999, Saunders, p. 453.)

- Holds the testes and epididymis
- Keeps the testes away from the body; body temperature is too high for sperm production
9. Penis
    - External male genitalia
    - Composed of 3 cylinders of erectile tissue
    - During sexual arousal, erectile tissue fills with blood and becomes erect
    - Contains the urethra
    - Distal end covered by the prepuce (foreskin), which is removed by circumcision

D. ORGANS/STRUCTURES OF THE FEMALE SYSTEM (see Figure 2-39)
    1. Ovaries
        - Essential organs (gonads)
        - Produce ova (female gamete)
        - Almond-shaped glands located in the pelvic cavity
        - Contain ovarian (Graafian) follicles where ova develop
        - Produce estrogen and progesterone
    2. Uterus
        - Pear-shaped muscular organ located in the pelvic cavity between the bladder and rectum
        - 3 divisions
            1) Fundus: upper region
            2) Body: large central region
            3) Cervix: lower neck region; opens to vagina
        - 3 layers
            1) Endometrium: inner layer; the fertilized ovum implants and grows here; shed monthly (menstruation; menses)
            2) Myometrium: middle muscular layer
            3) Epimetrium: outer layer
        - Contracts to deliver the fetus
    3. Fallopian tubes (oviducts)
        - Attached to the upper, outer sides of uterus
        - Serve as the site of fertilization; the fertilized ovum travels through the tube into the uterus for implantation
        - Distal ends contain fingerlike structures (fimbriae); gentle movement of fimbriae draws the ovum into the tube after release from the ovary
        - Site of female sterilization (tubal ligation)
    4. Vagina
        - Tubular structure that extends from cervix to the outside
        - Located between the rectum and urethra
        - Capable of great expansion
        - Serves as the birth canal and means of shedding menstrual tissues
    5. Vulva
        - External genitalia

- Includes
    a) Mons pubis: fat pad that covers the symphysis pubis
    b) Labia majora: two large folds of skin extending from the mons pubis to the anus
    c) Labia minora: two small folds of skin medial to the labia majora
    d) Clitoris: small nodule of erectile tissue superior to the labia majora; plays a role in sexual arousal
    e) Bartholin glands: located at the entrance to the vagina; secretes lubricating fluid during intercourse
6. Perineum
    - Region between the vaginal opening and the rectum; may be cut or torn during childbirth (episiotomy)
7. Breasts
    - Mammary glands
    - Fatty tissue and milk glands that overlie the pectoral muscles
    - Produces milk for offspring (lactation)
    - Nipple is protrusion for delivery of milk
    - Areola is dark area that surrounds nipple

E. REPRODUCTIVE CYCLE
    1. Ovarian cycle
        - Ovum develops and matures in the ovary
    2. Menstrual cycle
        a) Menses: days 1 to 5; if the ovum is not fertilized, the endometrium is shed
        b) Postmenstrual: days 6 to 13; the endometrium thickens as the ovum matures in the ovary; estrogen levels increase
        c) Ovulation: day 14; the mature ovum is released from the ovary
        d) Premenstrual: days 15 to 28; the corpus luteum develops on the ovary where the ovum was released and secretes progesterone; the endometrium thickens in preparation for a fertilized ovum

F. PREGNANCY
    1. Ovulation: release of ovum
    2. Insemination: sperm are released into the vagina and travel through the cervix and uterus into the Fallopian tube
    3. Conception: union of sperm and egg; occurs in the Fallopian tube; results in a zygote with 46 chromosomes (23 from ovum, 23 from sperm)
    4. Zygote divides and implants in the uterine wall; becomes an embryo at the third week of development until the end of the eighth week; becomes a fetus at the ninth week until birth
    5. Placenta: highly vascular disk-shaped organ; develops from embryonic and maternal tissues; attaches the developing fetus to the uterus; performs nutrition, excretory, and respiratory

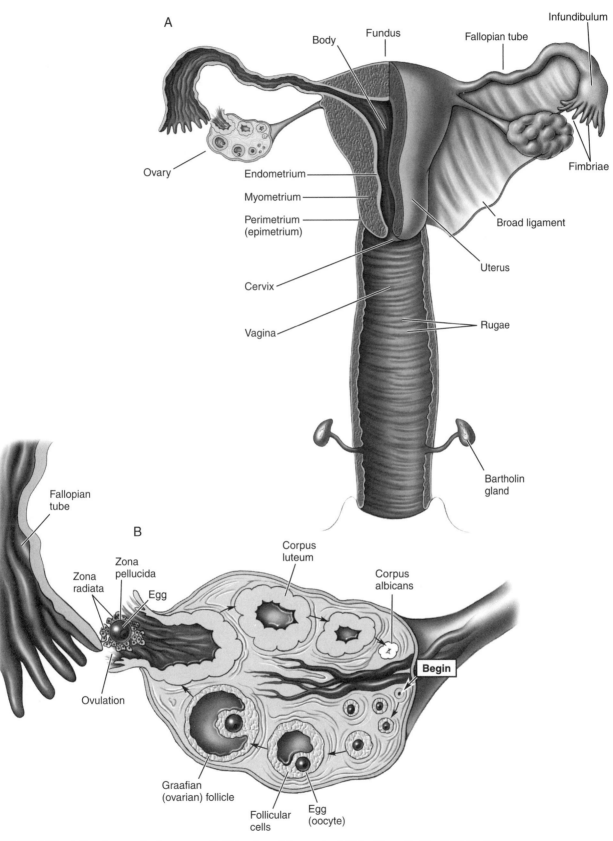

FIGURE 2-39 *A,* Female reproductive organs. *B,* Maturation of the ovarian follicle. (From Herlihy B, Maebius N: The Human Body in Health and Illness, Philadelphia, 1999, Saunders, p. 459.)

functions; excretes HCG for continued pregnancy

6. Gestation: lasts approximately 40 weeks; 3 three-month trimesters
7. Parturition: childbirth
   • 3 stages
      a) Onset of contractions to cervical dilation (10 centimeters)
      b) Dilation to birth of the fetus
      c) Expulsion of the placenta

G. DISEASES AND DISORDERS
   1. Abortion: termination of a pregnancy; can be spontaneous (miscarriage) or therapeutic
   2. Abruptio placenta: placenta prematurely separates from uterine wall
   3. Amenorrhea: absence of menstruation
   4. Benign prostatic hypertrophy (BPH): abnormal growth of prostatic cells causing enlargement of gland
   5. Cryptoichism: undescended testes; testes remain in abdomen
   6. Dysmenorrhea: painful menstruation
   7. Dyspareunia: painful intercourse
   8. Eclampsia (toxemia): serious condition of pregnancy characterized by hypertension, edema, and proteinuria; if untreated, may result in seizures and coma
   9. Ectopic pregnancy: implantation of fertilized ovum outside of uterus; usually in the Fallopian tube
   10. Endometriosis: growth of endometrial tissue outside of the uterus, usually within the pelvic cavity
   11. Hydrocele: accumulation of fluid in the scrotum
   12. Hyperemesis gravidarum: excessive vomiting during pregnancy
   13. Hypospodias: abnormal congenital opening of the urethra on the underside of the penis
   14. Impotence: inability to develop or sustain an erection
   15. Orchitis: inflammation of the testes
   16. Ovarian cyst: solid or fluid-filled cyst found on the ovary
   17. Pelvic inflammatory disease (PID): acute or chronic infection of the female reproductive tract
   18. Placenta previa: placenta implants over the cervix
   19. Premenstrual syndrome (PMS): various symptoms that occur before the menstrual period; can include fatigue, irritability, depression, swollen and tender breasts, edema, and/or cramping
   20. Prostatitis: inflammation of the prostate
   21. Sexually transmitted disease (STD)
      a) Trichomoniasis: parasitic infection caused by *Trichomonas vaginalis*
      b) Gonorrhea: bacterial infection caused by *Neisseria gonorrhea*
      c) Syphilis: bacterial infection caused by *Treponema pallidum*
      d) Genital herpes: viral infection caused by Herpes Simplex Type 2 virus
      e) Genital warts: growths caused by human papillomavirus
      f) Chlamydia: bacterial infection caused by *Chlamydia trachomatis*

Law and Ethics

I. Introduction to the Law

A. DEFINITION OF LAW
- System by which society gives order to our lives

B. FUNCTIONS OF LAW
1. Regulate: controls rules and standards
2. Punish: enforce penalties for infractions of rules and standards
3. Remedy: make wrongs committed right
4. Benefit: help society

C. SOURCES OF LAW
1. Common law: derives from the customs of society, court decisions
2. Administrative law: derives from agencies that enact state and federal law
3. Constitutional law: derives from the U.S. Constitution
4. Statutory law: derives from state and federal legislation

D. TYPES OF LAW
1. Civil law: a wrong, or perceived wrong, committed against a person or to property; civil law that affects the practice of medicine include
   a) Contract law: governs enforceable promises
   b) Tort law: governs intentional or accidental acts that bring harm to a person or damages property
   c) Administrative law: governs regulations set forth by governmental agencies
2. Criminal law: a wrong committed against a person or to property in violation of a statute or ordinance; criminal laws that may affect the practice of medicine include
   a) Infraction: a minor offense that usually results only in a fine
   b) Misdemeanor: violation of a law that includes as punishment a maximum imprisonment of no more than one year
   c) Felony: a major crime that includes punishment imprisonment of more than one year

II. Licensure, Registration, Certification

A. LICENSURE
1. Strongest form of administrative regulation
2. Mandatory credential to practice medicine
3. Granted by a state board, verifies that the person holding the license has met minimum standards; for doctors, defined by the Medical Practice Act; for licensed nurses, defined and governed by the Nurse Practice Act
   - State statute that defines what is included in the practice of medicine within that state
   - Governs the methods and requirements of licensure and establishes grounds for suspension and revocation of the license
4. Doctors can be licensed through
   a) Examination: passing a written and/or oral examination
   b) Endorsement: acceptance of a national examination score
   c) Reciprocity: one state accepts another state's license
5. Licenses may be revoked or suspended for
   a) Conviction of a misdemeanor or a felony
   b) Unprofessional conduct
   c) Personal or professional incapacity
   d) License must be periodically renewed (if not renewed, will be suspended from practice)

B. REGISTRATION
1. Medical assistants can be registered
2. Voluntary process
3. Professional listed on a state or national registry
4. Process similar to certification

C. CERTIFICATION
1. Medical assistants can be certified
2. Voluntary process
3. Identifies a professional as meeting minimum standards to be able to practice
4. Usually accomplished by written examination
5. Governed by a professional organization

III. Regulating Issues for the Medical Office

A. CLIA
1. Clinical Laboratory Improvement Acts of 1988
2. Identifies standards for lab testing
3. Any facility performing laboratory testing is subject to CLIA regulations

B. CON
1. Certificate of Need
2. Process of acquiring approval, based on need to the community, to expand service

C. JCAHO
1. Joint Commission of the Accreditation of Health Organizations
2. Accreditation of health care facilities

D. OSHA
1. Occupational Safety and Health Administration
2. Regulation of safety in the workplace

E. ADA
1. Americans with Disabilities Act
2. Sets up rules protecting people with physical or mental disability from being discriminated against

IV. Consent

■ Voluntary permission given by a capable person to receive medical care

A. TYPES
1. Express: oral or written expression of consent
2. Implied: actions or behavior that can be reasonably presumed to express consent

B. INFORMED CONSENT: PHYSICIAN, OR OTHER CAREGIVER, HAS AN AFFIRMATIVE DUTY TO EXPLAIN TO THE PATIENT INFORMATION NECESSARY TO ALLOW THE PATIENT TO EVALUATE THE MEDICAL CARE AND MAKE DECISIONS ON THAT INFORMATION BEFORE HAVING THE MEDICAL CARE PERFORMED.

■ Implies an understanding of
1. What procedure is to be done
2. Why the procedure should be done
3. The risks involved in performing the procedure
4. The expected benefits of having the procedure performed
5. Any alternative treatments that can be performed
6. The risks involved in performing the alternative treatment

C. WHO MAY/MAY NOT GIVE CONSENT
1. Persons who are mentally competent and of the age of majority can give consent
2. A parent, legal guardian, or someone legally charged with standing in place of the parent or guardian can give consent for a minor (a minor is a person not yet of legal age, which is often 18)
   - Consent can legally be given by a minor under the following circumstances
     ■ Minor serving in the armed forces
     ■ Emancipated minor
     ■ Testing for sexually transmitted diseases
     ■ Seeking contraception or abortion
3. Living will
   a) Advance directive
   b) Authorizes in advance the withholding of artificial life-support methods in case of terminal illness or accident
   c) Encouraged by the Patient Self-Determination Act of 1990
4. Uniform Anatomical Gift Act of 1968: allows for competent adults to give their body or body parts upon their death for research, transplantation, or placement in a tissue bank
5. Persons who are *non compos mentis* ("not of sound mind") cannot give consent, and these persons require some form of guardianship to give consent
6. In emergencies, consent to treatment is implied only as long as the emergency exists; Good Samaritan Act provides immunity from liability to (nonnegligent) volunteers at the scene of an accident
7. Mentally competent persons have the right to refuse medical treatment (refused consent)
   a) Patient's refusal must be documented
   b) Patient must sign a document ("release") absolving the caregiver of liability for not giving treatment
   c) Patient's "refused consent" can be overruled by a court of competent jurisdiction
8. Consent obtained by fraudulent means or misrepresentations is not binding
9. Without proper consent for treatment, a caregiver may be charged with
   a) Assault: intentional, unlawful attempt of bodily injury to another by force
   b) Battery: willful and unlawful use of force or violence (or touching) upon another person

V. Contracts

■ An agreement creating an obligation
■ Can be oral or written, expressed or implied

A. EXPRESS CONTRACT
1. Agreement between two or more parties
2. Contains the explicit terms of the agreement either orally or in writing

B. IMPLIED CONTRACT
1. Conclusion drawn from the actions of two or more parties
2. Patient/physician contract is implied

C. NECESSARY ELEMENTS OF A CONTRACT
1. Offer: one party makes an offer
2. Acceptance: another party agrees to the offer made
3. Consideration: mutual exchange of something of value between the parties
4. Capacity: all parties must be legally able to make the offer and to accept the terms
5. Legality: legal in nature and not against public policy

D. PATIENT/PHYSICIAN CONTRACT MAY BE TERMINATED BY
1. Patient: circumstances need to be fully documented in chart
2. Physician
   a) Must give patient notice (abandonment)
   b) Physician writes a certified letter with return receipt; copy in patient's record
   c) Letter should include:
      1) Reasons why care is being discontinued
      2) Assurance that physician will turn over patient records as directed
      3) Notice that patient should seek alternative care ASAP

VI. Torts
■ An act, intentional or accidental, that brings harm against another person or damage to another person's property

A. NEGLIGENCE
■ Unintentional (accidental) tort
■ Characterized by commission of an act that an ordinary, reasonable, and prudent person would not have done or omission of an act that an ordinary, reasonable, and prudent person, would have done
1. Forms of negligence
   a) Nonfeasance: failure to act when there was a duty to act causing or resulting in harm
   b) Misfeasance: improper performance of an act causing or resulting in harm
   c) Malfeasance: performance of an improper or unlawful act causing or resulting in harm
   d) Malpractice: negligence of a professional person, with the action or inaction compared to an ordinary, reasonable, and prudent, professional
2. "Four D's" of negligence
   a) Duty: exists when a patient/physician relationship has been established
   b) Derelict: neglect of professional obligation
   c) Direct cause: injury was directly caused by the physician's poor actions or by the physician's failure to act

   d) Damages: harm resulting to the patient
   —3 types
      1) Nominal: the damage exists in name only, token compensation
      2) Compensatory: actual damages suffered by the patient because of the physician's negligence
      3) Punitive: damages above the actual damage suffered by the patient, to punish the physician for the negligent act

B. *RES IPSA LOQUITUR*
1. "The thing speaks for itself"
2. Describes a situation in which the nature of the injury implicates negligence

C. INTENTIONAL TORTS
1. Assault: deliberate threat to make bodily contact
2. Battery: intentional physical contact
3. Abandonment: one-sided termination of the patient/physician relationship by the physician without proper notice to the patient
4. Invasion of privacy: giving out patient information without patient consent
5. Defamation: injury to a person's reputation caused by a false statement by another person
6. Libel: false or malicious writing against another person
7. Slander: false or malicious oral statement against another person
8. False imprisonment: unlawful restraint, or holding, of an individual against his or her will
9. Fraud: intentional misrepresentation that could cause harm

D. PRODUCT LIABILITY
■ Liability of a manufacturer of products for injuries due to defect of those products

E. VICARIOUS LIABILITY
1. *Respondeat superior* ("let the master answer")
2. Employers are liable for the conduct of their employees while the employees are performing within the scope of their employment

VII. Business Law
A. EMPLOYMENT PRACTICES
1. National Labor Relations Act of 1935 (NLRA): defines unfair labor practices and provides hearing/mediation of complaints
2. Fair Labor Standards Act of 1938 (FLSA): defines minimum wage, equal pay for equal work, child labor restrictions
3. Equal Pay Act of 1963 (EPA): amendment of FLSA that addresses wage disparities based on sex
4. Equal Employment Opportunity Act of 1972 (EEOA): prohibits employment discrimination

due to age, race, color, religion, sex, or national origin

5. Age Discrimination in Employment Act of 1967 (ADEA): prohibits discrimination based on age
6. Americans With Disabilities Act of 1990 (ADA): prohibits discrimination against persons with physical or mental disabilities
7. Workers' compensation laws: state-mandated programs to provide wage continuation and medical treatment compensation for persons with work-related injuries and/or illnesses

B. SEXUAL HARASSMENT

1. *Quid pro quo:* "something for something"; conditions of employment (raise, promotion) are based on a person's acceptance or rejection of unwelcome sexual conduct
2. Hostile work environment: creation of an intimidating, offensive, or hostile workplace due to unwelcome sexual conduct; interferes with a person's ability to perform job functions

C. PAYROLL

1. FLSA requires all employee records of hours worked to be continuously maintained
2. FICA (Federal Insurance Contributions Act): Social Security Tax; applied toward old age benefits
3. FUTA (Federal Unemployment Tax Act): tax to provide income during unemployment
4. Payroll Reports and Forms
   a) Form 944: Employer's Quarterly Federal Tax Return; filed each 3 months, with payment of quarterly tax due
   b) Form 8109: Federal Tax Deposit Book; used to pay FICA and federal income tax
   c) Form W-2: Wage and Tax Statement; given to employees yearly, itemizing the wages earned and all taxes deducted from wages for that year
   d) Form W-3: Transmittal of Income and Tax Statement; submitted to Social Security Administration; compares W-2 forms to Form 941
   e) Form W-4: Employee's Withholding Allowance Certificate; employee decides the number of withholding allowances for the company to take out of wages earned, based on the number of dependents claimed

VIII. Public Health Duties

■ States require physicians to report certain information
■ Reported information helps to provide for the health, safety and welfare of the public

A. BIRTHS: BIRTH CERTIFICATE COMPLETED BY BIRTH ATTENDANT

B. DEATHS: DEATH CERTIFICATE COMPLETED BY PHYSICIAN IN ATTENDANCE; MEDICAL EXAMINER MUST BE CALLED IN CASES OF

1. Violent or criminal activity death
2. Death without a physician present
3. Death from undetermined cause
4. Death within 24 hours of admission in a hospital or health care facility
5. Death without prior medical care

C. COMMUNICABLE DISEASES

1. Communicated to county health department
2. Includes smallpox, scarlet fever, rubella, measles, tuberculosis, plague, cholera, and sexually transmitted diseases

D. NATIONAL CHILDHOOD VACCINE INJURY ACT: REQUIRES PROVIDERS WHO ADMINISTER VACCINES TO REPORT THE FOLLOWING INFORMATION TO PUBLIC HEALTH AGENCIES

1. Date the vaccine was administered
2. Lot number and manufacturer of vaccine
3. Any adverse reactions to the vaccine
4. Name, title, and address of the person administering the vaccine

E. NEWBORN DISEASES: INBORN ERRORS OF METABOLISM (e.g., PKU)

F. ABUSE: IF SUSPECTED BY THE PROVIDER, THE PROVIDER HAS THE LEGAL DUTY TO REPORT SUSPECTED ABUSE TO THE AUTHORITIES

■ Types of abuse to be reported
1. Child abuse
2. Spouse/domestic abuse
3. Elder abuse
4. Drug abuse
5. Patient abuse in hospital and nursing homes

G. CRIMINAL ACTS: WHEN IDENTIFIED BY THE PROVIDER, THE PROVIDER HAS LEGAL DUTY TO REPORT SUSPECTED CRIMINAL ACTS TO AUTHORITIES

■ Types of criminal acts to be reported
1. Injuries by weapons
2. Assault
3. Attempted suicide
4. Rape (may require a release by the victim due to confidentiality)

IX. Introduction to Ethics

■ A set of moral principles or values
■ Concerns the thoughts, judgments, and actions on issues that have greater implications of moral right and wrong

A. DUTIES: OBLIGATIONS AND/OR COMMITMENTS TO ACT IN CERTAIN WAYS

■ Includes
1. Nonmalfeasance: not doing any harm
2. Beneficence: acting to create good

3. Fidelity: meeting the patient's expectations through respect, competence, adherence to laws, and honoring agreements
4. Veracity: telling the truth
5. Justice: sharing of benefits and burdens

B. RIGHTS: CLAIMS MADE ON A PERSON OR SOCIETY; CORRELATED TO DUTIES

C. VIRTUES: CHARACTER TRAITS THAT MAKE A PERSON ACT IN A CERTAIN WAY; PRINCIPLES ARE WRITTEN IN THE FORM OF A CODE OF ETHICS

X. AAMA Code of Ethics
■ As agent of physician, the medical assistant is governed by ethical standards
■ Decisions made in practice should be based on the professional nature of the professional and scope of practice
■ Code of Ethics is standard for all medical assistants to honor
■ Patterned after the AMA Code
■ NEVER practice medicine

XI. AMA Code of Ethics
■ Written code of conduct for medical practice
■ Includes 4 components:

A. PRINCIPLES OF MEDICAL ETHICS

B. FUNDAMENTAL ELEMENTS OF THE PATIENT/ PHYSICIAN RELATIONSHIP

C. CURRENT OPINIONS WITH ANNOTATIONS

D. REPORTS OF THE COUNCIL OF ETHICAL AND JUDICIAL AFFAIRS
■ Includes opinions on
1. Abortion: not prohibited by ethical standards
2. Abuse: legal and ethical requirement to report
3. Allocation of health resources: the physician must remain a patient advocate and allow institutional procedures to determine allocation
4. Artificial insemination: requires informed consent; deals with who has parental rights
5. Clinical investigation: the patient/physician relationship does not exist in clinical investigation
6. Cost: quality of patient care should be the physician's first consideration, not cost
7. Provision of adequate health care: an adequate level of health care for all persons
8. Genetic counseling: concerns for the quality of life
9. Organ donation: the donor should not receive payment for organ donation; protection of the right to privacy for both donor and recipient
10. Quality of life: primary consideration of what is best for the patient

11. Withholding/withdrawing life-prolonging treatment: the physician must be committed to saving life and relieving suffering; the patient may have his/her wishes known
12. Euthanasia: incompatible with the physician's role

XII. Professional Relationships

A. HOSPITAL RELATIONS
■ Privileges granted on the basis of competence and experience, not fees

B. ADVERTISING
■ Only restrictions are those that protect the public from deceptive practices; physicians can advertise fees, identification of educational background and specialty, but cannot include any statements as to the quality of their services

C. COMMUNICATION WITH THE MEDIA
■ Physician may not discuss a patient's condition with the press (unless a release has been granted); may release only authorized information that is in the public domain (births, deaths, accidents, police cases)

D. COMPUTERS
■ American Medical Association has developed guidelines for the use and sharing of computerized information

E. FEES AND CHARGES
1. Physician may not split patient fees with another physician for patient referral (fee splitting)
2. Physician's staff should assist in completing insurance forms without charge
3. Physician may request that the patient make payment at the time treatment is rendered
4. Insurance copayments may be waived or written off if access of care is threatened by inability to pay the copayment
5. Professional courtesy is a tradition

F. PHYSICIAN'S RECORDS
1. Physician owns the notes prepared by him/ her while treating a patient
2. Original medical records may not be released; records can be reproduced only on the physician's death, retirement, or sale of the physician's practice

XIII. Professional Rights and Responsibilities

A. DISCIPLINE
■ Physician should expose dishonest, corrupt, incompetent, or unethical colleagues

B. FREE CHOICE
■ Physician in private practice may decline to accept any individual as a patient

C. PATENT
 ■ Physicians may patent any device that he/she discovers or invents

D. PATIENT/PHYSICIAN RELATIONSHIP
 ■ Both parties are free to enter into, or decline to enter into, the relationship

E. INFECTIOUS DISEASE
 ■ Physician who is infected with an infectious disease should not engage in any patient contact or activity that may create a risk for the patient

F. SUBSTANCE ABUSE
 ■ Physician should not practice under the influence of any controlled substance, of alcohol, or of chemical agents that impair the ability to render treatment

Psychology

4

I. Major Theorists

A. SIGMUND FREUD

1. Provided the foundation from which all other psychological theories developed
2. Believed that infancy and childhood are the critical periods for psychological development
3. Psychoanalytical theory: theory of personality development includes
   a) Levels of awareness
      1) Conscious: experiences within one's immediate awareness; reality-based
      2) Subconscious: stores memories, thoughts, and feelings
      3) Unconscious: closed to one's awareness
   b) Components of the personality
      1) Id: body's basic primitive urges
      2) Ego: closely related to reality
      3) Superego: further development of ego; makes judgments; controls and punishes
   c) Psychosexual stages of development
      1) Oral stage: birth to end of first year of life; mouth is the source of all comfort and pleasure
      2) Anal stage: end of first year of life to third year; elimination gives pleasure and satisfaction
      3) Phallic stage: ages 3 to 6; associates pleasure and conflict with genital organs; Oedipus complex (boy's unconscious sexual attraction to his mother) and Electra complex (girl's unconscious sexual attraction to her father) develop
      4) Latency stage: ages 6 through 12; sexual urges are dormant; peer relationships develop with the same sex
      5) Genital stage: begins at puberty; body is preparing for reproduction; sexual attraction and heterosexual relationships begin

B. ERIK ERIKSON

1. Broadened Freud's theory of personality development
2. Identified eight stages (psychosocial theory)
   a) Trust versus mistrust: birth to 18 months; to develop a basic trust in the mothering figure and to be able to generalize it to others
   b) Autonomy versus shame and doubt: 18 months to 3 years; to gain self-control and independence within the environment
   c) Initiative versus guilt: 3 to 6 years; to develop a sense of purpose and the ability to initiate and direct our own activities
   d) Industry versus inferiority: 6 to 11 years; to achieve a sense of self-confidence by learning, competing, performing successfully, and receiving recognition from others
   e) Identity versus role confusion: 12 to 20 years; to integrate the tasks mastered in the previous stages into a secure sense of self
   f) Intimacy versus isolation: 20 to 30 years; to form an intense, lasting relationship or a commitment to another person, cause, institution, or creative effort
   g) Generativity versus stagnation: age 30 to 65; to achieve the life goals established for oneself while considering the welfare of future generations
   h) Ego integrity versus despair: age 65 to death; to review one's life and derive meaning from both positive and negative events while achieving a positive sense of self-worth

C. JEAN PIAGET

1. Cognitive development
2. Concerned with acquisition of intellect and development of thought processes
3. Believed that the child's cognitive abilities progress through four stages
   a) Sensorimotor stage: birth to 2 years; acquires knowledge through exploration of

the environment; attaches meaning and recognition of things

b) Preoperational stage: 2 to 6 years; develops language; child sees self as the center of the universe

c) Concrete operational stage: 6 to 12 years; begins to problem-solve and to think logically; becomes less egocentric and more social

d) Formal operational stage: 12 to 15 years; ability to think logically in hypothetical and abstract terms; cognitive maturity achieved

D. ABRAHAM MASLOW

1. Described human behavior as being motivated by needs that are ordered in a hierarchy

2. Believed people must meet their most basic needs before they can move up the hierarchy to any higher level

3. Hierarchy begins at the bottom with basic survival needs and moves to the top with more complex needs

a) Physiological needs: basic fundamental needs; includes food, water, elimination, air, sleep, exercise, shelter, and sexual expression

b) Safety and security: these needs are for avoiding harm and maintaining comfort, order, structure, physical safety, protection, and freedom from fear

c) Love and belonging: needs for giving and receiving affection, companionship, satisfactory interpersonal relationships, and identification with a group

d) Self-esteem: seeks self-respect and respect from others, works to achieve success and recognition within the group, and desires prestige from accomplishments

e) Self-actualization: possesses a feeling of self-fulfillment and the realization of the person's highest potential

E. LAWRENCE KOHLBERG

1. Introduced a theory of moral development

2. Expanded on Piaget's theory

3. Believed that the child progressively develops moral reasoning as he/she gains the ability to think logically

4. Identified 3 levels of moral development, subdivided into 6 stages of acquired moral reasoning

a) Level 1: preconventional thinking; ages 4 to 10; the child learns reasoning through parents' demands for obedience; begins to recognize right from wrong

■ Stage 1: obedience and punishment orientation

■ Stage 2: instrumental relativist orientation

b) Level 2: conventional thinking; ages 10 to 13; the child begins to seek approval from society; influenced by external forces such as peers and environment

■ Stage 3: interpersonal concordance orientation

■ Stage 4: law and order orientation

c) Level 3: postconventional thinking; postadolescence; develop our own moral code based on our own principles

■ Stage 5: social contract legalistic orientation

■ Stage 6: universal ethical principle orientation

F. ELIZABETH KÜBLER-ROSS

1. Identified stages of dying

2. Can also apply to the grieving process

3. Stages

a) Denial: direct denial and/or periods of disbelief

b) Anger: realization of what is happening; may display rage

c) Bargaining: attempts to make deals with a deity

d) Depression: may show signs and symptoms such as withdrawal, lethargy, periods of crying

e) Acceptance: comes to accept the facts and fate

II. Stages of Life Cycle

A. NEWBORN TO 1 YEAR

1. Physical characteristics

a) Head is larger in proportion to the rest of the body at birth; fontanelles close between 12 and 18 months

b) Birth weight doubles by 5 to 6 months and triples by the first year

c) Teething begins at about 5 to 6 months

d) Senses are present at birth and develop more fully during the first year

e) Blood pressure increases, pulse and respiration decrease as the child ages

2. Developmental milestones

a) Gross motor skills (involve large muscles of the arms and legs)

■ 2 months: controls head

■ 3 months: sits without support

■ 7 months: sits alone

■ 10 months: creeps

■ 9 to 11 months: stands without support

■ 12 to 15 months: walks alone

b) Fine motor skills (refined use of hands and fingers)

c) Psychosocial (Erikson's stages of growth and development)

d) Cognitive (mostly sensorimotor; heightened use of touch, taste, sight, hearing, and smell)

B. TODDLERHOOD (1 TO 3 YEARS)

1. Physical characteristics
   - Grows up to 3 inches each year
   - Gains 4 to 6 pounds each year
   - Extremities grow faster than the trunk
   - Face and jaw grow bigger to permit room for more teeth
   - Bones begin to ossify
   - Visual acuity developing; hearing is fully developed
2. Developmental milestones
   a) Gross motor skills
      - Depends on growth and maturation of muscles, bones and nerves
      - Can usually run, and walk up steps using both feet
   b) Fine motor skills
      - Puts simple puzzles together
      - Can turn knobs and open jar lids
   c) Psychosocial
      - Attached to mother, tolerates short separation
      - Dresses and undresses self
      - Nearly toilet-trained
   d) Cognitive
      - Searches for and finds toys
      - Locates body parts
      - Gives full name on request
   e) Language
      - Uses words and gestures to indicate needs
      - Uses two-word sentences
      - Initiates sounds and words
      - Can sing simple songs
      - Vocabulary of about 1,000 words

C. PRESCHOOL (3 TO 6 YEARS)

1. Physical characteristics
   - Trunk and body lengthen in proportion to rest of body
   - Gains 5 to 7 pounds each year
   - Grows 2½ to 3 inches each year
   - Deciduous teeth may begin to fall out; dental health is very important
   - Visual acuity improves to 20/20; frequent ear infections
2. Developmental milestones
   a) Gross motor skills
      - Able to walk and run on tiptoes
      - Able to hop and to balance on one foot
      - May begin certain sports such as soccer, baseball, skating, and dance
   b) Fine motor skills
      - Manages self-care activities
      - Manipulates clothing and clothing fasteners with ease
      - Handles eating utensils; can begin to learn table manners
      - Can draw faces, copy letters, and print own name
   c) Psychosocial
      - Learns to trust
      - Aware of genital organs and sexual identity
      - Needs discipline and limits
   d) Cognitive
      - Longer attention span than as toddler
      - Develops memory
      - Can pretend
   e) Language
      - Becomes talkative
      - May show some difficulty with pronunciation
      - Can recite full name, address, and telephone number
      - Imitates others

D. SCHOOL AGE (6 TO 11 YEARS)

1. Physical characteristics
   - Growth is steady but slows
   - Permanent teeth appear
   - Weight increases by 4½ to 6½ pounds each year
   - Height increases by 2 to 3 inches each year
   - Visual maturity achieved; peripheral vision and depth perception improve
   - Immune system matures
2. Developmental milestones
   a) Gross motor skills
      - Increase in muscle mass improves skills
      - Gender differences exist in motor skills
   b) Fine motor skills
      - Can print and begins to master script writing
      - Can throw and catch
      - Can begin to learn to play musical instruments
   c) Psychosocial
      - Outgoing, talkative, and enthusiastic
      - Fearlessness puts child at risk for injury
      - Sexual curiosity continues
      - Initiates a task and able to see it through to completion
      - Sibling rivalry can occur
      - Peers are more important than family
      - Privacy becomes important
      - Emotions have wide range of expression
   d) Cognitive
      - Has collections of stickers, books, sports cards

- Breaks things down into small parts and reassembles them
- Takes views of others into consideration
- Understands concepts of time, space, dimension
- Starts and continues formal education

   e) Language
- Use of language and communication techniques improve
- Language becomes important for socialization
- Can use proper parts of speech, proper tense of words

E. ADOLESCENCE (11 TO 19 YEARS)

1. Puberty (ages 11 to 14); puberty ends and adolescence begins with the onset of menses (menarche) in girls and sperm production in boys
   - Rapid physical growth
   - Changes in body proportions; trunk and limbs grow swiftly
   - Development of primary sexual characteristics
   - Development of secondary sexual characteristics

2. Physical characteristics
   - Puberty is the period of the greatest amount of rapid growth; growth slows after puberty
   - Muscular strength increases greatly
   - Trunk broadens at the hips and shoulders
   - Posture may be poor from the fast growth, slouching
   - Sexual growth and development are completed
   - Shows great concern about one's changing body
   - Sebaceous glands produce more oil and become larger
   - Changes in fat distribution

3. Developmental milestones
   a) Motor development
   - Comparable to adult
   - Hand-eye coordination improves

   b) Sexual development
   - Heightened emotions
   - Increased worries
   - Lack of self-confidence
   - Sex is given high priority; girls set limits on interactions
   - Good sex education enables responsible choices

   c) Psychosocial
   - Rebelliousness, argumentative, and/or rude
   - Egocentric
   - Need for privacy
   - Dishonesty
   - Responsibility
   - Curfews
   - Friends
   - Self-absorbed
   - Society places many demands
   - Discipline is very important

   d) Cognitive
   - Maturation of central nervous system leads to formal operational thought processes (logical thought)
   - School is at the center of development
   - Moral reasoning and spiritual awareness develop

   e) Communication
   - Vocabulary increases
   - Verbal communication allows thoughts and beliefs to be known
   - Development of common language typical to a group, time, and culture (slang)

F. EARLY ADULTHOOD (20 TO 40 YEARS)

1. Physical characteristics
   - Physical growth is completed
   - Men usually have more muscle mass
   - Wisdom teeth erupt; may need to be removed
   - Other body systems begin to decline at the end of this period

2. Developmental milestones
   - Major milestones include choosing and establishing a career, fulfilling sexual needs, establishing a family and a home, expanding social circles, and developing maturity

   a) Motor development
   - Peak physical efficiency reached
   - Physical efficiency declines toward the end of this period

   b) Sexual development
   - Sexuality established
   - Ability to experience and share love

   c) Psychosocial development
   - Strong sense of identity
   - Sharing of innermost thoughts
   - Career and work roles understood

   d) Cognitive development
   - No longer egocentric, as a rule
   - Can solve problems and process information
   - Attends college or vocational school

   e) Health concerns
   - Pap smear
   - Mammography and self breast exam
   - Self testicular exam
   - Cholesterol
   - Obesity
   - Stress
   - Family planning

G. MIDDLE ADULTHOOD (MID-40S TO EARLY 60S)

1. Physical characteristics
   - May lose height
   - Body contour changes; higher percentage of body fat
   - Visual and aural acuity decline
   - Skin becomes less elastic, wrinkles form
   - Gradual loss of taste
2. Developmental milestones
   a) Sexual development
      - Menopause and loss of reproductive capacity
      - Options, opportunities, and means of sexual expression may change
   b) Psychosocial development
      - Achievement of goals
      - Desire to serve the larger community
      - Family roles may change from child-centered to couple-centered
      - Grandparenting
      - Change in relationship with parents
      - Peak earning capacity
   c) Cognitive development
      - Capable of thinking in a concrete manner

H. LATE ADULTHOOD (AGE 65 TO DEATH)

1. Physical characteristics
   - Quality of life depends on the person's ability to perform activities of daily living (ADL)
   - Formation and composition of body changes
   - Body systems begin to decline
   - Sensory systems become less efficient
   - Problems with memory loss and learning difficulty
2. Developmental milestones
   a) Motor development
      - Movement slows
      - Fine motor skills affected by stiffening of the joints
   b) Sexual development
      - Capable of enjoying a satisfying sexual relationship
   c) Psychosocial development
      - Ego integrity achieved
      - Life review reassures about accomplishments and worth
      - Body image changes
      - Fear of loss of independence
      - Death of a spouse produces change of roles
      - Work and leisure activities change
      - Concept of death takes on a different meaning
   d) Cognitive development
      - Healthy persons retain cognitive abilities
      - Memory changes; short-term stores less than long-term

III. The Sick Role

■ Illness and/or injury forces the patient to adopt the "sick role"
   - Includes duties and rights (Parsons, 1951)

■ Duties include
1. Duty 1: make every effort to get well
2. Duty 2: seek professional help and cooperate to get well

■ Rights include
1. Right 1: exempt from responsibility for injury/illness
2. Right 2: exempt from normal social obligations

A. SICK ROLE MAY BRING BENEFITS
1. Financial protection: disability, workers' compensation
2. Social gain: sympathy and attention

B. SICK ROLE MAY BRING DETRIMENT
1. Uncertainty about the future
2. May create social stigmas
3. Loss of independence
4. Loss of privacy
5. Loss of income
6. Loss of body image and self-esteem
7. Loss of social role

C. TERMINALLY ILL OR DYING PATIENT HAS SPECIAL NEEDS
1. Kübler-Ross's stages of dying
2. Excessive stress

IV. The Provider Role

A. ROLE IS TO EMPOWER THE PATIENT, NOT TO UNDERMINE THE PATIENT'S PARTICIPATION IN CARE

B. PROVIDER/PATIENT RELATIONSHIP IS UNEQUAL

C. PROVIDER IS RESPONSIBLE FOR
1. Concern for the patient's well-being
2. Carrying out ethical duties
3. Respect for each patient as an individual
4. Knowing what is important to the patient
5. Assisting patient in adapting to the sick role
6. Assuming cooperation from the patient
7. Displaying confidence
8. Promoting and encouraging proper patient behavior

D. DIFFICULTIES IN PROVIDER/PATIENT RELATIONSHIP CAN OCCUR
1. Personal bias: describes a person's feelings toward a patient or a thing
2. Prejudice: strong adverse attitude toward a patient because of that patient's association with a particular group
3. Overidentification: "I know how you feel"; difficulty seeing the patient as an individual

4. Countertransference: response to the patient in a personal manner, such as a child or sibling

5. Transference: overdependence by the patient on the provider

E. CULTURAL DIFFERENCES ARE IMPORTANT; MEDICAL ASSISTANT NEEDS TO BE AWARE OF VARIOUS CULTURAL NORMS FOR OPTIMUM CARE AND OPTIMUM PATIENT COMFORT

F. PROVIDER NEEDS TO BE AWARE OF "DISTANCE" AND "PERSONAL SPACE" WHEN GIVING CARE; DISTANCE AND PERSONAL SPACE CAN BE CULTURAL

1. Intimate space: actual physical contact

2. Personal space: 1 to 4 feet

3. Social space: 4 to 12 feet

4. Public space: 12 to 25 feet

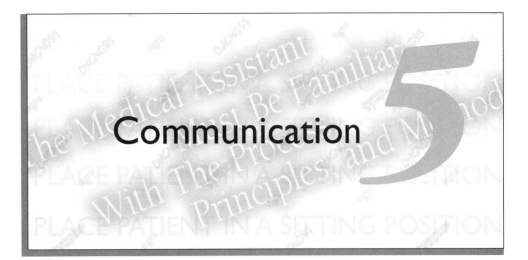

Communication 5

I. Communication
■ The process of sharing meaning

A. COMMUNICATION PROCESS
1. Source
   a) Sender of the message
   b) Can be a person, a group, or a company
   c) What is sent varies and is affected by the sender's present and past experiences
2. Message
   a) "What" is sent by the source
   b) Message has 3 parts
      1) Meaning: usually ideas or feelings
      2) Symbols: words or actions that represent the meaning; the process of turning words or actions into symbols is "encoding"
      3) Organization, or form: syntax and grammar of the message; putting the symbols in order
3. Channel
   a) Which symbols are given
   b) Can be visual, audio, print, or touch
4. Receiver
   a) Where the message is being sent
   b) Receiver processes into meaning ("decoding")
5. Feedback
   a) Response of the receiver
   b) Can be verbal or nonverbal
   c) Tells the source if the message was heard, seen, or understood
6. Noise
   a) Anything that interferes with the communication process
   b) Can be
      1) External: stimuli that draws attention away from the message
      2) Internal: personal thoughts and feelings that draw a person away from the message
      3) Semantic: message symbols that prevent the meaning from being understood (accents, dialect, grammar)

B. THERAPEUTIC COMMUNICATION
1. Process of relaying information from health provider to patient
2. Can be through verbal disclosure, touch, or gesture
3. Techniques include
   a) Acknowledgment: emphasizes the importance of the patient in the communication process
   b) Establishing guidelines: helps the patient to know what is expected of him/her
   c) Focusing: directs the communication toward important topics
   d) Listening: communicates interest in the topics raised by the patient
   e) Open-ended comments: helps the patient to decide what is relevant; encourages discussion ("Describe what you think is going to happen.")
   f) Reflecting: shows the importance of the patient's ideas and feelings
   g) Restating: lets the patient know how the provider interpreted the message the patient sent ("I hear you saying. . . .")
   h) Clarification: demonstrates the desire to understand what the patient is communicating (may ask who, what, where, when)
   i) Silence: communicates acceptance
4. Ineffective techniques include
   a) Advising: telling what the provider thinks should be done
   b) Minimizing: provider making light of the patient's situation
   c) Defending: provider protecting self from criticism
   d) Stereotyping: provider using cliches when responding
   e) Probing: provider discussing, or trying to discuss, topics the patient does not want to discuss
   f) Approval/disapproval: provider overly approving or disapproving of the patient's behavior

g) Agreeing/disagreeing: provider overly agreeing or disagreeing with the patient's perceptions, thoughts, or feelings

5. Barriers to communication
    a) Embarrassment: patient may be in awe of the provider, thereby being embarrassed to ask questions of the provider
    b) Discomfort: patient may be uncomfortable or ashamed to discuss patient's private body parts or symptoms
    c) Communication difficulties: patient can see disabilities as making the patient intellectually inferior
    d) Withdrawal: patient does not respond to provider's communication
    e) Ineffective techniques (see above) by provider may raise barriers

C. NONVERBAL COMMUNICATION
1. Messages conveyed without the use of words
2. Body language
3. Involves the provider's grooming, dress, eye contact, facial expressions, hand gestures, space, tone of voice, and posture

II. Patient Relationships
■ Medical assistant needs to understand the patient's concerns, needs, and reactions
■ Stress and anxiety are common patient responses

A. UNCONSCIOUS DEFENSE MECHANISMS
1. Compensation: overemphasizing a trait to make up for a failure
2. Denial: avoiding reality
3. Displacement: shifting an impulse from a threatening to a nonthreatening one
4. Dissociation: disconnecting the significance from an event
5. Identification: mimicking the behavior of another
6. Introjection: adopting the feelings of others
7. Projection: assigning one's own feelings to another as if those feelings had originated with the other person
8. Rationalization: justifying one's thoughts, feelings, or behavior
9. Regression: returning to a former behavior or more immature behavior
10. Repression: putting unpleasant thoughts or events out of one's mind
11. Sublimation: diverting unacceptable thoughts or feelings into acceptable behaviors
12. Substitution: making up for a deficiency by concentrating on another
13. Suppression: deliberately forgetting or avoiding dealing with an unpleasantness

B. INTERACTION WITH PATIENTS
■ Interaction is a therapeutic relationship
■ Assists patients to resolve problems and achieve goals
■ Maximizes patient comfort
1. Children
    a) Establish a friendly relationship
    b) Be aware of your own feelings toward children in general
    c) Speak in quiet tones, speak at the child's physical level (not looking down at the child)
    d) Use language appropriate for the child's age
    e) Allow the child to assist in his/her treatment
    f) Keep the child patient from experiencing long waits
    g) Understand that the child may regress when ill
    h) Be truthful with the child; this fosters trust
    i) Offer rewards for proper behavior
    j) Allow the child to play with the provider's equipment if that is safe and appropriate
    k) Infants should be held and comforted before any treatment procedures
2. Adolescents
    a) Patient demands independence yet requires comfort
    b) Permit patient's privacy
    c) Provider must allow examinations with the patient's parent present
    d) Treat the patient with respect and dignity
    e) Set fair limits for the patient
    f) Answer the patient's questions openly and honestly
    g) Explain the procedures to the patient in terms he/she will understand
3. Elderly patient
    a) Allow additional time with the patient; this may be a social interaction for a lonely patient
    b) Keep the patient physically and environmentally comfortable
    c) Patient may find comfort in a provider's routine
    d) Allow as much independence as possible
    e) Do not overprotect or be overattentive
    f) Speak slowly and precisely, but do not patronize
4. Terminally ill patient
    a) Help both the patient and the patient's family to adjust to the patient's loss in strength, sensation, mobility, and endurance
    b) Give support to the patient's family members

c) Be willing to listen
d) Patient will likely experience some, or all, of the stages of dying
5. Angry patient
    a) Patient's anger may be caused by the patient's medical condition
    b) Provider's goal is to calm the patient
    c) Provider must remain calm, firm, and direct
    d) Provider must not take the anger personally
    e) Provider must listen closely to the patient's concerns
    f) Provider must keep speaking tone calm and in control
    g) Keep the angry patient out of public areas of the office; escort the angry patient to a private room
6. Sensory-impaired patient
    a) Patient may need an interpreter (if hearing impaired or if speaks only a foreign language) to assist in communication
    b) Provider should be positioned directly in front of the patient and should speak slowly
    c) For the sight-impaired patient, the provider should ask how best to assist the patient
    d) Provider should be flexible, open, and supportive
7. Frightened patient
    a) A frightened patient may be uncooperative
    b) Provider should recognize fear and assist the patient in dealing with the fright
    c) Provider should maintain control of the situation
8. Depressed patient
    a) The depressed patient will experience feelings of gloom, hopelessness, and dread and may have feelings of no self-worth
    b) Provider should provide sympathy, support, and a friendly ear
    c) Provider should demonstrate an interest in the patient's needs
    d) Provider should keep the environment secure and nonthreatening
9. Suicidal patient
    a) Suicidal feelings can be the patient's final response to his/her depression
    b) Suicidal patient may disclose intentions to the provider
    c) All suicidal threats or attempts must be taken seriously
    d) Provider must listen closely to the suicidal patient
    e) Provider should demonstrate empathy
    f) Provider should seek professional advice and/or actions for the suicidal patient
10. Mentally impaired patient
    a) Patient may be confused and disoriented
    b) By correcting the patient's confusion, the provider may make the patient less frightened
    c) Provider must treat the patient kindly but must not be condescending
11. Abused patient
    a) Provider must treat the abused patient's physical injuries first
    b) Provider must focus on the patient as a victim; provider should express assurances of the patient's self-worth
    c) Refer the abused patient to existing social agencies
12. Drug-dependent patient
    a) Provider should not belittle the patient for the patient's behavior
    b) Provider should be compassionate, empathetic, and patient
    c) Provider should involve the patient's family in the patient's treatment
13. Significant others
    a) Part of the patient's emotional support group
    b) Provider should respect the wishes of the patient concerning the patient's loved ones
    c) Provider should keep any waiting relatives notified of progress and keep them informed of any delays
    d) Provider should address the concerns of the patient's family and friends
    e) Provider must be aware of confidentiality issues

Patient Reception 6

I. Reception

- Patient's first impression of the provider's office
- Influences patient's perception of the office
- Receptionist's attitude and appearance are important to set the tone of the office

II. Reception Area

1. Place to receive patients
2. Planned for patient comfort
3. Should be clean and uncluttered
4. Receptionist should be behind a counter that is high enough for provider privacy (of hard records, of patient information on computer screens, for patient financial records)
5. Colors should be calming and restful
6. Lighting should be adequate for reading and safety
7. Adequate ventilation is essential
8. Temperature should be regulated for patients' comfort
9. Play area for children, if it is appropriate
10. Spacious coat rack to store patients' outerwear
11. Furniture arranged for patients' comfort, movement, and safety
12. Periodicals should be up to date and appropriate

III. Receptionist

1. First professional person the patient comes in contact with, either in person or by phone
2. Medical Assistant should display pride in self and the job
3. Communication skills should demonstrate competence and a positive attitude
4. Clothing, hair, and makeup should be appropriate
5. Should have friendly, cheerful, caring, courteous, and respectful demeanor
6. Should be professional at all times
7. Greet every patient on arrival by name (correct pronunciation)

8. A friendly farewell can portray caring and courtesy
9. Duties may include
   a) Answering telephones
   b) Scheduling appointments
   c) Patient registration/taking history
   d) Handling complaints
   e) Preparing charts
   f) Handling nonpatient visitors (vendors, sales representatives, pharmaceutical representatives)

IV. Telephone Techniques

A. GENERAL
1. Majority of receptionist's communication occurs through the telephone
2. Telephone is the critical component of a successful health care provider's practice
3. Communication and listening skills are important
4. Incoming telephone calls may be from
   a) Established patients calling for appointments or advice
   b) Patient emergencies
   c) Other physicians making patient referrals
   d) Laboratories reporting information regarding provider's patient
   e) New patients making a first contact

B. EQUIPMENT
1. Six-button key set
   a) Several incoming lines
   b) Office intercom line
   c) Hold button
   d) Lights flash slowly for incoming calls, flash rapidly for reminder of call on hold
2. Two-line speakerphone
   a) Allows conversation without using the handset
   b) Last number redial
   c) Volume control
   d) Speed-dial and memory for frequent calls

107

e) Intercom paging

f) May have LCD display screen

3. Headset

a) Lightweight plastic earphone and microphone combination

b) Allows hands-free telephone use

4. Cellular phone

a) Mobile, transportable telephone

b) Permits communication outside an office or within a vehicle

5. Pager

a) Activated by calling the pager's number

b) Can leave a voice message or digital message

6. Facsimile machine (fax)

a) Transmits print material over telephone lines to other facilities that have fax capability

b) Can send and receive copies of printed documents

c) If sending sensitive patient information, call ahead to ensure that only the appropriate person receives the fax

7. Directories

a) White pages: alphabetical listing by last name, includes last name, first name, sometimes middle initial, address, and telephone number

b) Yellow pages: alphabetical listing by category of commercial business; in each category, alphabetical listing by company name (or businessperson's last name), includes company name (or businessperson's name), company address, and company telephone number(s)

c) Personal office directory: collection of frequently called telephone numbers within that office; can be stored in a Rolodex or in a 3 × 5 index card file

C. INCOMING CALLS

1. Answer promptly (ideally on the first ring, always by the third ring)

2. Hold the phone instrument correctly (with the mouthpiece about 1 inch from your mouth)

3. Develop a pleasing telephone voice

4. Identify the provider's office; identify yourself

5. Gain the identity of the caller (ask to whom you are speaking if the caller does not first identify self)

6. Offer assistance (proper words, proper tone)

7. Screen incoming calls (follow any office policies about how incoming calls are to be handled and categorized)

8. Minimize caller waiting time (caller should experience no more than 1 minute without voice contact of some type)

9. When answering a second call, ask the first caller to please hold, transfer to the second incoming line, identify the second caller, ask the second caller to please hold, and return to the first caller

10. End each call pleasantly and graciously (say, "thank you," some form of "good-bye")

D. TELEPHONE MESSAGES

1. May be recorded on message sheet or in an office telephone log

2. Message should include the following information

a) Name of the person to whom the call is directed

b) Name of the person calling

c) Caller's daytime telephone number (include pager and/or cell phone numbers)

d) Reason for the call

e) Action to be taken by the recipient

f) Date and time the call was received

g) Initials of the person taking the call

E. OUTGOING TELEPHONE CALLS

1. Know what needs to be said, how it is to be said, and have all pertinent information on hand before placing the call

2. Your voice should convey warmth, friendliness, confidence, and intelligence

3. Address the person by name

4. Use "please" and "thank you"

5. Do not rush the call

6. Use discretion when conveying personal or confidential patient or medical information

7. Long distance (check with office manager to verify this procedure, as different long-distance carriers have different calling requirements):

a) Direct dial: 1 + area code + seven-digit telephone number

b) Long-distance directory assistance: 1 + area code + 555-1212

c) Operator assisted: 0 + area code + seven-digit telephone number

1) Person-to-person (operator will not connect the line until the person to whom you requested answers the telephone)

2) Station-to-station (operator will connect the line as soon as anyone at the receiving phone number answers the telephone)

3) Collect call (operator will not connect the line until a recipient agrees to be billed for the long-distance telephone call)

4) Bill to third party (operator verifies that a third party [someone not a party to this long-distance phone call] will accept the charges for the phone call)

5) Request for time and charges (the operator, if asked before connecting the long-distance line, will call you back after the call is ended and will tell you the time of the long-distance call as well as the cost of the long-distance call; you will then be able to verify the long-distance charge against the next telephone bill)

d) Time zones

1) Pacific Time: 1:00 (WA, OR, NV, CA)

2) Mountain Time: 2:00 (MT, UT, ID, WY, CO, NM, AZ; parts of ND, SD, NE, KS)

3) Central Time: 3:00 (MN, WI, IA, MO, AR, OK, TX, LA, MS, IL, AL; parts of TN, KY, ND, SD, NE, KS)

4) Eastern Time: 4:00 (all other states, except for HI and AK)

e) Wrong number dialed

1) Verify the telephone number with the person answering

2) Apologize

3) If long distance, call the operator to credit the account

F. ANSWERING SERVICES

■ Provider must be able to be contacted at all times, to respond to emergencies (to prevent abandonment charges)

1. Answering services

a) Provides coverage when the office is closed

b) Answering services answer and screen incoming phone calls

2. Electronic answering devices

a) Recorded message that tells caller how to reach the provider (or provider's colleague) or invites the caller to leave a voice message

b) Messages can be retrieved directly from the machine or can be remotely accessed

c) Answering message may be changed as necessary

3. Voice mail

a) Computerized system used to record, send, or retrieve voice messages from the telephone system

4. Automatic routing

a) Telephone calls answered by automated operator that announces a list of options from which the caller selects one

b) This is a rather impersonal system but may be good for the larger clinic

V. Appointment Scheduling

■ Process that determines which patients will be seen by the provider ("appointment"), the dates and times for those appointments, and the allotted time for each appointment

■ Allotted time for each appointment is based on the patient's complaint as compared to the provider's availability

■ Important factor in the success of provider's practice

■ Many approaches to scheduling

A. GUIDELINES

1. Understand the nature of the practice

2. Know the personalities and habits of the medical staff

3. Be aware of the time needed to assess each patient complaint type

4. Plan realistically

B. MATERIALS NEEDED

1. Appointment book (see Figure 6-1)

a) May be for one or several providers

b) May show day, week, or month per page

c) May be blank or preprinted

d) May be loose-leaf or spiral bound

e) Each block of time must have sufficient space to record the patient's name, the patient's telephone numbers, and the purpose of patient's visit to the provider

f) Entire book must fit comfortably on the receptionist's desk and be easily accessible to all who are responsible for scheduling; the book must always be left in place

g) Appointment book is a legal document and must be preserved as such

2. Pen and/or pencil

a) Appointments should be written in black ink (as it is a legal document)

b) Must be corrected in the same manner as correcting the patient chart (no erasing, no scribbling, no white-out)

c) Use of pencil is more practical in anticipation of any appointment changes or cancellations

d) Occasional use of colored ink (or pencil) may denote new or special patient

3. Appointment card

a) Given to each patient after the follow-up appointment is made in the office

b) Often preprinted with the clinic name, address, and telephone number; space on the card for date, day and time of appointment, and patient name

C. METHODS OF SCHEDULING

1. Open-office hours

a) Clinic is open only for specified time period

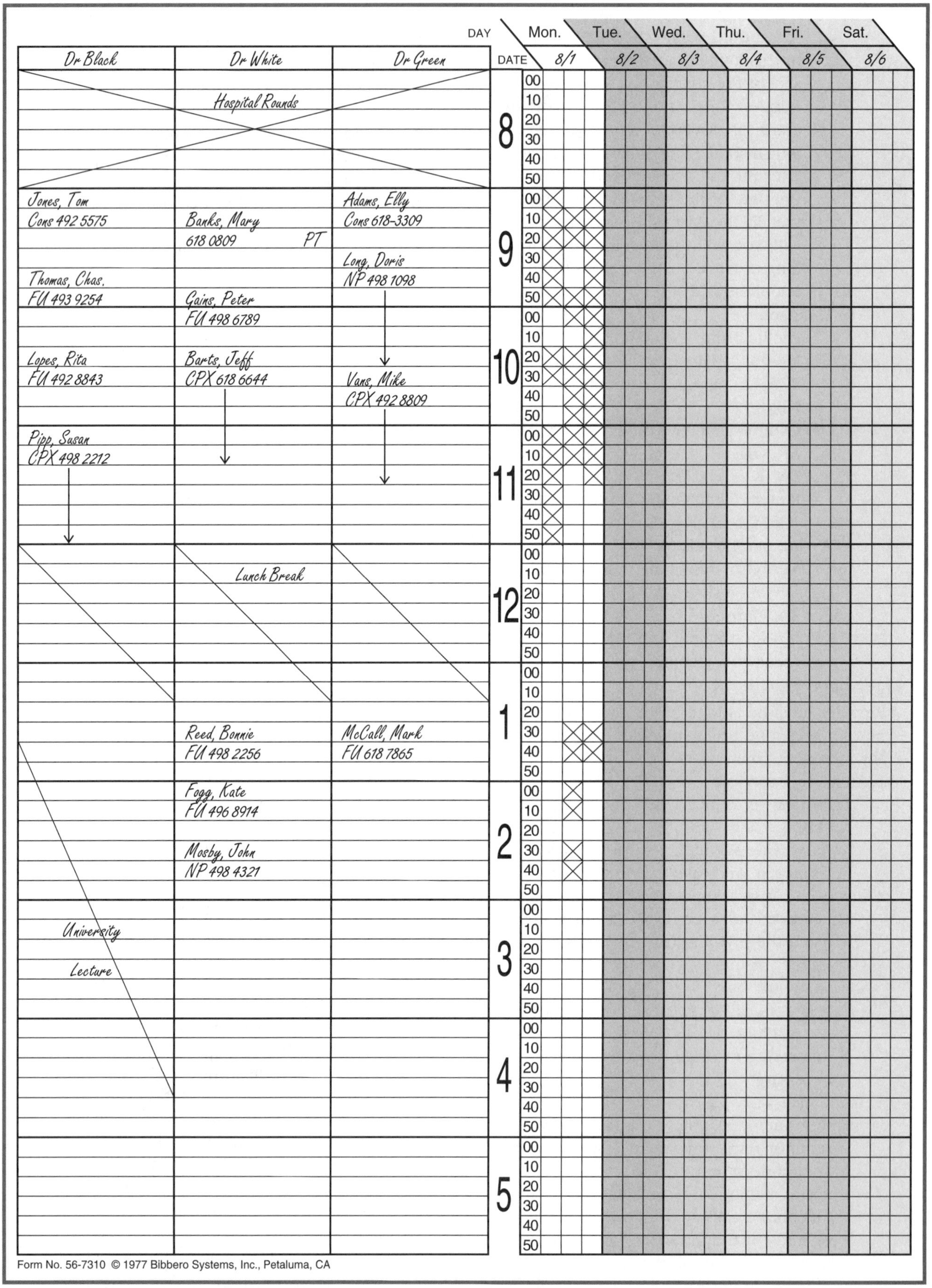

Dr Black	Dr White	Dr Green	DATE	Mon. 8/1	Tue. 8/2	Wed. 8/3	Thu. 8/4	Fri. 8/5	Sat. 8/6
	Hospital Rounds		8						
Jones, Tom Cons 492 5575	Banks, Mary 618 0809 PT	Adams, Elly Cons 618-3309	9						
Thomas, Chas. FU 493 9254	Gains, Peter FU 498 6789	Long, Doris NP 498 1098							
Lopes, Rita FU 492 8843	Barts, Jeff CPX 618 6644	Vans, Mike CPX 492 8809	10						
Pipp, Susan CPX 498 2212			11						
	Lunch Break		12						
	Reed, Bonnie FU 498 2256	McCall, Mark FU 618 7865	1						
	Fogg, Kate FU 496 8914		2						
	Mosby, John NP 498 4321								
University Lecture			3						
			4						
			5						

Form No. 56-7310 © 1977 Bibbero Systems, Inc., Petaluma, CA

FIGURE 6-1   Sample appointment book. (Courtesy of Bibbero Systems, Inc., Petaluma, California 94954-1180. 800-242-2376. Fax 800-242-8330. www.bibbero.com.)

b) Patients are seen in the order of their arrival in the clinic (patients sign into a logbook upon arrival), with provision that emergency treatment is given priority

c) Least efficient method of scheduling

d) Common among urgent care centers

2. Flexible office hours

a) Clinic is open at odd hours in addition to normal office hours (early morning or evening hours on certain days of the week)

b) Accommodates various work schedules of patients

c) Usually used in group practices

3. Time specified

a) Most common system

b) Each patient is given a specific time on a specific day for the appointment

c) Does not easily accommodate the unplanned illness or accident, does not allow any buffer time (unless one or two open appointments each day are kept for such use)

4. Wave

a) Gives short-term flexibility within each hour

b) Assumes that the average time needed for the appointments will average out over the course of the day

c) Each hour is divided into the average time the provider should spend with each patient (hour divided into 10-minute, 15-minute, or 20-minute blocks)

d) Patients are scheduled on the hour (6 per hour for 10-minute block, 4 per hour for 15-minute block, etc.) and are seen by the provider in the order in which they sign in with the receptionist

e) This system allows for late arrivals, allows for the patient whose accident or illness needs more (or less) time than the average, allows for the failed appointment, and allows for unscheduled interruptions of the provider

f) Variable waiting times may result from this method of scheduling

5. Modified wave

a) Appointments are staggered throughout the provider hour

6. Double booking

a) Scheduling 2 patients at the same time

b) Not an efficient way to schedule

c) Can be wavelike if 2 patients each needing 5 minutes are both scheduled in the same 15-minute block

7. Grouping

a) Similar procedures (such as Pap smears, well-baby checks, complete physicals) are all scheduled at a specific time of a specific day of the week or at specific hours

b) These like procedures can be color-coded for ease of view

D. SCHEDULING PROCEDURES

1. Establish a matrix

a) Block out times the provider is not available for appointments

b) Establish a buffer time both in the morning and in the afternoon, for catch-up

2. Chief complaint

a) Identify the reason for patient visit

b) Identify the level of urgency of the patient visit

c) Identify the provider resources available

3. Referral: determine whether the patient has been referred by another provider

4. Locate the first available time to see the patient, as well as one alternative time; offer the dates and times to the patient

5. Enter the patient's name, phone numbers, and complaint in the appointment book in the corresponding date and time block agreed to by the patient

6. Explain the pertinent office policies and instructions to the patient

7. Repeat the date and time to the patient for double-check before ending the call

E. APPOINTMENT PROBLEMS

1. Patient habitually late

a) Schedule this patient near the end of the day

2. Consecutive appointments

a) Schedule at the same time and day (different dates) for ease of remembering

3. Cancellations

a) Offer the patient an alternative appointment

4. Missed appointment/no-show

a) Prevent with a reminder phone call the day before the appointment

b) Patient may legally be charged for the missed appointment

c) Patient may be discharged from provider's care for habitual no-shows

d) Note all missed appointments in both the patient's chart and the appointment book

5. Emergencies

a) Follow office protocol

b) Emergencies take precedence over all other appointments

c) Call "911" if the emergency is outside of the office protocol

6. Acute needs

a) Provide the first available appointment to patient

b) Double-booking may be necessary

7. Referrals
   a) Process of sending patient to another provider (a specialist) for diagnosis and treatment
   b) Appointment may be made by the patient or by the referring provider
   c) Make sure all appropriate documents are provided to referred provider (necessary patient records, X-rays, insurance referral letter)

8. Delays
   a) Attempt to call affected patients about provider delays and request that they come later that day or reschedule for another date and time
   b) Explain courteously if the provider is called out of the office on an emergency
   c) Waiting patients should be given an explanation, an estimated time of the current delay, and the patients' option to wait on the provider or reschedule

Records Management

I. The Medical Record

A. GENERAL
1. The chart
2. Chronological system used to annotate patient's medical care rendered by the provider
3. Insures competent and necessary (nonredundant) medical care
4. Legal document

B. PURPOSE
1. Establishes the patient database
2. Serves as a communication link between the provider and the staff
3. Helps with the planning of effective patient care
4. Provides evidence of care given to the patient
5. Can provide data for research or education

C. CONTENT
1. Specific as to the type of practice
2. Usually includes
   - a) Chief complaint (CC): main reason for the patient seeking care
   - b) Past medical history (PH or PMH): gives information regarding UCD, past illnesses, surgeries, current health status; may be prepared by the patient, by the provider, or by the medical assistant
   - c) Family history (FH): information regarding the patient's parents and siblings; may include health status, age, cause of death, hereditary diseases
   - d) Present illness (PI): expanded chief complaint (CC)
   - e) Social history (SH): information on patient's personal habits; may include exercise, sleep, diet, tobacco/alcohol use, drug use, sexual history, sexual preference, hobbies
   - f) Occupational history (OH): information regarding patient's employment
   - g) Physical exam (PE): complete physical examination; gives information regarding each body system (review of systems:

ROS); may serve as a baseline against the future
   - h) Test results: diagnostic and laboratory tests; arranged with the most recent on top of the older
   - i) Consultations: reports on evaluations made by other providers as requested by this provider
   - j) Past medical records: records from other providers that have bearing on present treatment
   - k) Correspondence: all correspondence related to patient care
   - l) Progress notes: notes written in the chart by the provider regarding the patient's care, diagnosis, and/or treatment

D. ORGANIZATION
1. Source-oriented record
   - a) Observations and data are categorized according to their source (provider, laboratory, X-ray, nurse, technician)
   - b) Forms are filed in reverse chronological order (most recent on top)
   - c) Information is filed in separate sections (lab reports section, X-ray reports section, progress notes section, etc.)
2. Problem-oriented medical record (POMR)
   - Data is organized according to patient's disease or condition
   - Divided into 4 parts
   - a) Database: includes CC, PI, PE findings, and lab results; each condition will have its own page
   - b) Problem list: numbered and titled list of every problem complained of by patient; may include physical, psychological, and social problems related to the patient's condition
   - c) Plan: diagnostic and treatment decisions for the condition; each plan is titled and numbered

d) Progress notes: structured notes that correspond to each problem number uses SOAP
   1) S (subjective data): signs, symptoms, and feelings described by the patient in the patient's own words
   2) O (objective data): clinical evidence determined by health care provider
   3) A (Assessment = S + O): describes the physical impression and finally diagnosis
   4) P (plan = S + O + A): action needed to solve the problem; may include treatment, medications, consultations, surgery

E. DOCUMENTATION
   1. Chart in black ink
   2. All entries must be dated and initialed, or signed, by the technician making the entry
   3. All patient visits and phone calls must be documented
   4. No-shows must be recorded
   5. Patient's name should appear on each page
   6. Corrections are made by using the SLIDE rule
      a) SL: single line through the error
      b) I: initials of the person correcting the error
      c) D: date and correct the error
      d) E: write the word "error"
   7. Correspondence sent to the patient requires a note in the chart
   8. "If it wasn't charted, it wasn't done."

F. SIX "C's" OF CHARTING
   1. Current
   2. Complete
   3. Concise
   4. Correct
   5. Confidential
   6. Clean

G. LEGALITIES AND THE MEDICAL RECORD
   1. The chart is a legal document
   2. The chart belongs to the provider or the clinic, but the patient owns the information found on the chart
   3. Records requested by patients or third parties may be released only if the provider and the patient give consent, usually by a medical records release form
   4. Records can be withheld from patients if the information can reasonably expected to cause harm to the patient (doctrine of professional discretion)
   5. Patient information is confidential and privileged (this patient confidentiality can be waived in writing by the patient or overruled in a courtroom)

6. Release of confidential patient information without the patient's written consent could lead to a charge of invasion of privacy by the patient
7. Medical records must be kept up to date, complete, and accurate
8. Records are retained according to the requirements of each state's statutes; medical records are usually retained permanently, until the patient's death
9. Medical records are destroyed by shredding or burning
10. Entries into medical records should be typewritten or written in black ink

II. Records Management

A. PURPOSE
   ■ To classify, arrange, and store documents in an efficient, orderly, and accessible manner
   1. Records to be stored include
      a) Medical records (charts)
      b) Financial records
      c) Correspondence
      d) Business records
      e) Research records
   2. Records can be stored as
      a) Hard, printed, copies of the records
      b) Computer documents
      c) Microfiche/microfilm

B. EQUIPMENT AND SUPPLIES FOR RECORDS MANAGEMENT
   1. Storage cabinet
      a) Vertical: file cabinet style
      b) Lateral: chest of drawers style
      c) Shelf: open or closed storage
   2. Guides
      a) Plastic or cardboard dividers; permit grouping of similar type files
      b) Outguide: guide used to replace a file taken from the cabinet, enables technician to replace the file in the proper place when ready
   3. Folders
      a) Cardboard or plastic holders that contain the patients' medical records
      b) Have tabs within them for separating contents
   4. Labels
      a) Small stickers placed onto folders to identify the contents or folder identity

C. PROCESS
   1. Condition
      a) Check for damage and, if found, repair it before refiling the record
      b) Date your work on the record, if required

2. Inspect and release
    a) Documents cannot be filed until the responsible parties have seen the document and have taken action on the record
    b) Release mark of some sort (office protocol) must be noted on the file

3. Index and code
    a) Determine where the document should be filed
    b) Identify the caption to be used in filing the document

4. Sort
    a) Arrange the documents according to the office protocol (system) used

5. Store
    a) Place the documents in the appropriate file folder and place in the filing cabinet

D. FILING METHODS

1. Alphabetical
    a) Used with names of persons, businesses, or organizations; oldest, simplest, and most commonly used method
    b) Rules include
        1) Names are divided into units and filed left to right
        2) Surname is unit 1, given name is unit 2, middle name (initial) is unit 3, and so on
        3) Names are alphabetized according to first unit letter; second unit considered if first units are the same; third unit considered if first two units are the same
        4) Initials filed before complete names starting with the same letter
        5) Units having no name filed before those that do (nothing before something)
        6) Hyphenated name is considered a single unit; if business name, each name is a separate unit
        7) Apostrophes are disregarded
        8) Abbreviations are indexed as if written in full
        9) Numbers as part of a name are indexed as if written out
        10) Titles and degrees are indexed last
        11) Married women are indexed by their own given name (first name)
        12) If two names are identical, patient's address is used as an index unit
        13) For names of organizations:
            (a) Index in order as written, except when organization name includes a person's name (surname first, then given name)
            (b) Numbers are indexed as if written out

            (c) Disregard punctuation
            (d) Directional terms are indexed as separate units
            (e) Articles, conjunctions, and prepositions are disregarded unless "the" is the first word (if so, "the" is indexed as the last unit)

2. Numerical
    a) Used when each patient is assigned a number that is used on the patient's chart
    b) Patient number is cross-referenced with the patient's name and filed alphabetically
    c) Numerical filing is used in large clinics, group practices, and hospitals
    d) Types include
        1) Consecutive numeric system
            (a) Simplest system
            (b) Patients are assigned consecutive numbers in the order of the date of their first visit to the facility
        2) Terminal digit system
            (a) Patients assigned consecutive numbers as they visit the facility
            (b) Digits in the patient number are separated into groups of twos or threes
            (c) Read in groups from right to left, instead of left to right, and filed backwards in groups
        3) Social Security Number
            (a) Patient's Social Security Number is patient's filing number
            (b) Not every patient has a Social Security Number

3. Subject
    a) Documents indexed by subject matter and then filed alphabetically, then filed numerically, or both
    b) Generally not used for medical records

4. Color Coding
    a) Colored tabs are used to represent patient information at a glance
    b) Used on letters of the patient's surname
    c) Can help keep files from being misfiled
    d) Selection of colors and division of the alphabet are determined by the practice's needs
    e) Can be used as colored folders, adhesive labels, or a combination
    f) Can be filed alphabetically or numerically

5. Tickler File
    a) System that organizes items chronologically for follow-up
    b) Can be notations on the daily calendar, or a card file divided into months, with months divided into days
    c) Must be checked daily for effectiveness

Administrative Practices

8

I. Computer Basics

A. GENERAL: ELECTRONIC DEVICE THAT ACCEPTS, PROCESSES, EXPORTS, AND STORES DATA; CLASSIFIED ACCORDING TO SIZE
   1. Mainframe: large computer that can handle many users at the same time
   2. Microcomputer: personal computer (PC)
   3. Laptop: personal portable computer

B. HARDWARE: COMPUTER EQUIPMENT
   1. Central processing unit (CPU)
      a) Control unit: supervises data processing operations
      b) Arithmetic logic unit (ALU): carries out arithmetic and logic operations
      c) Primary storage unit: stores data and program instructions
         ■ 1) RAM: random access memory; computer's temporary memory
         ■ 2) ROM: read-only memory; computer's permanent memory
   2. Input devices: allows communication between the user and the computer hardware; allows data to be entered into the computer
      a) Keyboard: the "typewriter"; allows input of alphanumeric data
      b) Mouse: handheld pointing device; contains a ball that is moved when the mouse is rolled on a flat surface; movement of the mouse, and of the ball, moves the cursor on the computer screen
      c) Scanner: device that "reads," or converts, printed matter directly into computer-readable format
   3. Output devices: allows data to be displayed or recorded
      a) Monitor: device that resembles a television set; displays computer-generated information
      b) Printer: device that records computer-generated information onto paper (hard copy)

   4. Storage: methods of saving the information input for future reference or for printing
      a) Hard drive: part of the computer hardware inside the computer box; contains the computer-operating information
      b) Floppy disk: part of the computer software; "diskette"; thin disk of magnetic material that can be inserted into the computer's disk drive
      c) Disk drive: loads a program or data that is stored on a diskette into the computer; also can be used to transfer stored information from the computer onto a diskette for safekeeping; each microcomputer may have more than one drive

C. SOFTWARE: DISKETTES OR CD DISK ON WHICH COMPUTER INFORMATION MAY BE STORED; TYPICALLY REFERRED TO AS A PROGRAM, WHICH PROVIDES PROCESSING INSTRUCTIONS TO THE COMPUTER
   1. Systems software: manages the overall operations of the computer system; program instructions that control, interface with, and communicate between the applications software and the workstation
   2. Applications software: mainly commercially prepared programs that perform specific data processing functions

D. DATA PROCESSING: TRANSFORMS RAW INFORMATION (DATA) INTO USEFUL INFORMATION; THE SMALLEST PIECE OF INFORMATION PROCESSED IS A BIT (BINARY DIGIT); AN 8-BIT UNIT IS A BYTE
   ■ 1 byte is required to represent 1 character
   ■ 1 kilobyte (K) equals 1,024 bytes
   ■ 1 megabyte (M) equals 1,000 kilobytes
      • All data is processed in a cycle
   1. Input: data is entered into the computer by an input device
   2. Processing: data is manipulated

3. Output: processed information is accessed from an output device

4. Storage: information is stored for future use

II. Word Processing

■ Use of computer to produce documents

■ Software programs that allow the preparation of written documents

A. KEYBOARD KEYS

1. Alphanumeric: keys that represent letters, numbers, symbols

2. Backspace: allows the cursor to be moved to the left; erases characters backspaced over

3. Caps Lock: keeps the alphabet keys in uppercase

4. Ctrl and Alt (control and alternate keys): used in combination with other keys to increase the number of functions on the keyboard

5. Cursor control arrows: allows the cursor (the blinking arrow [or dash] on the screen that identifies where the data will be placed on the screen) to be moved up, down, to the left, or to the right

6. Del (delete): erases characters to the right of the cursor

7. End: moves the cursor to the end of a line of printing

8. Enter/Return: returns the cursor to the beginning of the next blank line

9. Esc (escape): allows the exit of a program or window

10. F1 through F12 (function keys): perform special program-directed moves

11. Home: moves the cursor to the upper, lower, left, or right margin

12. Page Up, Page Down: moves the cursor 1 page up or down

13. Print screen: allows only the displayed screen to be printed (if allowed by the program)

14. Shift: places the alphabet key in uppercase when the Shift key is pressed simultaneously

15. Space bar: allows blank spaces to be placed between letters or words

16. Tab: moves the cursor a predetermined number of blank spaces; used to indent

B. FORMATTING

■ Determines the physical layout of the document

1. Margins: the amount of blank space at the edges of the document

2. Tab Set: sets a specific number of blank spaces to be used in each tab

3. Line spacing: sets a specific number of blank lines between each line of input text (usually set for single or double spacing)

4. Pitch: number of characters per inch of type

5. Justification: alignment of text to the left and/or right margin

6. Header/Footer: information to be included at the top (header) or bottom (footer) of each page

7. Pagination: positions and prints the page numbers on each page

8. Widows/Orphans: eliminates a last paragraph line that appears alone at the top of the next page (widow), or eliminates a first paragraph line that appears at the bottom of the previous page (orphan)

9. Font: style of the print used

C. EDITING

■ Allows changes to be made within a document

1. Highlight/Block: text can be highlighted for manipulation by using the cursor

2. Delete: erases the highlighted text block

3. Copy and Paste: copies the highlighted text block for placement (Paste) elsewhere in the document, at the new cursor location, without erasing

4. Cut and Paste: takes (Cut) the highlighted text block and places (Paste) it elsewhere in the document, at the new cursor location, without erasing

5. Print: allows the document to be recorded (Print) on paper (hard copy)

6. Save: allows data to be placed in storage on a diskette, on a CD, or on the hard drive

7. Retrieve: allows data that has been previously stored to be brought onto the screen

D. TERMS FOR WORD PROCESSING

1. Default: predefined settings automatically loaded by the program used, unless changed by the user

2. Directory: index of files on a floppy or hard drive

3. Grammar check: application that identifies input grammar and/or punctuation errors

4. Help screen: provides explanations and/or instructions about a particular task within a particular program

5. Menu: display on the screen that gives a list of options for word processing

6. Page break: places the beginning of a new page where the cursor is positioned

7. Prompt: a message displayed on the screen that gives the user helpful information and/or instructions

8. Reveal codes: normally invisible word processing codes are made visible for quick editing

9. Sort: organizes a list in alphabetical or numerical order

10. Spell check: application that checks for misspelled words (a medical spell check program is available for separate purchase)

11. Thesaurus: identifies synonyms and antonyms for the word on which the cursor sits
12. Window: an application that allows more than one program to be in use at the same time
13. Word wrap: automatically moves the beginning of a line to the next line without having to press Enter/Return

III. Written Communication Skills

A. TYPES OF WRITTEN COMMUNICATION WITHIN THE MEDICAL OFFICE

1. Transcription from machine dictation
2. Formal handwritten consultation and/or surgical reports
3. Composition of letters to patients, consulting physicians, suppliers
4. Replies to inquiries
5. Responses to requests for information
6. Written collection letters
7. Ordering of supplies
8. Documentation of treatment instructions for patients
9. Processing other types of office communication

B. LETTERS

1. Parts of a letter
    a) Heading
        1) Printed letterhead at the top of the page
        2) Dateline: 3 blank lines below the letterhead; name of the month written in full, followed by the day and year
    b) Opening
        1) Inside address
            > 4 blank lines below the dateline
            > Title, name, and address of receiver
            > Street, avenue, boulevard; east, west, north, south are all spelled out
            > Street numbers 1 through 10 are spelled out
            > Street numbers 11 and above are identified by numerals
            > City is spelled out, followed by a comma
            > State uses the standard 2-letter abbreviation without any period
            > Zip code uses the 5, or 9 if available, numerals one space after the state
        2) Attention line
            > Optional
            > Placed 2 blank lines below the inside address

> Directs the letter to a particular department or person when the letter is addressed to an organization
        3) Salutation
            > Opening greeting to the letter
            > 2 blank lines below the inside address
            > Recipient's title and name followed by a colon (personal correspondence allows use of a comma)
            > Use the courtesy title (Dr., Mr., Mrs., Ms.) when the letter is addressed to a specific individual
            > Use the phrase "To Whom It May Concern:" or "Dear Sir or Madam:" when the letter is addressed to an unidentified individual within an organization
    c) Body
        1) Placed 2 blank lines below the salutation
        2) Contains the message of the letter
        3) Each line is single-spaced; there is a double-space between paragraphs
    d) Closing
        1) Complimentary closing
            > Placed 2 blank lines below the body of the letter
            > Only the first letter of the first word in the closing is capitalized
            > Comma follows the complimentary closing
            > May be formal ("Truly yours," or "Very truly yours,") or common ("Sincerely," or "Sincerely yours,")
        2) Signature line
            > Placed 4 or 5 blank lines below the complimentary closing
            > Typed name of the person authoring the letter
            > Author's title follows author's name, separated by a comma
            > Author signs name above the signature line
        3) Reference notation
            > Placed 2 lines below the signature line
            > Identifies the letter's author and the transcriber ("DH:gm" or "DH/gm"), with the author's initials in capital letters, the transcriber's initials in lowercase letters
            > If the author types own letter, no reference notation is necessary
        4) Enclosure notation
            > Placed 1 or 2 blank lines below the reference notation (or signature line)

> Identifies any printed material accompanying the correspondence ("Enc:", "Enclosure:", "Enclosures:")

5) Copy notation
> Placed 1 to 2 lines below enclosure notation
> Indicates that a copy of the correspondence, with any enclosures, was also forwarded to a third party ("cc: Rob David")
> If there is more than one third party recipient, the recipients are listed alphabetically or in order of authority
> Blind carbon copy ("bcc: Rob David") allows a short note to be typed on the copy to be sent to one third party; the short note is placed only on the one copy of the letter that is sent to the blind carbon copy recipient

6) Postscript
> An afterthought
> Placed 2 lines below the last typed line ("P.S.:")

2. Letter styles
a) Full block (see Figure 8-1)
■ All lines begin flush at the left margin
■ Most efficient style, although the least attractive on paper

b) Modified block (see Figure 8-2)
■ All lines begin flush at the left margin except for the dateline and the complimentary close (these 2 lines begin at the center of the page)

c) Semi-block (see Figure 8-3)
■ Same as modified block, except the beginning of each new paragraph of the body of the letter is indented 5 blank spaces

d) Hanging indentation
■ Same as the modified block, except that all lines of each new paragraph of the body of the letter are indented 5 blank spaces, except the first line of each paragraph

e) Simplified
■ Same as the full block, except that there is no salutation and there is no complimentary close

3. Margins
a) Short letter (>100 words in the body): 2-inch margins
b) Medium letter (100–200 words): 1½-inch margins
c) Long letter (<200 words): 1-inch margins

4. Multiple pages
a) Use plain paper in same stock (weight) as letterhead
b) Type the recipient's name 7 blank lines from the top of the page; type the page

---

Elizabeth Blackwell, M.D.
223 Orange Avenue, N.W.
Cottonwood, UT 84121

January 26, 20—

Mr. Richard Fluege
3678 North Willow Avenue
Palm Beach, FL 33480

Dear Mr. Fluege:

Please send me full particulars on the professional suites you expect to offer for sale or rent in the Medical Arts Professional Annex.

In about six months, I will be ready to open my practice, and I am interested in locating in Florida. My preference is a street-level suite of approximately 2,000 square feet.

After I have had an opportunity to study the information you send me, I will write or telephone you if I have further questions.

Very truly yours,

Elizabeth Blackwell, M.D.

EB:mek

FIGURE 8-1 Block letter style. (From Kinn ME, Woods MA: The Medical Assistant, Administrative and Clinical, ed 8, Philadelphia, 1998, Saunders, p. 146.)

MEDICAL ARTS PROFESSIONAL ANNEX
3678 North Willow Avenue
Palm Beach FL 33480

January 29, 20—

Elizabeth Blackwell, M.D.
223 Orange Avenue, N.W.
Cottonwood, UT 84121

Dear Doctor Blackwell:

We have two remaining street-level suites available for occupancy about July 1. These are marked on pages 3 and 4 of the enclosed descriptive brochure. If one of these suites appeals to you, we will be pleased to customize it for your practice.

Please feel free to call me collect at the number on the brochure for further discussion of your needs.

Sincerely yours,

Richard Fluege
Business Manager

RF:ab
Enclosure

FIGURE 8-2 Modified block letter style. (From Kinn ME, Woods MA: The Medical Assistant, Administrative and Clinical, ed 8, Philadelphia, 1998, Saunders, p. 147.)

WILLIAM OSLER, M.D.
1000 South West Street
Park Ridge, NJ 07656

January 26, 20—

Robert Koch, M.D.
398 Main Street
Park Ridge, NJ 07656

Dear Doctor Koch:

Mrs. Elaine Norris

Thank you for referring your patient, Mrs. Elaine Norris, for consultation and care. She was examined in my office today.

FINDINGS: The patient complained of pain in the left lower quadrant and some abdominal tenderness. She had a temperature of 100.2 degrees.

RECOMMENDATIONS: The patient was placed on a soft, low-residue, bland diet, antibiotics, and bed rest for a few days. Upper and lower gastrointestinal x-rays will be performed next week.

TENTATIVE DIAGNOSIS: Diverticulitis of large bowel.

Mrs. Norris has been asked to return here for reevaluation in about ten days.

Sincerely yours,

William Osler, M.D.

WO:gm

FIGURE 8-3 Modified block letter style with indented paragraphs. (From Kinn ME, Woods MA: The Medical Assistant, Administrative and Clinical, ed 8, Philadelphia, 1998, Saunders, p. 147.)

number 1 line below the recipient's name; type the current date 1 line below the page number

c) The body of the letter continues 3 blank lines below the page heading

d) The same page heading (with corresponding page number) on all subsequent pages

C. ENVELOPES

1. Sizes
   a) #6¾: 6½ × 3⅝ inches
   b) #10: 9½ × 4⅛ inches
2. Folding letters for insertion (see Figure 8-4)
   a) #6¾ envelope
      - Fold the page in half, bottom up, and crease
      - Fold the right one third over the left, and crease
      - Fold the left one third over the right, and crease
      - Insert the last-creased edge into the envelope first
   b) #10 envelope
      - Fold the bottom one third, bottom up, and crease
      - Fold the top one third, top down, and crease
      - Insert the last-creased edge into the envelope first
3. Return address
   • Placed 3 blank lines from the top edge, 5 spaces from the left edge (if the return address is not preprinted on the envelope)
   • Always place the complete return address on the envelope

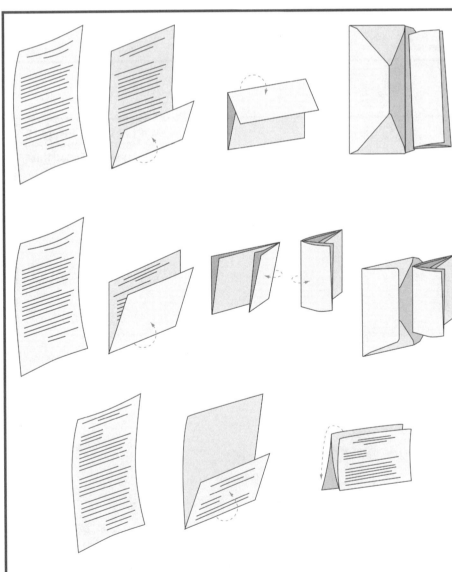

FIGURE 8-4 Correct methods of folding letters. (From Kinn ME, Woods MA: The Medical Assistant, Administrative and Clinical, ed 8, Philadelphia, 1998, Saunders, p. 155.)

4. Mailing address (see Figure 8-5)
- #6¾ envelope: placed 2 inches down from the top edge and 2½ inches to the right of the left edge
- #10 envelope: placed 2 inches down from the top edge and 4 inches to the right of the left edge
- Type the address in block format; capitalize all letters; no punctuation used (copy the inside address from the letter to insert onto the envelope)
- Use standard 2-letter state abbreviation

5. Notations
   a) Directed to the recipient ("Personal and Confidential")
      ▪ Typed 2 blank lines below the return address

   b) Directed to the post office ("Special Delivery," "Certified Mail")
      ▪ Capitalize all letters in upper-right side, below the area of stamp placement

D. MEMORANDA (see Figure 8-6)
   1. Written communication within an office or organization
   2. Use headings, including Receiver, Sender, Date, and Subject of Memo; each office will have a shell to be used in all memoranda
   3. Information pertaining to the headings should be on the same line and 2 or 3 spaces after the heading, separated by a colon
   4. Message should begin 3 blank lines below the last line of the headings
   5. Can have a reference notation, and a copy notation (use the same format as for letters)

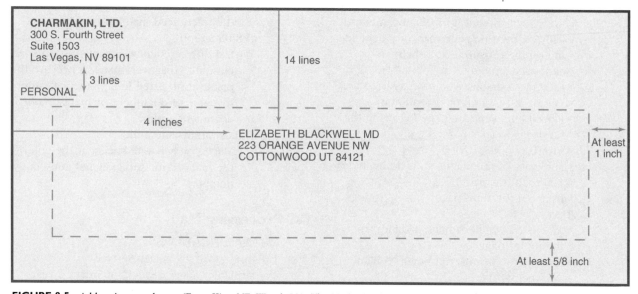

FIGURE 8-5 Addressing envelopes. (From Kinn ME, Woods MA: The Medical Assistant, Administrative and Clinical, ed 8, Philadelphia, 1998, Saunders, p. 154.)

INTEROFFICE MEMORANDUM

TO   All Staff

FROM   Office Manager

DATE   December 1

SUBJECT   Holiday Schedule

Our entire facility will be closed on December 24, December 25, December 31, and January 1. The office will be on reduced staff during the days of December 26, 27, 28, 29, and 30. Assignments will be based on seniority of staff members. Please submit your preferences as soon as possible.

A

MEMO TO: George Walker

FROM: Stanley Barr

DATE: February 8, 20XX

SUBJECT: Office rental

We are experiencing unexpectedly rapid growth in our business office and will soon need additional space for our increased number of employees. Do you have a larger facility available in this building? If so, I would like to hear from you regarding the location, square footage, and anticipated rental costs.

B

FIGURE 8-6 Examples of memoranda. (From Kinn ME, Woods MA: The Medical Assistant, Administrative and Clinical, ed 8, Philadelphia, 1998, Saunders, p. 145.)

E. MANUSCRIPTS

1. Written document submitted for publication
2. Different professional organizations require different standard formats (shells) for manuscript preparation and submission (each will forward its shell on request)
3. Includes:
   a) Title page
      - Identifies the title or theme of the manuscript
      - Title, author, and author's credentials are normally centered horizontally and vertically on the title page (can vary depending on the organization's shell)
   b) Acknowledgments
      - Identifies persons who have assisted the author in research or preparation
      - Placed on a separate page following the title page
   c) Abstract
      - Summary of the manuscript, normally in 100 to 200 words
      - Place on the third page
   d) Text
      - Title is typed, all capitals, 13 lines from the top of page
      - Body of the manuscript begins 3 blank lines below the title
      - Text of the manuscript is double-spaced
   e) References
      - Identifies published works of others referenced within the text
      - Each reference is indicated by numerical superscripts or numbers in parentheses after each citation; references are listed in numerical order at the end of the manuscript
   f) Footnote
      - Cites references and their explanations near the bottom of the page on which the referenced material is written
   g) Bibliography
      - List of reference books, manuscripts, articles, etc., that were used to prepare the manuscript; listed in alphabetical order by name of document or by last name of document author
   h) Illustrations and tables
      - Placed on separate sheets at the end of the manuscript and assigned consecutive numbers

IV. Processing Mail

A. MAIL CLASSIFICATIONS

1. Express Mail, Next-Day Service
   - Available 7 days a week, 365 days a year
   - Cost is normally one standard price per item

2. First Class
   - Sealed or unsealed material
   - Includes letters, postcards, business-reply mail
   - Cost is based on weight (in 1-ounce increments)
3. Priority Mail
   - First class mail weighing more than 11-ounces (maximum weight is 70 pounds)
   - Postage calculated on the combined basis of weight and destination
4. Second Class
   - Regular rates
   - Available to newspapers and periodicals pre-authorized by the post office
5. Third Class
   - Includes catalogs, circulars, books, photographs, and other preprinted materials
   - Must be marked "Third Class"
6. Fourth Class
   - Merchandise, books, and preprinted material not included in First or Second Class and that weigh 16 ounces or more
7. Registered Mail
   - First Class mail additionally protected by registration
   - Post office receives an additional fee for this service
   - Post office verifies delivery of the material
   - Recipient may be required to sign a form to acknowledge receipt, if the sender requests
   - Registered Mail request form must be filled out prior to mailing
8. Certified Mail
   - Delivery of mail requiring the recipient's signature as proof of delivery
   - Certified Mail request form must be filled out prior to mailing

B. EQUIPMENT AND SUPPLIES
1. Postage scale
   - Used to weigh mail to determine the correct postage
2. Postage meter
   - Machine used to print prepaid postage directly on the envelope or on an adhesive label, depending on the weight of the material
   - The date and the amount of postage are set by pressing the appropriate buttons
3. Stationery
   - Standard size and weight, as determined by the office manager
   - Normally light-colored paper with darker imprinting
4. Rubber stamps
   - Can indicate the date of receipt of mail
   - Can be used to endorse checks for deposit

C. INCOMING MAIL
1. Schedule a set time during which to sort and distribute received mail
2. Date-stamp the front (or the back) of each piece of paper within each envelope, and date-stamp the envelope, depending on the office method (except for checks)
3. "Personal" or "Personal and Confidential" noted mailings are delivered directly to the addressee without being opened
4. Any mail that is opened by mistake muse be re-sealed with tape and noted on the envelope that it was opened by mistake
5. All checks received must be endorsed immediately and forwarded to the accounts receivable clerk

V. Transcription

A. GENERAL
1. Process of listening to voice-recorded dictation and translating it into written form
2. Can also be the typing into standard format of consultation or surgical notes
3. Standard office formats and styles should be followed
4. Main requirements of the transcription are appearance, clarity, and legibility
5. Three definite stages within the transcription
   a) Author speaks into a dictating (recording) unit
   b) Transcriptionist listens to (or deciphers what has been written) the record
   c) Transcriptionist keyboards the text into a printed document, using the office-standard format and punctuation

B. EQUIPMENT
1. Audiocassettes: contain recorded notes
2. Transcriber: machine used by transcriptionist
3. Headphones: used to hear the recorded tapes
4. Foot pedal: allows the transcriptionist to manipulate the recorded tapes while keeping both hands free for keyboarding

C. FORMAT
1. Title of document
   - Centered on first line of page
   - All capitalized letters; underlining is optional to the office
2. Identifying information
   - Patient name, patient record number, physician name, date of admission/treatment
   - Typed at the left margin, used as header titles
   - Capitalize the first letter of each name; each different name or number is separated by a colon

- Each header should be double-spaced
- Narrative information is begun 2 blank spaces after the colon
3. Headings
    a) Major headings, typed in all-capital letters, followed by colon
        1) History
        2) Chief Complaint
        3) History of Present Illness
        4) Family History
        5) Social History
        6) Past Medical History
        7) Review of Systems
        8) General
        9) Physical Exam
        10) Diagnosis ("Impression") ("Conclusion")
        11) Admitting Diagnosis
        12) Surgical Procedures
        13) Lab Data
    b) Secondary headings, typed in all-capital letters, followed by a colon
4. Format styles
    a) Full block
        ■ All headings, except title, are flush with the left margin
        ■ Headings are double-spaced from the last line of the previous narrative
        ■ Narrative begins 2 spaces after the colon following the heading
    b) Indented
        ■ Subheadings are indented 3 to 5 spaces under the main headings
        ■ Headings are double-spaced from the last line of the previous narrative
        ■ Narrative begins on the same line as the heading, with the first 2 lines indented 23 to 27 spaces from the left margin
        ■ Third and subsequent lines begin at the left margin
    c) Modified block
        ■ All headings begin at the left margin
        ■ All headings are double-spaced from the last line of the previous narrative
        ■ Narrative begins on the same line as the headings
        ■ Second and subsequent lines are 23 to 27 spaces from the left margin
    d) Run-on
        ■ All headings begin at the left margin
        ■ No double-spaces between any headings
        ■ The narrative begins on the same line as the headings
        ■ Second and subsequent lines are flush with the left margin

5. Signature line
    - Type solid line from the center page to the right margin, 4 to 6 blank lines following the end of the narrative
    - Type the physician's full name immediately below the solid line
6. Notations and date
    - Typed 2 lines below the physician's name at the left margin
    - Identify the dictator and the transcriptionist
    - Type the dictator's initials in all capital letters, followed by a colon, followed by transcriptionist's initials in all lowercase letters ("DH:gm")
    - Immediately below the initials, insert the date the report was dictated (use "D:" followed by 2 spaces and the relevant date)
    - Immediately below the date, insert the date the report was transcribed (use "T:" followed by 2 spaces and the relevant date)
7. Multiple pages
    - Type the word "(continued)" in parentheses 2 lines below the last line of the narrative on the page, at the left margin
    - Begin the next page with patient's name, the reporting physician's name, the date of treatment, and the page number
    - Do not begin a new page with only the physician's signature line; include at least 2 lines of narrative from the preceding page (this is a legal requirement)
8. Syntax
    - Uses sentence fragments; type as dictated, and punctuate accordingly
    - Follow the instructions stated by the dictator

D. STYLE
1. Eponyms are capitalized
2. Drug product names are capitalized; generic names are not capitalized
3. Underline or italicize scientific names of organisms; genus is capitalized; species is not capitalized
4. Capitalize proper names of religions, languages, races
5. Patient allergies are in all-capital letters and are underlined
6. Capitalize acronyms
7. Numbers from 1 to 10 are spelled out; use numerals for 11 and higher
8. Use numerals for numbers in measurements
9. Use numerals when using symbols with the numbers ("100%")
10. Numbers less than 1 expressed as a decimal must be preceded by "0" ("0.25")
11. Spell out ordinals except with a date ("second," but "May 2")

12. Vertebrae are abbreviated ("C1 to C7," "T1 to T12," "L1 to L5")
13. Cranial nerves are written as Roman numerals
14. Titers/ratios include a colon ("1:2")
15. Patient temperature readings include indication of "F" or "C"
16. Suture material is indicated as "2-0" or "00"
17. Use subscripts or superscripts, as noted by dictator
18. Use numbers for cancer grades, EKG leads, and military time
19. Abbreviate metric without a period
20. Pharmacological abbreviations are written in lowercase without periods

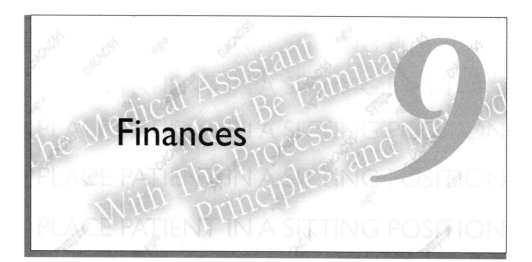

Finances

I. Accounting

A. GENERAL
- Process of recording, classifying, summarizing, reporting, analyzing, and interpreting financial data
- Provides financial information about the business operation

B. ACCOUNTING ELEMENTS
1. Asset: property owned or controlled by a business
   - Includes
     a) Land, buildings, fixtures, furnishings
     b) Medical or office equipment
     c) Money
     d) Accounts receivable
     e) Stocks, bonds, investments
2. Liability: debt obligation of the business
   - Includes
     a) Accounts payable
     b) Bank debts
3. Owner's equity: amount by which assets exceed liabilities; "net worth"
   - Includes
     a) Revenue (assets in)
     b) Expense (assets out)
     c) Drawing (personal use of assets)
4. Accounting equations
     a) Assets = Liabilities + Owner's Equity
     b) Liabilities = Assets − Owner's Equity
     c) Owner's Equity = Assets − Liabilities

II. Bookkeeping

A. SYSTEMS
1. Single-entry system (see Figure 9-1):
   - All transactions recorded at one time, using a pegboard system
   - Uses the following materials
     a) Pegboard
       - Plastic board with pegs along the left edge
       - Pegs hold perforated accounting entry pages
     b) Daysheet
       - Page size of pegboard
       - Keeps record of all daily charges and receipts
     c) Ledger card
       - Record of all charges and payments for each individual patient
     d) Charge slip, charge receipt
       - Form used to record a charge
       - Serves as a bill or receipt if payment is made by the patient
       - May be in the form of a "superbill" (a multipage, carbonless charge slip; one copy of the form is given to the patient, one copy is kept by the office; one copy of the form is forwarded to the patient's insurance company)
   - Daysheet is affixed to the pegboard (perforations on the sheet are placed over the pegs on the pegboard)
   - Each patient ledger card is placed over the daysheet, hooked onto the pegs, so that the columns and rows line up with the daysheet
   - Charge slip/charge receipt is placed over the patient ledger card
   - Bookkeeping entries are made and recorded simultaneously on all forms on the pegboard
2. Double-entry system:
   - Each transaction is recorded in a way that keeps a balance of accounting equation
   - Each transaction affects two accounts: one is debited, the other is credited

B. ACCOUNTS RECEIVABLE
1. Fees owed by patients for services performed
2. Most receipts come from third-party payments (as insurance carrier); payments might not be received for 30 to 90 days after service
3. Accounts are classified according to the amount of time that the balance remains unpaid (current, 30 days, 60 days, over 90 days, past due)

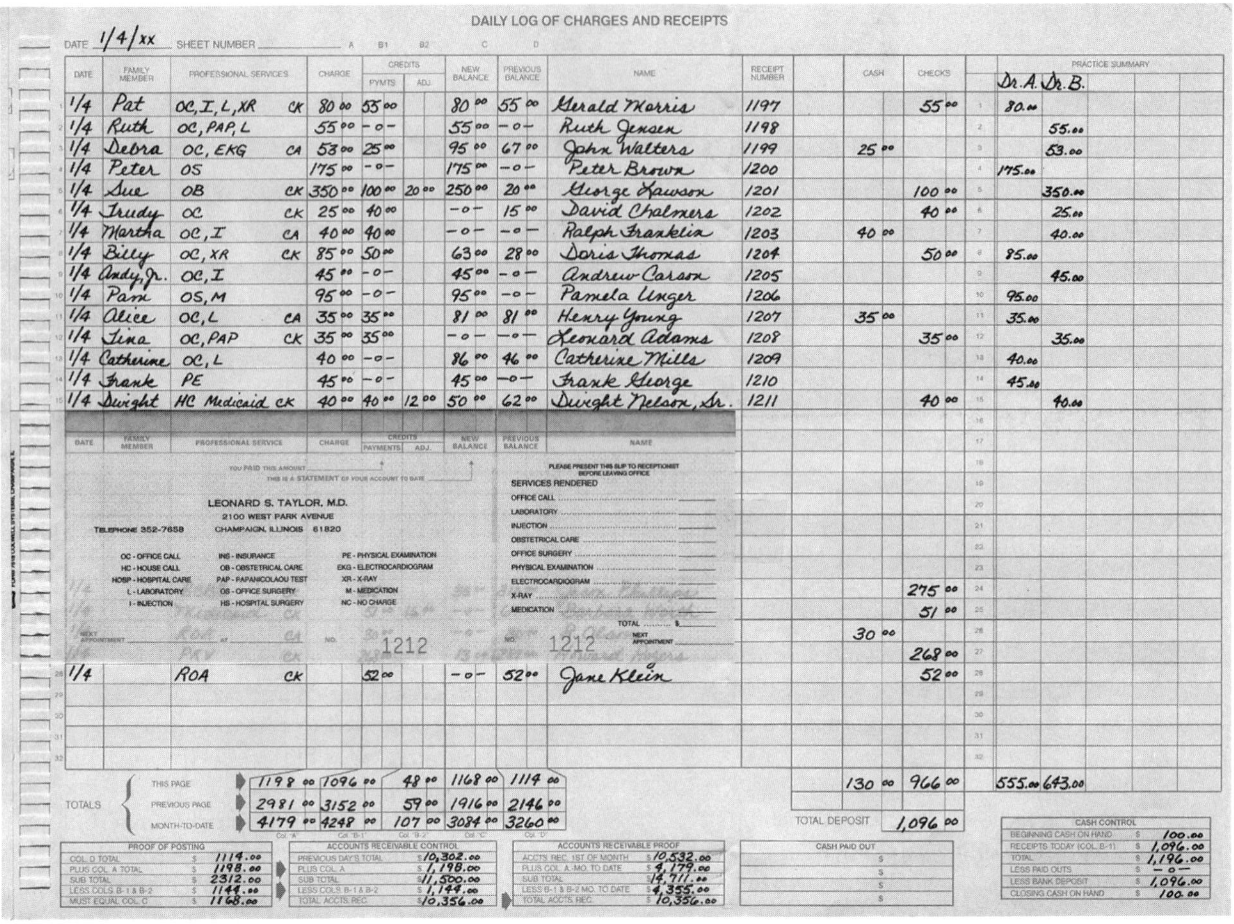

FIGURE 9-1 Sample day sheet for pegboard bookkeeping system, with deposit list of checks and optional business analysis summaries. (As printed in Kinn/Woods: *The Medical Assistant: Administrative and Clinical*, 8/e, Philadelphia, 1999, Saunders, p. 243. Courtesy of Colwell, a division of Patterson Dental Supply, Inc., Phone 800-637-1140.)

C. ACCOUNTS PAYABLE

1. Money owed to outside businesses
2. Payments to outside businesses for purchases and services
3. Invoice normally accompanies the purchase
4. Record of payments kept by making an entry into the appropriate accounts payable record

D. PETTY CASH

1. Cash kept within the office to cover minor purchases
2. Eliminates the need to write a check for minor purchases
3. Fund is established by writing a check on the office account; that check is cashed by the bank, and the cash is placed in a safe place within the office
4. One person is designated to make disbursements from the petty cash fund
5. A voucher is normally required to draw cash out of the fund; the voucher should show the name of the person taking the cash, the amount of cash taken, and the purpose of the petty cash draw; this voucher is used to balance out the account
6. A register should be maintained to track the vouchers
7. The petty cash fund is replenished by again writing and cashing a check

III. Billing

A. FEES

1. Should reflect the revenue necessary to maintain the financial stability of the practice
2. Influenced by the time to be spent and the degree of difficulty in providing the service
3. Set up by a schedule that includes code numbers, detailed description, and cost of each particular service rendered within the practice
4. The schedule must be available to all patients
   a) Usual fee: fee most frequently charged for a particular service
   b) Customary fee: range of usual fees charged for the particular service by practitioners of similar training and experience

c) Reasonable fee: fee assigned to an unusual service or a service that has complex features; meets the criteria of usual and customary fees

B. FORMS
1. Patient information form
   • Used to collect and maintain general information about the patient for billing purposes
   • Includes the patient's name, home address, home phone number, occupation, business address, business phone number, Social Security Number; the insured's name, insurance carrier, and policy number; the spouse's name, occupation, business address, and business phone number; and an emergency contact phone number
2. Release of information form
   • Used to request information gathered by other medical providers
   • Patient's signature authorizes a third party (insurance company) to be given information about the patient's treatment
3. Assignment of benefits form
   • Patient's signature requests the insurance company to send insurance proceeds directly to the provider

C. BILLING METHODS
1. Time-of-service
   • Fee collected when the service is provided
   • Reduces collection costs
   • Increases cash flow
2. Monthly billing
   • Send a bill to each patient on a monthly basis
3. Cycle billing
   • Certain segments of the patient population are sent bills at a consistent time each month, with each segment being sent at a different time during the month
4. Billing service
   • The office may contract with an outside agency to prepare and send the bills to the patients

D. STATEMENTS
1. Typed
   • Each patient bill is individually typed
2. Ledger cards
   • Copies made of the patient's ledger card entries and mailed to the patient
3. Superbill (see Figure 9-2)
   • Presented to the patient at each visit
   • Payment is made at the time of the office visit or mailed in at a later date
4. Computerized
   • Data is keyed into an accounting computer program; statements are automatically generated by the accounting software

IV. Collections
■ Revenue from services rendered must be collected to cover expenses
■ It is illegal to harass debtors

A. TELEPHONE COLLECTIONS
■ It is illegal to make threatening or abusive calls when attempting to collect a debt
■ Call between 8:00 A.M. and 8:00 P.M., only to the patient's home phone when attempting to collect a debt
■ Determine the identity of the person with whom you are discussing debt collection, by using the debtor's full name
■ Be positive and assertive
■ State the purpose of your call
■ Attempt to obtain a commitment by the debtor before ending the debt collection call; attempt to get the debtor to promise to deliver a certain sum on by a certain date
■ After this initial debt collection contact, follow up with another confirmation call

B. MAILINGS
■ Use letters within opaque envelopes for debt collection, never postcards
■ Prepare correspondence to meet the situation (begin debt collection process with a friendly tone, progressing to a more assertive tone as debt collection lags)
■ Debt collection letters should be signed by the office manager
■ Inform the patient by Certified Mail, Return Receipt Requested, of possible collection agency action or legal action to collect the debt

C. PROGRESSIVE COLLECTION PROCESS
■ Office should have developed a color-coded or written stage-by-stage process by which the office can keep track of debt collection efforts (with the process identified first by friendly tones, progressing to more assertive tones as debt collection lags)

D. COLLECTION AGENCY
■ Forward the past-due account to the collection agency once the account has been determined uncollectable by office personnel
■ Once the account is given to a collection agency, the clinic may not continue collection efforts on that debt
■ Patients should make payments on their debt only to the collection agency once the account has been turned over to the agency
■ The collection agency will keep a percentage of the amount collected as their fee

V. Payroll
■ Affected by federal and state laws and regulations

LIC. # 181181
S.S. # 052-56-3472
UPIN # F29065

MARGARET J. NACHTIGALL, M.D.
Reproductive Endocrinology
251 EAST 33RD STREET
NEW YORK, N.Y. 10016

TELEPHONE: (212) 683-0519
FAX: (212) 779-8432

PATIENT INFORMATION

PATIENT'S LAST NAME		FIRST		INITIAL	BIRTHDATE / /	SEX ☑FEMALE	TODAY'S DATE / /
ADDRESS	CITY	STATE	ZIP	RELATION TO SUBSCRIBER		REFERRING PHYSICIAN	
SUBSCRIBER OR POLICYHOLDER				INSURANCE CARRIER			
ADDRESS	CITY	STATE	ZIP	INS. ID		COVERAGE CODE	GROUP

OTHER HEALTH COVERAGE? ☐ NO ☐ YES IDENTIFY

DISABILITY RELATED TO: ☐ IND. ☐ ACCIDENT ☐ PREGNANCY ☐ OTHER

DATE SYMPTOMS APPEARED, INCEPTION OF PREGNANCY, OR ACCIDENT OCCURRED: / /

ASSIGNMENT & RELEASE: I hereby assign my insurance benefits to be paid directly to the undersigned physician. I am financially responsible for non-covered services. I also authorize the physician to release any information required to process this claim.
SIGNED: (Patient, or Parent, if Minor)   DATE: / /

✔ DESCRIPTION	CODE	FEE	✔ DESCRIPTION	CODE	FEE	✔ DESCRIPTION	CODE	FEE
OFFICE VISIT			**OFFICE PROCEDURES**			**LABORATORY - IN OFFICE**		
New Patient			Sperm Wash	58323		Pregnancy Test	85160	
Consultation	99204		Cauterization of Cervix	57510		Urinalysis	81002	
Comprehensive	99205		Cervical Biopsy	57500		Stool Occult Blood	82270	
OFFICE VISIT			Endocervical Curettage	57505		Lyme Titer	86317	
Established Patient			Endometrial Biopsy	58100		Estradiol	82670	
Limited	99211		Office Endometrial Curettage	58102		Chemistry	80019	
Intermediate	99212		Post Coital Test	89300		CBC, pit., Diff.	85024	
Extended	99213		Artificial Insemination	58310		T3 Uptake	84479	
Comprehensive	99214		Pelvic Sonogram	76856		T4	84435	
Comprehensive	99215		Vulvar Biopsy	56600		TSH	84443	
SURGERY			Bilateral Mammogram	76091		ESR	85650	
D & C	58120		Unilateral Mammogram	76090		Pregnancy Test	84702	
Pregnancy Termination	59840		Breast Ultrasound	76645		FSH	83000	
Laparoscopy	56305		Abdominal Ultrasound	76700		Prolactin	84146	
Hysteroscopy	56351		Polypectomy	57500				
Laporotomy	49000							
Myomectomy	58140							
Hysterectomy	58150							

DIAGNOSIS: ICD-9
☐ Abortion, Incomplete 634.71
☐ Abortion, Spontaneous 634.90
☐ Alopecia 704.09
☐ Amenorrhea 626.0
☐ Anemia 285.9
☐ Anovulation 628.0
☐ Atrophic Vaginitis 627.3
☐ Breast Cyst 610.1
☐ Breast Mass 611.72
☐ Breast Pain 611.71
☐ Cervical Polyp 622.7
☐ Cervicitis 616.0
☐ Condyloma 091.3
☐ Cyclic Adrenal Hyperplasia .255.2
☐ Cystocele 618.0
☐ Cystitis 595.9

☐ Diabetes Mellitus 250.0
☐ Dysmenorrhea 625.3
☐ Dyspareunia 625.0
☐ Dysuria 788.1
☐ Ectopic Pregnancy 633.9
☐ Edema 782.3
☐ Endometrial Hyperplasia .621.3
☐ Endometriosis 617.0
☐ Fatigue 780.7
☐ Fibrocystic Breast Disease .610.1
☐ Galactorrhea 676.6
☐ Headache 784.0
☐ Hemorrhoids 455.6
☐ Herpes 054.1
☐ Hypercholesterolemia ...272.0
☐ Hyperprolactinemia 253.1
☐ Hypertension 401.9

☐ Hyperthyroidism 242.9
☐ Hypothyroidism 244.9
☐ Infertility 628.9
☐ Luteal Phase Insufficiency .628.8
☐ Menometrorrhagia 626.2
☐ Menopausal Syndrome ..627.2
☐ Menorrhagia 626.2
☐ Monilial Vaginitis 112.1
☐ Obesity 278.0
☐ Osteoarthritis 715.9
☐ Osteopenia 733.9
☐ Osteoporosis 733.0
☐ Ovarian Cyst 620.2
☐ Ovarian Insufficiency ...256.3
☐ Pelvic Pain 625.9
☐ Polycystic Ovary Syndrome 256.4
☐ Postmenopausal Bleeding .627.1

☐ Pregnancy V22.2
☐ Pregnancy Termination ...V72.4
☐ Premature Ovarian Failure .256.3
☐ Premenopausal Menorrhagia .627.0
☐ Prolactinoma 253
☐ Prolapsed Uterus 618.1
☐ Rectocele 569.1
☐ Thyroiditis 245.2
☐ Trichomonas 131.0
☐ Urinary Tract Infection ...599.0
☐ Uterine Fibroids 218.9
☐ Vasomotor Instability 780.2
☐ Vaginitis 616.1
☐ Vulvitis 616.1

DIAGNOSIS: (IF NOT CHECKED ABOVE)   ADDITIONAL INFORMATION: DOCTOR'S SIGNATURE

SERVICES PERFORMED AT: ☐ OFFICE ☐ University Hospital ☐ Day Surgery / University Hosp.
560 First Avenue   530 First Avenue
N.Y., N.Y. 10016   N.Y., N.Y. 10016

REFERRING PHYSICIAN:

ACCEPT ASSIGNMENT? ☐ YES ☐ NO

TOTAL TODAY'S FEE	
PREVIOUS BALANCE	
AMT. REC'D. TODAY	
NEW BALANCE	

INSTRUCTIONS TO PATIENT FOR FILING INSURANCE CLAIMS:

1. COMPLETE UPPER PORTION OF THIS FORM; SIGN AND DATE.
2. MAIL THIS FORM DIRECTLY TO YOUR INSURANCE COMPANY. YOU MAY ATTACH YOUR OWN INSURANCE COMPANY'S FORM IF YOU WISH, ALTHOUGH IT IS NOT NECESSARY.
PLEASE REMEMBER THAT PAYMENT IS YOUR OBLIGATION, REGARDLESS OF INSURANCE OR OTHER THIRD PARTY INVOLVEMENT.

INSUR-A-BILL ® BIBBERO SYSTEMS, INC. • PETALUMA, CA • © 5/95 (SB M-N)   (REV. 9/96)

FIGURE 9-2 Superbill. (Courtesy of Bibbero Systems, Inc., Petaluma, California 94954-1180. 800-242-2376. Fax 800-242-8330. www.bibbero.com.)

■ Income tax, FICA, and FUTA amounts withheld from employee checks must be paid to the Internal Revenue Service (IRS) and to the state tax commissioner at regular intervals
■ Payroll procedures must be explained to all new employees

A. LAWS AND REGULATIONS
  1. Detailed records must be kept in the office for each employee
     • Name, address, Social Security Number
     • Amount and date of each wage payment and period covered by the payment

- Amount of wages subject to taxes
- Amount and type of taxes withheld from employee's pay
- Date when employee begins work; date when employee leaves the employment

2. Fair Labor Standards Act
   - Sets minimum wage
   - Requires employers to pay 1½ times employee's regular wage for time worked over 40 regular hours.

3. Title VII, Civil Rights Act of 1964
   - Prohibits discrimination based on employee's race, color, religion, or gender in hiring, firing, or promoting employees

4. Age Discrimination in Employment Act
   - Prohibits unfair practices in employment decisions regarding people over 40 years

5. Americans with Disabilities Act
   - Prohibits unfair practices in employment decisions (and in many other areas) regarding people with physical, mental, or medical disabilities

B. TAXES
   1. Income tax
      - Employers are required by law to withhold employee income tax
      - Amount withheld from the employee's paycheck is based on a graduated rate table
   2. Federal Insurance Contributions Act (FICA)
      - Social Security and Medicare Tax
      - Employers are required to withhold (collect) these taxes from employee wages
      - Employer submits amounts withheld to the IRS when the employer pays the employer's taxes
      - Taxes are deducted from the employee's earnings each pay period
      - Every dollar paid by the employee is matched, dollar for dollar, by the employer
   3. Unemployment compensation (FUTA)
      - Federal law requires employers to withhold tax to support the unemployment insurance programs
      - Amount of tax withheld is computed on a graduated rate table, based on employee earnings

C. FORMS AND REPORTS
   1. Form SS-4
      - Federal Tax Identification number application form
      - Required for employers who hire employees and who withhold taxes from employee pay
   2. Form SS-5
      - Social Security Number application form

- All employees are required to have a Social Security Number

3. Form W-2
   - Wages and Tax Statement
   - Given to all employees
   - Lists the wages earned (by one employee) and taxes withheld on those wages for the preceding year
   - Used to prepare personal income tax return
   - Must be provided to employees by January 31 of the following year
   - Consists of 6 parts
     a) Copy A: sent to the Social Security Administration
     b) Copy 1: sent to the state tax department
     c) Copy B: filed with the employee's federal tax return
     d) Copy C: kept by the employee
     e) Copy 2: filed with employee's state tax return
     f) Copy D: retained by the employer

4. Form W-3
   - Transmittal of Income and Tax Statement
   - Used to report the total amount of income and FICA tax withheld during the year
   - Filed by the employer with the Social Security Administration

5. Form W-4
   - Employee's Withholding Allowance Certificate
   - Identifies the total number of withholding allowances claimed by the employee

6. Form 940
   - Employer's annual federal unemployment tax return

7. Form 941
   - Employer's quarterly federal tax return
   - Filed quarterly to report FUTA and income tax amounts to the federal government

8. Form 8109
   - Federal Tax Deposit Coupon Book
   - Used to make quarterly federal income tax and FUTA payments

D. PAYROLL SYSTEMS
   1. Manual
      - Most common for smaller organizations
      - Payroll is computed and processed by hand
   2. Computerized
      - Data is entered into accounting management computer program
      - Payroll calculations automatically prepared by the software
      - Detailed records and reports are automatically prepared by the software

3. Payroll services
   • Payroll data is sent to the payroll service
   • Service prepares the payroll and delivers detailed records, reports, and the payroll checks to the office

VI. Checking Accounts

A. GENERAL (see Figure 9-3)
   ■ The majority of money transactions out of the office are conducted by check
   ■ A check is a commercial paper drawn on funds deposited in a bank account
   ■ A check is a written order for the bank to pay a person a specific amount of money
   ■ A check is negotiable; anyone who properly endorses the check is entitled to receive the money
   ■ Parties involved in a check:
      1. Drawer: the person writing the check
      2. Drawee: the bank
      3. Payee: the person who is to receive the money from the check

B. OPENING A CHECKING ACCOUNT
   1. Requires approval from a bank official
   2. Requires an initial deposit, in accordance with the bank's rules
   3. Requires a signature card
      • The signature card contains the names and signatures of all persons who are authorized to access the checking account

C. DEPOSITS
   ■ Can be made by using
      1. Paper money
         • Arranged in order of denomination (smallest value bill on top)
         • All bills should be arranged face up and top up
      2. Coins
         • A large quantity of coins should be wrapped in coin wrappers before deposit
      3. Checks
         • Office personnel should verify each check for completeness
         • Each check must be endorsed (in writing or by stamp), directing how the check is to be applied
      4. Deposit slip (see Figure 9-4)
         • Preprinted with account information, it identifies all items being deposited
            a) Enter the date of the deposit
            b) Enter the total amount of coins and currency being deposited
            c) Enter and note separately each check to be deposited
            d) Record the total amount of the deposit
            e) Withdraw cash by entering the amount to be withdrawn on the designated space on

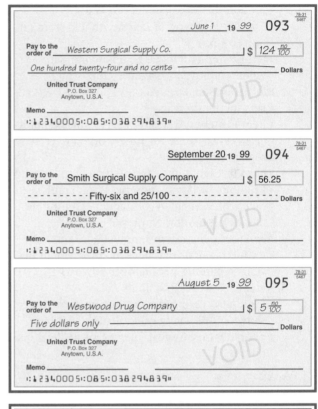

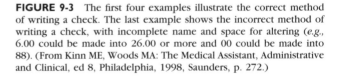

FIGURE 9-3 The first four examples illustrate the correct method of writing a check. The last example shows the incorrect method of writing a check, with incomplete name and space for altering (*e.g.,* 6.00 could be made into 26.00 or more and 00 could be made into 88). (From Kinn ME, Woods MA: The Medical Assistant, Administrative and Clinical, ed 8, Philadelphia, 1998, Saunders, p. 272.)

the deposit slip and subtracting that amount from the deposit total; if a withdrawal of cash is needed, the deposit slip must be signed

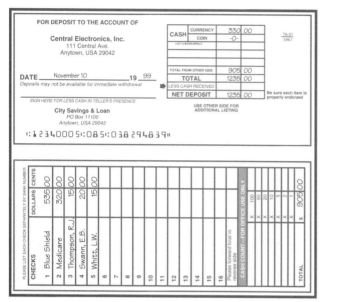

FIGURE 9-4 Front and back of a deposit slip. (From Kinn ME, Woods MA: The Medical Assistant, Administrative and Clinical, ed 8, Philadelphia, 1998, Saunders, p. 276.)

D. DISHONORED CHECKS
- A check that the bank refuses to pay
- Usually due to insufficient funds in the account ("NSF": not sufficient funds)
- If a check is deposited and not accepted by the bank it is written on, the payee's bank will return the dishonored check back to the payee, will deduct the amount of that check from payee's account, and normally will assess the payee a fee for the work caused
  1. Overdraft
     - Issuing a check without sufficient funds in the writer's account
     - Illegal to knowingly issue NSF check
  2. Postdated check
     - Issuing a check but putting a date in the future on the check; a bank may not honor a check until the date on the check

E. BANK STATEMENTS
- Statement of account sent to each depositor once a month by the bank
- Gives the account holder the following information:
  1. Account balance at the beginning of the period
  2. Amount of deposits made during the period
  3. Amount of checks paid during the period
  4. Other items paid or credited during the period
  5. Account balance at the end of the period
- Canceled checks may be enclosed with the statement
- Statement needs to be reconciled (to ensure that the bank's balance agrees with the office's balance)
  1. Compare the deposited amounts recorded in the office files with the amounts recorded on the statement
  2. Compare the canceled check amounts with those on the statement and on the office check register
  3. Identify all debits and credits to the account between the bank's and the office's records
  4. Identify any errors found on the bank statement or on the office register
  5. Add and subtract all adjustments made to the bank statement and to the office register; both balances should be equal

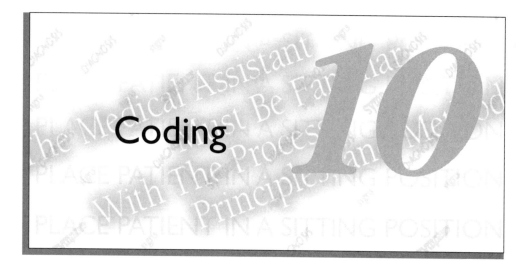

Coding

I. Introduction to Coding

A. PURPOSE

- Coding system translates descriptions of diseases, illnesses, injuries, and procedures into numerical codes
- Helps insurance company quickly and accurately review what services the patient received and how they are related to the illness or injury
- Facilitates the use of computers in insurance claim processing
- Developed for
  1. Tracking disease processes
  2. Classification of medical procedures
  3. Medical research
  4. Evaluation of hospital utilization

B. TYPES OF CODING SYSTEMS

1. ICD-9-CM
   a) International Classification of Diseases, 9th Revision, Clinical Modification
   b) Used to code disease conditions or diagnosis
2. CPT
   a) Current Procedural Terminology
   b) Used to code procedures and medical services provided by practitioner
3. HCPCS
   a) Health Care Finance Administration (HCFA) Common Procedural Coding System
   b) Used to report services performed to Medicare program
4. RVS
   a) Relative Value Scale
   b) Assigned unit value given to commonly performed medical procedures
   c) Based on time, knowledge, and skill required by the practitioner
   d) Point value is multiplied by a dollar factor to find a final fee amount

5. RBRVS
   a) Resource-Based Relative Value Scale
   b) Fee schedule for Medicare for services based on level of resources needed to provide the service
6. DRG
   a) Diagnosis Related Groups
   b) Medicare-fixed fee structure for hospital billing of inpatient services
   c) Based on principal diagnosis

II. ICD-9-CM

- Assigns numeric codes to illnesses, diseases, injuries, and health-related condition

A. ICD-9-CM SYSTEM

1. Volume I (Tabular List of Diseases): numerical arrangement of conditions
   a) 110 to 799: codes that refer to specific conditions by body systems
   b) 800 to 959, 990 to 999: codes that refer to injury
   c) 960 to 989: codes that refer to poisoning
   d) V-codes (V01 to V82): codes that refer to factors that influence health status (such as well-baby checks, annual physicals)
   e) E-Codes: external causes of injury or poisonings
   f) M-Codes: morphology of neoplasms
2. Volume II (Disease: Alphabetical List): three-part index for Volume I
   a) Section I: alphabetical index of disease and injury
   b) Section II: table of adverse reactions to drugs and chemicals
   c) Section III: index of external causes (E-Codes)
3. Volume III (Tabular List and Alphabetical Index of Procedures)
   a) Used primarily in hospitals
   b) Procedures are arranged both alphabetically and numerically

B. ORGANIZATION OF VOLUMES

1. Volume I
   a) Codes 001 through 999 use a 3-digit main number, with a specificity to etiology identified with a fourth digit; a fifth digit may be required
   b) Chapter headings in bold uppercase letters
   c) Notes following the chapter headings give guidelines for coding within the chapter
   d) Major topic headings are in uppercase letters followed by inclusive codes in parentheses
   e) Exclusion statements tell what is NOT included in the specific code number
   f) Category headings further divide major topic headings
   g) Subcategory headings are indented and include a fourth-digit modifier
   h) Fifth-digit modifiers further subdivide the subcategory heading; generally flagged in some way (a section mark)

2. Volume II
   a) Alphabetical listing of conditions
   b) May be expressed as nouns, adjectives, or eponyms
   c) Main terms are highlighted in bold type, followed by the code number
   d) Modifiers in parentheses may be present between the main term and the code number
   e) Subterms are indented, giving further subclassifications

C. CONVENTIONS

1. Volume I
   a) Colon (":"): modifiers after the colon complete the statement before the colon
   b) Brace (}): term after the brace is a required modifier
   c) Section mark: identifies a code that needs a fifth-digit modifier
   d) Excludes: enclosed in a rectangle; conditions following this mark do not qualify for code assignment
   e) Includes: clarifies a description

2. Volume II
   • Diagnoses are organized by main terms printed in boldface type
   a) Modifiers: specific factors that influence a diagnostic code
      1) Nonessential: main term followed by terms in parentheses; may be included with the main term
      2) Subterm: specific manifestations of a condition; these have a specific code number; indented below the main term
      3) Adjectives: appear as main terms with no code numbers; reference to "see condition"
   b) "See also": directs researcher to another code number
   c) "See category": directs the researcher to look into a synonym for the condition
   d) "See condition": directs the researcher that the wrong word is being looked up

3. Volumes I and II
   a) Brackets ("[ ]"): enclosed terms are synonyms, explanatory phrases, or alternative words
   b) Parentheses ("( )"): enclosed terms may or may not affect a main term
   c) NEC (Not Elsewhere Classified): used for ill-defined terms for which more precise information is not available
   d) NOS (Not Otherwise Specified): general diagnosis term that may require more specific information
   e) Note: defines terms, or provides directions (fifth-digit modifier)
   f) "See": directs researcher to look at another code

D. CODING STEPS

1. Locate the term in the alphabetical index of Volume II
2. Read and act on the notes printed after the term
3. Consider modifiers of the term
4. Follow cross-references
5. Verify the code number in Volume I and make modifications as instructed
6. Record the code assignment

E. TABLE GUIDELINES

■ Two coding tables in Volume II:
1. Hypertension table: 3 main column headings
   a) Malignant: severe; vascular damage; diastolic >130 mmHg
   b) Benign: mild; in control
   c) Unspecified: no note of malignant or benign
2. Neoplasm table
   • Arranged by site
   • 6 classifications
   a) Primary malignancy: original tumor site
   b) Secondary malignancy: tumor metastasized
   c) Carcinoma in situ: localized: noninvasive malignant tumor
   d) Benign: nonspreading, noninvasive tumor
   e) Uncertain behavior: impossible to predict behavior or morphology

f) Unspecified: tumor with no indication of histology

III. CPT-4

- Lists and codes procedures and services performed by practitioners
- Each procedure is identified by a 5-digit code
- Simplifies reporting to insurance carriers
- CPT book is divided into 6 sections; subsections include anatomic, procedural, conditions, and descriptors:
  1. Evaluation and Management (E&M): 99200 to 99499
  2. Anesthesia: 00100 to 01999
  3. Surgery: 10000 to 69999
  4. Radiology, Nuclear Medicine, and Diagnostic Ultrasound: 70000 to 79999
  5. Pathology and Lab: 80000 to 89999
  6. Medicine: 90701 to 99199

A. FORMAT AND CONVENTIONS

1. Main statement followed by semicolon; subordinate statement describes procedure or extent of services
2. Terms: indented below main statement giving additional statements
3. Guidelines: specific directions at the beginning of each section; necessary to code correctly
4. Modifiers: 2-digit, terminal code; represents an alteration of the procedure or circumstances
5. Major headings are boldface
6. Notes: provide coding instructions
7. Descriptive qualifiers: descriptions surrounding a code provide more detailed information; sometimes in parentheses

B. CODING STEPS

1. Review the guidelines beginning each section
2. Turn to the index and locate the main term
3. Locate the subterm and follow the cross-references
4. Read the code descriptors of all code numbers
5. Record the proper code

C. EVALUATION AND MANAGEMENT (E&M)

- Includes basic diagnostic and treatment services
- E&M section divided into broad categories with 2 or more subdivisions
  1. New patient: patient who is new to the practice or who has not received any professional services by the practitioner for 3 or more years
  2. Established patient: patient who has received professional services from the practitioner within the past 3 years
  3. Concurrent care: rendering of similar services to the same patient by more than one practitioner on the same day
  4. Counseling: discussion with the patient and/or family regarding diagnosis, treatment, and patient education
- The following MUST be determined within each category to select the correct E&M code
  1. History
     a) Problem-focused: chief complaint and brief history of problem
     b) Expanded problem-focused: chief complaint, brief history, and review of system affected by the problem
     c) Detailed: chief complaint, expanded history of the problem, expanded review of system affected and pertinent past, family, and/or social history
  2. Examination
     a) Problem-focused: examination is limited to the affected body area or system
     b) Expanded problem-focused: examination is limited to the affected body area or system and other closely related systems
     c) Detailed: extended examination of the affected body area or system and other closely related systems
     d) Comprehensive: complete single-system specialty examination or a complete multi-system examination
  3. Complexity of Medical Decision-Making (diagnosis and/or management)
     a) Straightforward: all three criteria are minimal
     b) Low complexity: low degree in each criterion
     c) Moderate complexity: moderate degree in each criterion
     d) High complexity: high degree of complexity in each criterion
- Criteria to be considered at each complexity level
     a) Number of diagnoses or management options available
     b) Amount and/or complexity of data
     c) Risk of complication, morbidity, and/or mortality

IV. HCPCS

- HCFA: Health Care Financing Administration; government agency that regulates Medicaid and Medicare
- Coding system that expands the CPT system
- Provides a temporary list of new codes prior to inclusion in the CPT system

■ 3 levels
1. Level I: existing CPT codes
2. Level II: additional codes that provide greater precision in CPT categories
   - 5-character alphanumeric system (A0000 to V5999)
   - Includes:
     a) Nonphysician services
     b) Codes not found within the existing CPT system
3. Level III: codes used by private insurance companies contracted to process government claims (Medicare)

Health Insurance 11

I. General

■ Protection against financial loss by unplanned events

A. TYPES OF HEALTH INSURANCE PROGRAMS

1. Commercial
   - Policies created and sold by general companies
2. Health Maintenance Organization (HMO)
   - Organization that provides a comprehensive range of services for a prepaid fee
3. Preferred Provider Organization (PPO)
   - Agreement between employers and physician to provide services to employee subscribers at a discount

B. INSURANCE TERMS

1. Beneficiary: person designated to receive the benefits of the insurance policy
2. Carrier: insurance company; insurer
3. Copayment: portion of the cost of service to be paid by the insured
4. Deductible: annual amount to be paid by the insured toward the cost of service before insurance policy benefits will be paid
5. Exclusion: treatment or conditions not covered by the insurance policy
6. Explanation of benefits: document prepared by the carrier that identifies the services covered by the policy, the amount billed by the provider, and the amount paid by the carrier
7. Fee-for-service: provider bills for each service rendered
8. Group policy: policy purchased by an organization for the benefit of its members
9. Insured: policyholder; subscriber
10. Managed care: health care program that designates a primary care physician
11. Preexisting condition: medical conditions present and/or being treated at the time a health insurance application is made
12. Premium: the fees paid for the health insurance coverage
13. Provider: health professional who provides services

14. Rider: clauses to the health insurance policy designating coverage items in addition to those included within the standard contract

C. PLAN OPTIONS

1. Basic benefits include the following
   a) Diagnostic studies
   b) Hospitalization
   c) Surgical treatments
   d) Obstetrical care
   e) Intensive care
   f) Chemotherapy
2. Major medical; services not normally covered by a basic plan may include the following
   a) Outpatient visits
   b) Minor surgery
   c) Physical and occupational therapies
   d) Cost of medical equipment
   e) Mental health care
   f) Dental care
   g) Prescriptions
3. Companion plan: policy that pays in addition to health insurance policies carried, pays the fees not covered by conventional plans

D. METHODS OF PAYMENT

1. Physician fee profile: usual, customary, and reasonable charges
2. Assignment of benefits
   a) Gives the carrier instructions to send insurance payments directly to the provider
   b) Most commercial carriers will reimburse patient unless instructed not to
   c) Assignment of benefits is accomplished by the patient (insured) signing the appropriate box on insurance claim form or completing a separate assignment of benefits form
   d) Patient is responsible for paying the difference between the provider charge and the insurance benefits paid
   e) If the provider accepts the assignment, the carrier makes payment to the provider (in accordance with the policy lan-

guage); if a government plan claim, the provider must indicate on the claim form whether or not the assignment is accepted or rejected

    f) If the provider rejects the assignment of benefits, the provider may bill the patient the difference between the fee charged and the fee reimbursed

3. Medicaid and workers' compensation: provider must accept government reimbursement as payment in full if the provider agrees to treat Medicaid and/or workers' compensation patients

4. Deductibles and copayments: patients are responsible to pay any deductible or copayment according to the terms of the insurance policy

II. Sources of Insurance

A. MEDICARE: FEDERAL PROGRAM ADMINISTERED BY HCFA; ESTABLISHED IN 1965 AS TITLE 18 OF THE SOCIAL SECURITY ACT

    1. Eligibility
      a) Age 65 or older
      b) Disabled under Medicare rules

    2. Benefits
      a) Part A: covers inpatient care after applicable deductible is satisfied
      b) Part B: voluntary program; covers certain outpatient services

    3. Medigap: commercial insurance policies available to cover the Medicare deductible, the co-insurance, and some specific treatments not covered by Medicare

B. MEDICAID: FEDERAL PROGRAM ADMINISTERED BY EACH STATE; ESTABLISHED IN 1965 AS TITLE 19 OF THE SOCIAL SECURITY ACT

    1. Eligibility
      a) Determined by the state
      b) Available to persons with income levels below the federal poverty level
      c) Eligible patients receive an official identification card for their periods of eligibility
      d) Persons may be covered by both Medicare and Medicaid (Medi/Medi); Medicare is the primary carrier and is always billed first

C. CHAMPUS (CIVILIAN HEALTH AND MEDICAL PROGRAM OF THE UNIFORMED SERVICES), CHAMPVA (CIVILIAN HEALTH AND MEDICAL PROGRAM OF THE VETERANS ADMINISTRATION): BOTH ARE FEDERAL MEDICAL CARE PROGRAMS BENEFITING MILITARY DEPENDENTS AND VETERANS; THESE PROGRAMS ARE SECONDARY PAYERS TO ALL

COMMERCIAL AND GOVERNMENT INSURANCES, EXCEPT FOR MEDICAID

    1. Eligibility for CHAMPUS: military dependents and military retirees who are normally eligible to be treated in a military health care facility but must seek civilian care owing to lack of availability

    2. Eligibility for CHAMPVA
      a) Dependents of service-related permanently disabled veteran
      b) Dependents of military personnel who died in the line of duty

D. WORKERS' COMPENSATION: STATE-ADMINISTERED PROGRAM; ESTABLISHED TO HELP PAY THE COST OF MEDICAL CARE AND LOST WAGES ASSOCIATED WITH WORK-RELATED INJURIES OR ILLNESSES; PATIENTS ARE COMPENSATED IN FULL FOR THEIR RELATED MEDICAL EXPENSES AND FOR A PORTION OF THEIR LOST WAGES

    1. Eligibility: patients must sustain an injury or illness while carrying out their job duties

    2. Classification of cases
      a) Claim with no disability: filed for minor injuries or illnesses; patient returns to work in a few days
      b) Temporary disability: filed for injuries and illnesses requiring more than a few days of recuperation before returning to work
      c) Permanent disability: filed for injuries and illnesses resulting in diminished capacity of the patient; ranges from 10% to 100% disability
      d) Vocational rehabilitation: filed for permanently or temporarily disabled persons who require training or education to return to work

III. Insurance Claims

A. HCFA-1500 CLAIM FORM (see Figure 11-1)

    1. Universal health claim form developed by HCFA

    2. Standardizes data required by most carriers so that claims can be processed

    3. Before submitting a claim for payment, make sure patient information release forms are current

    4. Type information onto the form using upper-case letters

    5. Do not use periods, hyphens, commas, dollar signs, or slashes

    6. Use two zeros ("00") in the cents column for whole dollar amounts

    7. Dates should be filled in using 6 digits (mmddyy)

PLEASE
DO NOT
STAPLE
IN THIS
AREA

APPROVED OMB-0938-0008

CARRIER

| | PICA | | | **HEALTH INSURANCE CLAIM FORM** | PICA | | |

1. MEDICARE   MEDICAID   CHAMPUS   CHAMPVA   GROUP HEALTH PLAN   FECA BLK LUNG   OTHER

☐ (Medicare #) ☐ (Medicaid #) ☐ (Sponsor's SSN) ☐ (VA File #) ☐ (SSN or ID) ☐ (SSN) ☐ (ID)

1a. INSURED'S I.D. NUMBER   (FOR PROGRAM IN ITEM 1)

2. PATIENT'S NAME (Last Name, First Name, Middle Initial)

3. PATIENT'S BIRTH DATE
MM DD YY   SEX
M ☐   F ☐

4. INSURED'S NAME (Last Name, First Name, Middle Initial)

5. PATIENT'S ADDRESS (No., Street)

6. PATIENT RELATIONSHIP TO INSURED
Self ☐   Spouse ☐   Child ☐   Other ☐

7. INSURED'S ADDRESS (No., Street)

CITY   STATE

8. PATIENT STATUS
Single ☐   Married ☐   Other ☐
Employed ☐   Full-Time Student ☐   Part-Time Student ☐

CITY   STATE

ZIP CODE   TELEPHONE (Include Area Code)
(   )

ZIP CODE   TELEPHONE (INCLUDE AREA CODE)
(   )

9. OTHER INSURED'S NAME (Last Name, First Name, Middle Initial)

10. IS PATIENT'S CONDITION RELATED TO:

11. INSURED'S POLICY GROUP OR FECA NUMBER

a. OTHER INSURED'S POLICY OR GROUP NUMBER

a. EMPLOYMENT? (CURRENT OR PREVIOUS)
☐ YES   ☐ NO

a. INSURED'S DATE OF BIRTH
MM DD YY   SEX
M ☐   F ☐

b. OTHER INSURED'S DATE OF BIRTH
MM DD YY   SEX
M ☐   F ☐

b. AUTO ACCIDENT?   PLACE (State)
☐ YES   ☐ NO

b. EMPLOYER'S NAME OR SCHOOL NAME

c. EMPLOYER'S NAME OR SCHOOL NAME

c. OTHER ACCIDENT?
☐ YES   ☐ NO

c. INSURANCE PLAN NAME OR PROGRAM NAME

d. INSURANCE PLAN NAME OR PROGRAM NAME

10d. RESERVED FOR LOCAL USE

d. IS THERE ANOTHER HEALTH BENEFIT PLAN?
☐ YES   ☐ NO   *If yes*, return to and complete item 9 a-d.

READ BACK OF FORM BEFORE COMPLETING & SIGNING THIS FORM.

12. PATIENT'S OR AUTHORIZED PERSON'S SIGNATURE I authorize the release of any medical or other information necessary to process this claim. I also request payment of government benefits either to myself or to the party who accepts assignment below.

SIGNED _____   DATE _____

13. INSURED'S OR AUTHORIZED PERSON'S SIGNATURE I authorize payment of medical benefits to the undersigned physician or supplier for services described below.

SIGNED _____

14. DATE OF CURRENT: ◄ ILLNESS (First symptom) OR INJURY (Accident) OR PREGNANCY(LMP)
MM DD YY

15. IF PATIENT HAS HAD SAME OR SIMILAR ILLNESS. GIVE FIRST DATE MM DD YY

16. DATES PATIENT UNABLE TO WORK IN CURRENT OCCUPATION
MM DD YY   MM DD YY
FROM   TO

17. NAME OF REFERRING PHYSICIAN OR OTHER SOURCE

17a. I.D. NUMBER OF REFERRING PHYSICIAN

18. HOSPITALIZATION DATES RELATED TO CURRENT SERVICES
MM DD YY   MM DD YY
FROM   TO

19. RESERVED FOR LOCAL USE

20. OUTSIDE LAB? $ CHARGES
☐ YES   ☐ NO

21. DIAGNOSIS OR NATURE OF ILLNESS OR INJURY. (RELATE ITEMS 1,2,3 OR 4 TO ITEM 24E BY LINE)

1. L___ . ___   3. L___ . ___

2. L___ . ___   4. L___ . ___

22. MEDICAID RESUBMISSION
CODE   ORIGINAL REF. NO.

23. PRIOR AUTHORIZATION NUMBER

24. A				B	C	D		E	F	G	H	I	J	K	
DATE(S) OF SERVICE				Place of	Type of	PROCEDURES, SERVICES, OR SUPPLIES (Explain Unusual Circumstances)		DIAGNOSIS	$ CHARGES	DAYS OR	EPSDT Family	EMG	COB	RESERVED FOR	
From		To		Service	Service	CPT/HCPCS	MODIFIER	CODE		UNITS	Plan			LOCAL USE	
MM	DD	YY	MM	DD	YY										
1															
2															
3															
4															
5															
6															

25. FEDERAL TAX I.D. NUMBER   SSN EIN
☐ ☐

26. PATIENT'S ACCOUNT NO.

27. ACCEPT ASSIGNMENT? (For govt. claims, see back)
☐ YES   ☐ NO

28. TOTAL CHARGE
$

29. AMOUNT PAID
$

30. BALANCE DUE
$

31. SIGNATURE OF PHYSICIAN OR SUPPLIER INCLUDING DEGREES OR CREDENTIALS (I certify that the statements on the reverse apply to this bill and are made a part thereof.)

SIGNED _____ DATE _____

32. NAME AND ADDRESS OF FACILITY WHERE SERVICES WERE RENDERED (If other than home or office)

33. PHYSICIAN'S, SUPPLIER'S BILLING NAME, ADDRESS, ZIP CODE & PHONE #

PIN#   GRP#

(APPROVED BY AMA COUNCIL ON MEDICAL SERVICE 8/88)   **PLEASE PRINT OR TYPE**   FORM HCFA-1500 (12-90)
FORM OWCP-1500   FORM RRB-1500

PATIENT AND INSURED INFORMATION

PHYSICIAN OR SUPPLIER INFORMATION

FIGURE 11-1   HCFA-1500 insurance claim form.

8. Boxes that should be checked are filled in with an "X"
9. Type corrections are made by permanent correction methods (white-out)
10. Completed forms should be maintained in provider files for 6 years

B. MEDICARE
1. Requires the provider to report to the primary carrier on HCFA form
2. Filing deadline is December 31 of the year following service

C. MEDICAID
1. File this claim as soon as possible after service
2. Providers treating Medicaid patients must accept the assignment and accept Medicaid reimbursements as payment in full for the service
3. Patients cannot be billed for qualified services, regardless of the Medicaid amount reimbursed to the provider
4. Services not covered by Medicaid may be billed directly to the patient
5. Keep a copy of the patient's Medicaid ID card within his/her chart

D. WORKERS' COMPENSATION
1. Form completed in quadruplicate at patient's first visit to report the injury; copies are sent to the state workers' compensation board, compensation carrier, employer, and a copy inserted in patient's chart
2. Filing deadlines may vary by state
3. Progress reports should be a narrative and should indicate any significant changes on the patient's current status
4. If an established patient seeks treatment for a work-related condition, create a separate chart and separate ledger card for the work-related condition
5. Provider must accept assignment and reimbursement as payment in full

IV. Reasons Claims Can Be Delayed or Rejected
1. Coding errors
2. Typographical errors
3. Missing dates
4. Incorrect identification or policy numbers
5. Diagnosis does not support treatment rendered
6. Patient names do not match the policyholder's names
7. Dates of treatments do not correspond with the dates on the documents
8. Missing attachments
9. Defacement of bar code area of the claim form
10. Submission of claim to the wrong carrier
11. Patient ineligible for benefits
12. Fee total calculated incorrectly

Office Management 12

I. Introduction
- Process of developing, implementing, and achieving organizational goals
- Administration (nonhuman resources) and leadership (human resources) work together to achieve goals
- Chain of command is the line of authority in clinics

A. PROCESS OF MANAGEMENT
1. Planning: development of goals
2. Organizing: assembling resources needed to achieve the goals
3. Coordinating: bringing various resources together to achieve the goals
4. Directing: supervising the use of resources to achieve the goals
5. Controlling: making necessary adjustments to achieve the goals

B. SUPERVISION
1. Begins with leadership
2. Leadership is the process of working with and through employees to achieve goals
3. Leadership requires two types of behavior
   a) Task behavior: leader tells the person what, when, how, where, and who is to perform a specific task
   b) Relationship behavior: the way the leader communicates, listens, supports, and facilitates in assisting employees in performing a specific task
4. Leadership styles
   a) Telling: makes decisions and supervises employee performance
   b) Selling: makes and explains decisions to employees
   c) Participating: shares ideas and facilitates employee decision making
   d) Delegating: turns responsibility for making and implementing decisions over to the employees

C. HUMAN RESOURCES
1. Hiring process
   a) Recruiting: potential candidates are notified of an available position through advertisement
   b) Interviewing: face-to-face meeting and discussion with employee candidate
   c) Checking references: calling the references indicated by the employee candidate to verify the candidate's information
   d) Selection: choosing the best employee candidate on the basis of the candidate's education, experience, references, and ''fit''
   e) Offer: formally offering the position to the employee candidate, including wage and benefit information
   f) Negotiation: negotiating the specific terms of the employment offered
   g) Acceptance/rejection: employee candidate accepts the job offer and begins employment, or the candidate rejects the offer and the employer again begins the process (or offers the position to the next-best candidate)
2. Job description: should include
   a) Job title
   b) Job summary
   c) Supervisor's title
   d) Job duties and employee responsibilities
   e) Job specifications
3. Orientation
   a) Transition from candidate to employee
4. Probation
   a) Time needed to determine whether the newly hired employee is a good fit
   b) Usually 60 to 90 days
5. Performance appraisal
   a) Objective employee performance assessment
   b) Should assess the employee's work, dependability, teamwork, appearance, and attitude

c) Should be done regularly

d) Result must be discussed with the employee

6. Discipline

a) All actions on employee performance should be recorded in the employee's personnel file

7. Professional development

a) Encourage and subsidize professional development

b) Encourage membership in professional organizations

c) Promote the employee attendance at seminars, workshops, and conventions

d) Enable the employee to obtain continuing education units (CEUs)

D. POLICY MANUAL

■ Information about the office for employees, includes

1. Office or clinic mission statement

2. Orientation information

3. Dress code

4. Job descriptions

5. Holidays, leaves, vacations, sick days

6. Payroll and benefits

7. Disciplinary actions

II. Meetings

■ Keep a calendar of all scheduled meetings (with date, time, place, and topic)

■ Meetings conducted in accordance with Robert's Rules of Order

■ Person chairing the meeting is responsible for all portions of the meeting process to ensure that objectives are met

■ Agenda should be typed and distributed to meeting members

■ Minutes are the record of the meeting; should include the date, time, place, and topic of the meeting, those in attendance, those absent, issues discussed, and time of adjournment

III. Employer Travel

■ Travel arrangements may be made by the medical assistant, a travel agent, or both

■ Itinerary should be typed; must include departure and arrival times and locations, contact telephone numbers, destination ground transportation, hotel accommodations, and a schedule of events and activities involved in the travel function; a copy of the travel itinerary must be kept in the office; a copy of the itinerary is given to the traveler

■ If the travel function is a speaking arrangement, confirm the time, place, and topic; confirm the honorarium (payment)

■ Check with the airlines before leaving for the airport in case of flight delay

■ Confirm ground transportation at the destination location (courtesy car, taxi service, hotel shuttle, rental car)

■ Confirm hotel accommodations; copy the reservation confirmation number onto the travel itinerary

IV. Resource Management

A. FACILITY

1. Temperature: 68 to 74 degrees, with proper ventilation

2. Lighting: fluorescent lighting in all examination and working areas

3. Floor covering: carpeting in waiting room, office, and hallways; sheet vinyl flooring in all examination, bathroom, and laboratory areas

4. Walls: soft or pastel colors, paint or wallpaper

5. Storage: locked space for supplies, equipment, and patient charts; locked and secure cabinets for drugs

6. Noise control: examination rooms and physician offices should be arranged to keep sounds at a minimum

7. Patient rooms: arranged so that the patient cannot be seen by others when the door is opened

8. Offices: separate from the patient exam areas

9. Clinical areas: checked between patients to maintain cleanliness and to keep neat and well stocked with supplies

10. Lab area: well-ventilated, ensure that contamination is well-controlled

11. Bathrooms: clean and well-stocked; patient bathrooms should be separate from staff facilities

12. Janitorial services: staff should keep all areas neat, clean, and repaired; staff should schedule janitorial services for the remainder of cleaning duties

13. Safety: continually monitor the office for hazards; smoke alarms and fire extinguishers should be strategically placed and checked often to ensure that they are properly functioning; fire exits should be clearly marked and kept free of obstacles

14. Security: an adequate number of security personnel should be readily available

15. Waste disposal: schedule regular waste removal and sharps biohazard waste removal

B. OFFICE EQUIPMENT

1. Keep warranties filed for future reference

2. Maintain a file for service agreements

3. Maintain a file with service technician telephone numbers
4. Keep inventories reports on file, with a physical inventory completed at least once a year; inventory should include
    a) Name of item
    b) Model and serial number
    c) Date of purchase or lease (and price)
5. Inventory should be made of the following property
    a) Laboratory equipment
    b) Clinical equipment
    c) Clinical instruments
    d) Office equipment
    e) Office furniture
    f) Anything of value that is not consumed in the treatment of patients

C. SUPPLIES
1. Includes consumable items that are needed to operate the office, housekeeping supplies, medical supplies
2. Ordered on an ongoing basis
3. One person within the office should be designated to order supplies and to maintain and inventory the supplies
4. Supply inventory (separate from office equipment inventory) should be kept up to date so that supplies never run out
5. Contents of supply deliveries should be checked in and verified against the purchase order and packing slip
6. Supplies must be stored in a neat and orderly fashion

Infection Control and Asepsis

I. Chain of Infection (see Figure 13-1)
- Growth of microorganisms in cycle
- Break the cycle, break the process

A. RESERVOIR HOST
1. Start of chain
2. May be insect, animal, or human
3. Supplies nutrition to microorganism
4. May not cause disease in the reservoir

B. MEANS OF EXIT
1. How the organism escapes the reservoir host
2. Exits include mouth, nose, eyes, ears, intestines, urinary tract, reproductive tract, and open wounds

C. MEANS OF TRANSMISSION
1. Way organisms are spread
   a) Direct transmission: occurs from contact with an infected person or discharges of an infected person
   b) Indirect transmission: occurs from droplets in the air, vectors (insects) that harbor pathogens, contaminated food or drink, fomites (contaminated objects)

D. MEANS OF ENTRY
1. How the organism gains entry into a new host
2. Entries include mouth, nose, eyes, intestines, urinary tract, reproductive tract, and open wounds

E. SUSCEPTIBLE HOST
1. One that is capable of supporting the growth of microorganism
2. Factors that affect susceptibility include
   a) Location of entry
   b) Dose of organisms
   c) Physical condition of individual
3. If conditions are right, susceptible host becomes reservoir host; the chain or cycle begins again

F. INFLAMMATION
1. Trauma to the body alerts the protective mechanisms
2. The body responds
   a) Blood vessels at the site dilate; the number of white blood cells in the area increases, which causes redness
   b) White blood cells overpower and consume microorganisms (phagocytosis), which causes swelling
   c) Fluids in tissues increase and put pressure on nerves, which causes pain
   d) Increased blood supply to area causes heat
3. The process creates four classic signs of inflammation: redness, swelling, pain, heat

II. OSHA Standards
- Occupational Safety and Health Administration
- Sets standards and protocols for health and safety

A. BLOOD-BORNE PATHOGENS
1. Disease-causing microorganisms that may be present in the blood or bodily fluids
2. Concerned mainly with hepatitis B virus (HBV) and human immunodeficiency virus (HIV)
3. Blood-borne pathogens are transmitted when infected blood comes into contact with nonintact skin or mucous membranes

B. STANDARD PRECAUTIONS
1. Concept of treating all blood and bodily fluids as if they are infected
2. Includes blood, bodily fluids, excretions, and secretions

C. PREVENTION OF EXPOSURE
1. Immunization: all persons who come in contact with blood or bodily fluids should receive hepatitis B series
2. Engineering controls: mechanical devices designed to minimize exposure; include
   a) Eyewash stations
   b) Sharps containers
   c) Biohazard waste containers and labels
   d) Handwashing stations

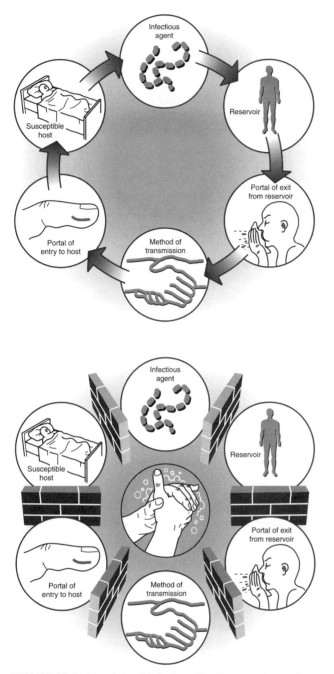

FIGURE 13-1 The chain of infection. The disease cycle continues to repeat unless measures are taken to purposely stop the cycle. (From Polaski A, Warner J: Saunders Fundamentals for Nursing Assistants, Philadelphia, 1994, Saunders, p. 232.)

3. Personal protection equipment: equipment that minimizes exposure beyond engineering controls; includes
   a) Gloves
   b) Lab coats
   c) Eye and/or face shields

D. EXPOSURE CONTROL
  1. Contaminated sharps placed in sharps container (puncture-resistant, leak-proof container) immediately after use

2. Do not bend, break, or recap used needles
3. Work surfaces and equipment should be cleaned and decontaminated with disinfectant after each use
4. Contaminated waste (except sharps) should be disposed of in a clearly labeled biohazard waste container ("red bag trash")
5. Employee exposure incidents should be reported as directed and properly followed up to ensure that they do not again occur

III. Handwashing
■ Single most important defense against transmission of microorganisms
■ Proper handwashing depends on friction and running water
■ Hands should be washed
  1. Between patients
  2. After handling specimens
  3. Before and after using bathroom
  4. After handling contaminated materials
  5. Before leaving the clinic at the end of the day
■ Handwashing procedure
  1. Remove all jewelry except plain wedding band
  2. Using warm water, thoroughly wet the hands
  3. Apply soap; lather while keeping the fingers pointed downward
  4. Rub, using friction for 30 seconds; wash between the fingers
  5. Rinse; allow water to flow from the wrist to the fingertips
  6. Thoroughly dry the hands with paper towels, and turn off the faucet(s) with the paper towels
  7. Apply lotion if desired

IV. Sanitization
■ Process of cleaning or removing materials from objects
■ Requires scrubbing objects with detergents and brushes
■ First step in the sterilization process
■ Methods include
  1. Detergents: agents that remove bacteria, fats, oils, and protein substances (blood)
  2. Ultrasound: machine that uses sound waves through a liquid to cause a vibration
  3. Antiseptic: agent that sanitizes skin

V. Disinfection
■ Process of removing infectious material from objects
■ Processes include
  1. Chemical
    a) Surface germicide

b) Used on inanimate objects that are sensitive to heat
   1) Soap: mechanically removes bacteria but does not destroy them unless the soap is germicidal
   2) Alcohol: commonly used on skin
   3) Acids: solutions containing phenol
   4) Alkalis: bleach; used in the laboratory on flat surfaces
   5) Formalin: solution requires rinsing
2. Ultraviolet radiation: ultraviolet light can have an effect on surfaces but does not penetrate surfaces
3. Desiccation: drying; does not kill spores
4. Boiling: kills most bacteria; does not kill some spores and viruses

VI. Sterilization
■ Complete destruction of microorganisms
■ Processes include
1. Chemical
   a) May be used for heat-sensitive materials
   b) Objects must be completely submerged for long periods
   c) Glutaraldehyde solutions commonly used
2. Steam under pressure
   a) Autoclave
   b) Most common and effective sterilization method
3. Gas: special chamber that uses a gas
4. Oven: dry heat

VII. Use of the Autoclave

A. PREPARING INSTRUMENTS AND SUPPLIES
1. Instruments are sanitized and dried before wrapping
2. Wrapping materials include
   a) Muslin
   b) Disposable paper
   c) Peelback pouches
3. Open any hinged instruments to allow steam to reach all surfaces
4. Items to be wrapped are placed in the center of the wrapping material, with corners of the wrap at the top, bottom, and sides; bring the bottom of the wrapper up over the instrument, folding back a small corner for a "handle"; bring in the sides, one at a time, also folding back the small corners; the top of the wrapper is brought around the object and secured with sterilizer tape
5. Label the tape with the identity of the contents, date, and operator's initials
6. Packs should be no larger than $12 \times 12 \times 20$ inches
7. Sterilization indicator should be included in the pack to show that the proper time and temperature were achieved

B. LOADING THE AUTOCLAVE
1. Packs should be placed vertically, 1 to 3 inches apart, away from the sides of the chamber
2. Place hard goods underneath soft goods
3. Open glassware should be placed on its side

C. AUTOCLAVE PROCEDURE
1. Autoclave is a piece of equipment that provides steam under pressure
2. Autoclave is normally run at 250 degrees Fahrenheit, 20 to 30 pounds pressure, for 15 to 30 minutes
3. Moist heat in the form of steam circulates in a pattern throughout the autoclave chamber
4. Check the autoclave water level; add distilled water if necessary
5. Properly load the autoclave
6. Close the autoclave door securely; turn the unit on
7. Begin timing when the proper temperature and pressure are achieved
8. After the autoclave cycle is completed; vent the autoclave chamber
9. Open the autoclave door just slightly to allow the contents to dry
10. Remove the items and check the indicator on the sterilizer tape; wrapped items may be handled with clean hands
11. Store sterilized items in a clean, dust-proof area; the shelf life of sterilized items is about 28 days (resterilize the items after 28 days)

Vital Signs and Anthropometric Measurement

I. Vital Signs

- Measurements that indicate the patient's general state of health and homeostasis
- Can indicate a change in health and/or the presence or disappearance of a disease
- Accuracy is essential
- Includes temperature, pulse, respiration (TPR), and blood pressure (BP)

A. TEMPERATURE

- Balance between heat lost and heat produced by the body
- Heat is produced by metabolism
- In illness, metabolism increases, increasing internal heat production, increasing the body temperature
- Variation in patient's baseline temperature may be the first warning of an illness or change in condition
- Body temperature is regulated by hypothalamus
  1. Factors affecting body temperature
     a) Age: body heat decreases with age
     b) Environment: exposure, windchill, temperature
     c) Activity: physical activity increases body temperature
     d) Diurnal variation: body temperature is lowest in the morning, highest in the evening
     e) Emotions: agitation increases body temperature; depression lowers body temperature
     f) Physiological processes: body temperature increases with digestion, ovulation, pregnancy
  2. Normal values
     a) Oral: 97 to 99 degrees Fahrenheit; 36 to 37.8 degrees Celsius
     b) Rectal: 1 degree higher than oral (most accurate measurement)
     c) Axillary: 1 degree lower than oral (least accurate measurement)
     d) Tympanic (aural): same as oral

  3. Characteristics
     a) Fever: temperature >100 degrees Fahrenheit; pyrexia; temperature ≥105 degrees Fahrenheit can cause brain damage or death if untreated
     b) Febrile: having fever
     c) Afebrile: without fever
     d) Intermittent: fluctuation between normal, abnormal, and fever
     e) Remittent: elevated fluctuations that do not return to normal
     f) Lysis: gradual return to normal
     g) Crisis: sudden return to normal
  4. Equipment: thermometer: device used to measure body temperature
     a) Oral: glass with mercury column; long, slender bulb; can be placed under the tongue or axilla; color-coded blue
     b) Rectal: glass with mercury column; short, squat bulb; color-coded red
     c) Electronic: consists of a battery-powered unit and a probe covered by a disposable plastic cover; temperature is displayed digitally; unit has blue (oral) and red (rectal) probes
     d) Tympanic (aural): handheld processor unit with a tympanic probe covered by a disposable cover: picks up infrared energy from the tympanic membrane: proper technique is important for correct results
  5. Charting
     a) Record the patient's temperature within the patient chart
     b) Indicate (after the number) whether it was recorded by oral (O), rectal (R), axillary (A), or tympanic (T)
  6. Procedure
     a) Oral: place the thermometer under the patient's tongue, instruct the patient to keep the lips closed around the thermometer

and to breathe through the nose; leave in place for 5 minutes

    b) Axillary: wipe the axilla dry; place the thermometer under the patient's arm; leave in place for 10 minutes

    c) Rectal: apply lubricating jelly to the thermometer; insert into the rectum about 1 inch; leave in place for 2 to 3 minutes

    d) Tympanic (see Figure 14-1)

        1) For adult: gently pull the pinna up and back; insert the probe into the ear canal

        2) For child: gently pull the pinna down and back; insert the probe into the ear canal

B. PULSE

■ Palpable beat of arteries as they expand with the beat of the heart

■ Pulse in any artery will usually be the same as the heartbeat

■ Rate and characteristics can give information about the cardiovascular system

  1. Factors affecting pulse

    a) Increased pulse rate: pain, fever, infection, hyperthyroidism

    b) Decreased pulse rate: chronic pain, central nervous system disorders, hypothyroidism

  2. Characteristics

    a) Rate: number of beats per minute (bpm)

    b) Rhythm: time between beats

    c) Volume: force of beats

    d) Condition of the arterial wall: springy, resilient, and elastic

  3. Normal values

    a) Birth: 70 to 190 bpm

    b) 1 to 4 years: 80 to 120 bpm

    c) 6 to 12 years: 70 to 110 bpm

    d) 12 to 16 years: 75 to 90 bpm

    e) Adult: 60 to 80 bpm

  4. Pulse sites (see Figure 14-2)

    a) Radial: most common; located on the thumb side of the wrist

    b) Carotid: located in the groove of the neck between the larynx and the sternocleidomastoid muscle; used in emergencies and during CPR

    c) Brachial: located in the antecubital space; reference for blood pressure

    d) Femoral: located in the groin

    e) Temporal: located over the temporal bone

    f) Popliteal: located at the back of the knee

    g) Dorsalis pedis: located on the top of the foot

    h) Apical: located just below the right nipple on the left side of the chest; taken with a stethoscope for 1 full minute; used for infants, young children, and cardiac patients

  5. Procedure

    a) Radial pulse

        1) Have the patient in a sitting or lying position

        2) Gently press on the radial artery until the pulse is felt

        3) Count the beat for 30 seconds and multiply by 2; if the beat is irregular, count for the full minute

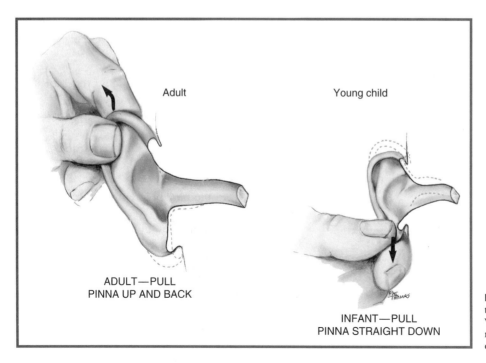

Adult   Young child

ADULT—PULL PINNA UP AND BACK

INFANT—PULL PINNA STRAIGHT DOWN

FIGURE 14-1 Positioning the ear for temperature taking. (From Kinn ME, Woods MA: The Medical Assistant, Administrative and Clinical, ed 8, Philadelphia, 1998, Saunders, p. 587.)

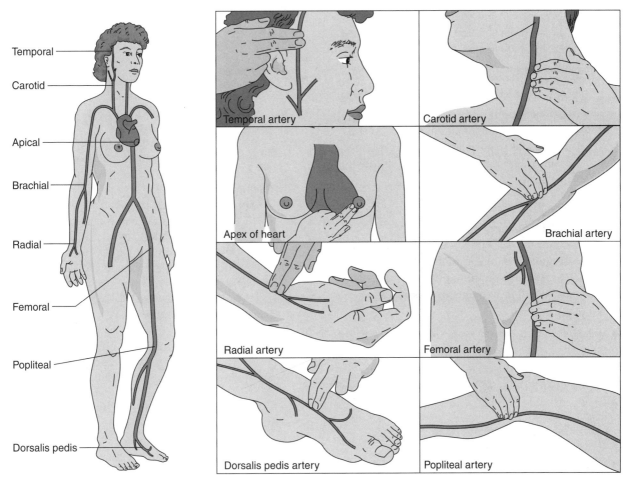

FIGURE 14-2 Pulse sites. (From Kinn ME, Woods MA: The Medical Assistant, Administrative and Clinical, ed 8, Philadelphia, 1998, Saunders, p. 459.)

4) Chart the pulse; note the rate, rhythm, and strength
  b) Apical pulse
    1) Have the patient in a sitting or lying position
    2) Warm the stethoscope; place the stethoscope below the patient's right nipple at the fifth internal space
    3) Count for 1 minute
    4) Chart the pulse; note the rate, rhythm, and strength and indicate that the pulse was taken apically ("A")

C. RESPIRATION
■ Involves the exchange of oxygen and carbon dioxide
■ Cycle consists of 1 inspiration and 1 expiration
■ Controlled by the medulla oblongata; the breathing rate is determined by the carbon dioxide level in the blood
  1. Factors affecting respiration
    a) Disease
    b) Age
    c) Physical activity
    d) Emotional status
    e) Medications and drugs
    f) Body position
  2. Characteristics
    a) Rate: number of respirations per minute
    b) Rhythm: breathing pattern
    c) Depth: amount of air being inhaled
  3. Normal values
    a) Newborn: 30 to 40 bpm
    b) 1 to 6 years: 20 to 40 bpm
    c) 7 to 14 years: 15 to 25 bpm
    d) Adult: 16 to 20 bpm
  4. Breathing patterns
    a) Eupnea: normal breathing
    b) Dyspnea: difficult, painful, or labored breathing
    c) Apnea: absence of breathing; temporary condition
    d) Orthopnea: difficulty breathing while lying down
    e) Hyperpnea: increased rate of breathing
    f) Tachypnea: excessively rapid breathing
    g) Rales: gurgling sounds due to secretions

h) Rhonchi: rattling sounds
i) Cheyne-Stokes: alternating periods of apnea and tachypnea; can indicate impending death
5. Procedure
a) Respiration can be consciously controlled; the respiration rate should be counted without the patient's knowledge; so that the patient is unaware of your respiration count, continue to act as if you are taking the pulse
b) Watch the rise and fall of the patient's chest; count 1 inhalation and 1 exhalation as 1 respiration
c) Count for 30 seconds and multiply by 2; if irregular, count for a full minute
d) Chart the respiration; note the rate, depth, and rhythm; note any irregularities

D. BLOOD PRESSURE
■ Measurement of the pressure of the blood against the walls of the arteries
■ Two readings
1. Systolic pressure (systole): highest pressure; occurs when the heart contracts
2. Diastolic pressure (diastole): lowest pressure; occurs when the heart relaxes
■ Systole + diastole = 1 cardiac cycle
■ Measured in millimeters of mercury (mmHg)
■ Recorded as a fraction: systolic/diastolic
1. Factors affecting blood pressure
a) Age: blood pressure increases with age
b) Activity: blood pressure increases with physical activity
c) Gender
d) Diurnal variation: blood pressure is lower in the morning
e) Stress
f) Disease state
g) Medication
2. Normal values
a) Newborn: 50/30
b) 1 to 6 years: 95/65
c) 6 to 12 years: 100/65
d) 16 to adult: 118/75
e) Adult: 120/80 (average); normally ranges from 90/60 to 140/90
f) Elderly: 140/90
3. Characteristics
a) Hypertension (HTN): high blood pressure
1) Blood pressure >140/90
2) Essential HTN: unknown etiology
3) Secondary HTN: associated with other disease processes
b) Hypotension: low blood pressure
1) Blood pressure <90/60

c) Orthostatic hypotension
1) Temporary fall in blood pressure that occurs when the patient rapidly changes from a lying or sitting position to a standing position
d) Pulse pressure
1) Difference between systolic and diastolic pressure
2) Average is 40 mmHg
3) Ratio of systolic to diastolic pulse is 3 : 2 : 1
4. Equipment
• Sphygmomanometer
a) Consists of an inflatable cuff (various sizes for sizes of patient) with an inflation bulb (with control valve) and pressure gauge (mercury column or aneroid dial)
b) Stethoscope; instrument used to listen to pulse
5. Procedure (see Figure 14-3)
a) Objective
■ Use of the inflatable cuff causes circulation in the artery to disappear
■ As the cuff is slowly deflated, blood flow resumes, and cardiac cycle sounds are heard through the stethoscope
■ Gauge readings are taken when the first sound is heard (systolic) and when the last sound is heard (diastolic)
b) Palpate the brachial artery in the antecubital space
c) Place the cuff snugly around the patient's arm about 1 to 2 inches above the arm fold with the arrow on the cuff pointing to the brachial artery
d) Place the stethoscope over the brachial artery
e) Close the valve and inflate the cuff to about 200 mmHg
f) Slowly release the valve to deflate the cuff; the gauge needle should drop 2 mmHg per second for proper release rate
g) Note the gauge reading when the first beat is heard (systolic)
h) Continue deflating the cuff until the last beat is heard (diastolic)
i) Fully release the bulb valve, deflate the cuff, and remove it from the patient
j) Record the result in the patient's chart; indicate which arm was used for reading ("R" or "L"); may also indicate the patient's position (sitting, standing, lying)
6. Korotkoff sounds: sounds heard during the measurement of blood pressure
a) Phase I: first sound heard as the cuff deflates; systolic reading
b) Phase II: swishing sound; blood is flowing through the artery, and sounds may com-

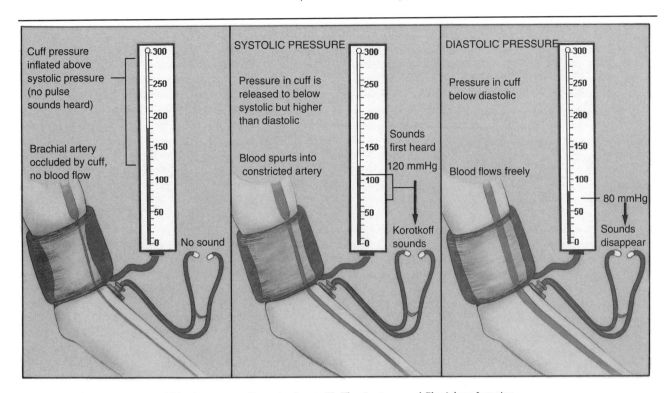

FIGURE 14-3 Measurement of blood pressure. (From Applegate EJ: The Anatomy and Physiology Learning System, ed 2, Philadelphia, 2000, Saunders, p. 268.)

pletely disappear and reappear later (auscultatory gap)

c) Phase III: sharp, tapping sounds return and continue rhythmically

d) Phase IV: soft tapping sound that becomes muffled and begins to grow fainter; may be recorded as the fading sound and recorded between the systolic and diastolic (e.g., 130/85/70)

e) Phase V: sounds disappear; last sound heard; diastolic reading

II. Anthropometric Measurement
- Deals with the measurement of size, weight, and proportion of the human body
- Often included with vital signs

A. WEIGHT
- May be measured in pounds or kilograms
1. Place a paper towel on the base of the scale if the patient removes his/her shoes; the patient should be weighed consistently with or without shoes depending on office procedure
2. Have the patient stand erect in the center of the base of the scale
3. Move the large weight to the 50-pound notch nearest to, but under, the patient's weight
4. Move the smaller weight to the right until the balance needle is in the middle of the frame

5. Add the large and small weights together; record the result, in pounds, on the patient's chart to the nearest one-quarter pound
6. Return both weights to "0" after the patient leaves the scale

B. HEIGHT
- May be measured in inches or centimeters
1. Place a paper towel on the base of the scale if the patient removes his/her shoes (per above)
2. Have the patient stand erect in the center of the base of the scale
3. Lower the height bar until it rests on the top of the patient's head
4. Note the height indicated on the height bar; record the result, in inches, on the patient's chart to the nearest one-quarter inch
5. Return the height bar to the lowest position

C. BODY FAT
- Measures percentage of body fat; percentage of body fat may be an indicator of cardiovascular disease, health, vitality, and appearance
- Three methods
1. Body density measurement method
   a) Patient is submerged under water
   b) Most accurate and most difficult
2. Electroimpedence method
   a) Electrodes are placed on the patient

b) Computer determines body fat percentage on an impedance monitor

3. Caliper method

  a) Measures the thickness of a fold of tissue

  b) Measurements are taken in three areas of the body

    1) Triceps

    2) Subscapular

    3) Suprailiac

  c) Indicates total percentage of body fat

  d) Generally 15% to 19% for men

  e) Generally 22% to 25% for women

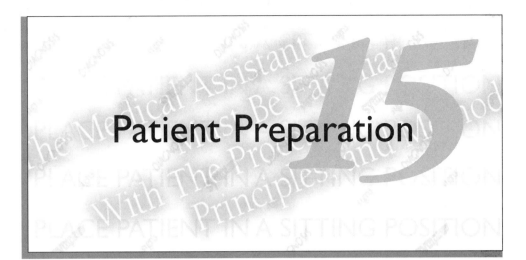

Patient Preparation

■ The medical assistant prepares the patient for examination by gowning, positioning, and draping

I. Gowning
■ Patient must undress and put on a gown that makes performing the procedure easier for the surgical team
■ Principle of gowning: expose only the body part that needs to be examined or exposed

A. CONSIDERATIONS OF GOWNING
1. Patient's need for privacy and comfort
2. Type of exam or procedure to be performed
3. Patient's age and gender
4. Accessibility of the body part to be examined or exposed

B. TYPES OF GOWNS
■ Usually all patient clothing is removed under the gown
■ Gown will have an opening either in back or in front
1. Full gown
   a) Knee length
   b) Opening extends the full length of the gown
   c) Closures of Velcro or ties
   d) Can be paper or cloth material
2. Partial gown
   a) Covers only the chest, back, and shoulders
   b) Opening extends the full length of the gown
   c) Can be paper or cloth material

II. Positioning and Draping
■ Patient generally positioned on an examination table
■ Table should be long and wide enough to support any size patient
■ Table covered with a paper covering or cloth sheet; the covering is changed after each patient

A. POSITIONS (see Figure 15-1)
1. Erect
   a) Standing
   b) Patient upright with arms at sides
   c) Used to examine musculoskeletal system and nervous system
2. Sitting
   a) Patient sits upright on the table with legs dangling over the end
   b) Used to examine the head, chest, heart, lungs, breasts, axilla, and upper extremities
   c) Draping: drape the sheet across the lap
3. Supine
   a) Horizontal recumbent
   b) Patient lies flat on the back with arms at the sides
   c) Used to examine the chest, abdominal area, heart, and extremities
   d) Draping: the drape sheet extends from under the arms
4. Dorsal recumbent
   a) Patient is supine with legs bent at the knees and feet flat on the table
   b) Used to examine the genital and rectal areas
   c) Draping: drape sheet is placed over that patient in a diamond-shaped fashion with side corners wrapped around each leg; upper and lower corners cover the chest, abdominal, and pubic areas
5. Lithotomy
   a) Patient is in dorsal recumbent position, except that the feet are placed in stirrups; knees are bent; buttocks are moved to the end of the table
   b) Used for vaginal examination, pelvic examination, and Pap smear procedure
   c) Draping: same as for dorsal recumbent
6. Sims'
   a) Lateral position
   b) Patient lies on the left side with the left arm behind the body and the right arm forward; both legs are flexed at the knees, but the right leg is sharply bent and positioned next to the left leg

Visualization of upper body parts; provides full expansion of lungs

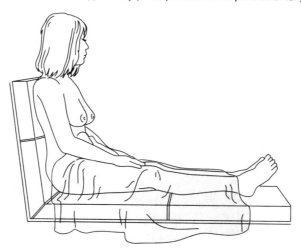

Most relaxed position; prevents contracture of abdominal muscles; provides pulse sites; facilitates breast examination

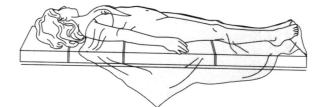

Provides more comfortable position for patients with painful disorders

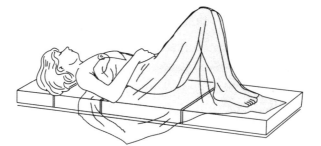

FIGURE 15-1   Positions for examination. (From Lane K: Saunders Manual of Medical Assisting Practice, Philadelphia, 1993, Saunders, pp. 320–22.)

Provides maximum exposure of genitalia; facilitates insertion of vaginal speculum

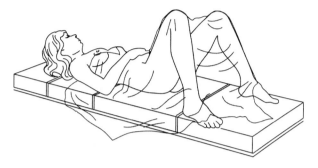

Facilitates assessment of hip joint

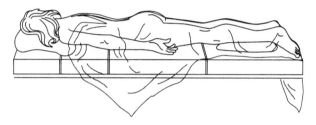

Improves exposure of the rectal area

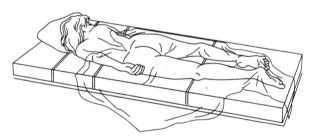

Provides maximum exposure of rectum and facilitates insertion of proctological instruments

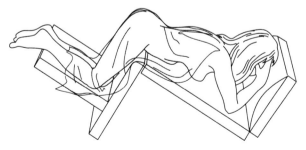

FIGURE 15-1 *Continued*

Illustration continued on following page

Is the same as proctological in the absence of a special table for examination

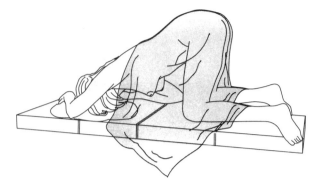

FIGURE 15-1 *Continued*

c) Used to examine the rectal area, perform enemas and douches, and insert suppositories
d) Draping: drape sheet covers the patient from the shoulders to the toes; adjust to expose the necessary area

7. Prone
   a) Patient lies flat on the abdomen with the head turned to the side; arms are positioned above the head or at the sides of the body
   b) Used to examine the back, spine, and lower extremities
   c) Draping: drape sheet covers the patient from the waist to the knees; adjust to expose the necessary area

8. Knee-chest
   a) Genupectoral
   b) Patient assumes a kneeling position with the buttocks elevated, with head and chest on the table
   c) Used for proctological examinations
   d) Draping: drape sheet covers the buttocks; adjust to expose the necessary area

9. Proctological
   a) Knee-chest position facilitated by the use of a special table
   b) Used for a proctological examination
   c) Draping: same as for knee-chest

10. Fowler's
    a) Patient sits on the examination table with the back supported at a 90 degree angle

b) Used for examination and treatment of the head, neck, and chest; helpful for patients with breathing difficulties
c) Draping: drape sheet covers the patient from the shoulders down; adjust to expose the necessary area

11. Semi-Fowler's
    a) Modification of Fowler's; back supported at a 45 degree angle
    b) Used for postsurgical examinations and for patients with head trauma or head pain
    c) Draping: same as for Fowler's

12. Trendelenburg
    a) Patient is supine with the foot of the table elevated 45 degrees (head lower than feet)
    b) Used for shock or abdominal surgery
    c) Draping: drape sheet covers the patient from underarms to below the knees; neck, head, and hands are left uncovered

B. GENERAL CONSIDERATIONS
   1. Expose only the body part being examined/treated
   2. Keep the patient as comfortable as possible
   3. Provide a blanket for comfort and warmth
   4. Modify the position to accommodate a weak or painful body part
   5. Prevent the patient from falling from the table
   6. Medical assistant should be present when a male physician examines a female patient

Assisting with Patient Examinations

I. Complete Physical Examinations
- Normally performed on new patients to assess their health status and to establish the patient's base
- Also performed on established patients for health maintenance
- Medical assistant must be familiar with the process, principles, and methods to prepare the patient and to assist the provider

II. Diagnosis (see Figure 16-1)

A. SYMPTOMS
- Conditions and feelings experienced by the patient

B. SIGNS
- Observable characteristics by health care providers
- May also be noticed by patient

C. DIFFERENTIAL DIAGNOSIS
- Comparing certain diseases with others that have similar signs and symptoms
- Process of ruling out (R/O)

D. IMPRESSION
- Working diagnosis
- Subject to change as the provider adds data from other diagnostic tools

E. DIAGNOSTIC TOOLS
1. Patient history
2. Physical examination
3. Vital signs
4. Laboratory and diagnostic tests
5. Patient's communications
6. Physician's perceptions

F. FINAL DIAGNOSIS
- The provider's final conclusion

III. Methods of Examination

A. INSPECTION
- Process of visual observation
- Includes looking for abnormalities in size, shape, color, continuity, symmetry, and/or position

B. PALPATION
- Process of touching and feeling
- Can detect abnormalities of size, shape, texture, and tenderness

C. PERCUSSION
- Process of tapping or striking the body
- Done with fingers or small hammer
- Aids in determination of size, position, or density of an organ or body cavity

D. MANIPULATION
- Forceful passive movement of a joint to determine range of motion

E. AUSCULTATION
- Process of listening to the body using a stethoscope

F. MENSURATION
- Process of measurement

IV. Commonly Used Equipment (see Figure 16-2)

A. OPHTHALMOSCOPE
- Instrument used to illuminate the internal eye for visual inspection
- Runs off a power source (battery or wall unit)

B. OTOSCOPE
- Instrument used to illuminate the external and internal ear for visual examination
- Runs off a power source (battery or wall unit)

C. POCKET FLASHLIGHT OR HEADLIGHT
- Instrument used to illuminate the mouth, throat, and nose for visual examination

D. TAPE MEASURE
- Instrument used to measure body structures

E. TONGUE DEPRESSORS
- Instrument used to control tongue movement while examining the mouth and throat

F. STETHOSCOPE
- Instrument used to listen to the sounds of the body

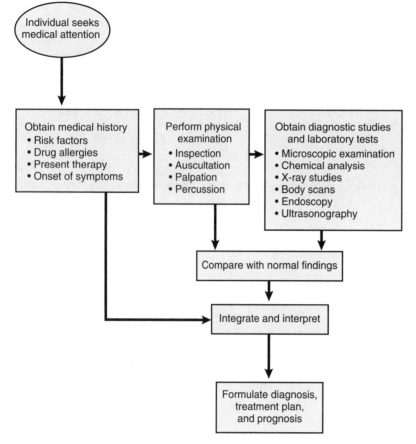

FIGURE 16-1 Essential steps in diagnosis. (From Frazier MS, Drzymkowski JW: Essentials of Human Diseases and Conditions, Philadelphia, 2000, Saunders, p. 16.)

G. GLOVES AND LUBRICANT
   ■ Used for rectal and/or pelvic examinations

H. VAGINAL SPECULUM
   ■ Instrument inserted into the patient's vagina to allow visualization of the cervix and vagina

I. PERCUSSION HAMMER
   ■ Rubber-tipped hammer used to test patient's reflexes

J. TUNING FORK
   ■ Instrument used to test the patient's hearing; vibrates when struck to produce sound

K. MISCELLANEOUS
   1. Cotton-tipped applicators
   2. 2 inch × 2 inch gauze squares
   3. Glass slides
   4. Specimen/slide fixative
   5. Tissues

V. Sequence of Events

A. PATIENT HEALTH HISTORY

B. SPECIMEN COLLECTION
   ■ Includes urine, blood, or other body fluids
   ■ Exam may be more comfortable if the patient's bladder is empty

C. VITAL SIGNS AND ANTHROPOMETRIC MEASUREMENTS

D. PHYSICAL EXAMINATION

E. DIAGNOSTIC TESTS
   ■ Includes EKG, X-ray, spirometry, immunizations

F. PATIENT CONSULTATION/DISCUSSION WITH PROVIDER

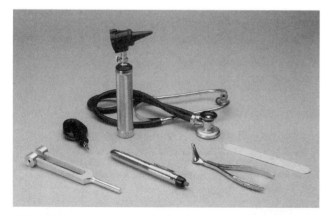

FIGURE 16-2 Physical examination instruments. (From Kinn ME, Woods MA: The Medical Assistant, Administrative and Clinical, ed 8, Philadelphia, 1998, Saunders, p. 490.)

VI. Physical Examination Sequence

A. PRESENTING APPEARANCE (PATIENT'S GENERAL APPEARANCE)
- General assessment of patient's state of health
- Includes
  1. Signs of distress
  2. Appearance of skin
  3. Posture, gait, and motor activity
  4. General grooming
  5. Presence of odors
  6. Speech patterns
  7. Body language and facial expressions

B. HEAD—PATIENT IN SITTING POSITION
  1. Hair, scalp, and face
  2. Eyes
     - Use an ophthalmoscope to visually examine the retina and vessels
  3. Ears
     - Use an otoscope to examine the external ear and tympanic membrane
  4. Nose and sinuses
     - Use an otoscope or nasal speculum to examine the nares and sinus cavities
  5. Mouth and throat
     - Lips, gums, teeth, and tongue
     - Use a light source, tongue depressor (blade), and laryngeal mirror to visually examine the throat
  6. Neck
     - Inspect and palpate the thyroid, trachea, and lymph nodes

C. THORAX—PATIENT IN A SITTING POSITION
  1. Back
     - Spine and muscles of the back are visually inspected
     - Lungs are auscultated with a stethoscope
  2. Chest
     - Visually inspected for symmetry and expansion
     - Inspirations auscultated
     - Axillary nodes palpated
  3. Heart
     - Stethoscope used to listen to heart sounds
     - Complete silence in the exam room is necessary to interpret the sounds
  4. Breasts
     - Examined for masses, tenderness, and discharge
     - May also be examined with the patient in supine position

D. ABDOMEN—PATIENT IN THE SUPINE POSITION
- Auscultated for the presence or absence of bowel sounds
- Visually inspected for symmetry and contour
- Manipulated and palpated for contours of the organs
- Area needs to be relaxed for proper examination

E. GENITAL/RECTAL—PATIENT IN THE SUPINE POSITION
  1. Inguinal area
     - Palpated for lymph nodes and hernias
  2. Male genital and rectal
     - Penis, scrotum, prostate, and anus palpated and inspected
  3. Female genital and rectal—patient in the lithotomy position
     - External genitalia, vagina, cervix, and anus inspected
     - a) Pelvic exam
        - Speculum inserted into the vagina to visualize the vaginal wall and cervix
        - Bimanual exam done with a gloved hand inserted into the vagina and the other hand palpating the external abdomen to examine the uterus, ovaries, and fallopian tubes

F. LEGS—PATIENT IN THE STANDING POSITION
- Inspected for pulse and varicosities

VII. Integumentary System (Dermatology)
- Deals with disorders of the skin, hair, glands, nails, and subcutaneous tissue
- Specialized physician: dermatologist

A. GENERAL EXAMINATION
- Skin, hair, and nails
- Examined for
  1. Color
  2. Consistency and texture
  3. Eruptions, lesions, growths
  4. Tenderness
  5. Irregularities

B. DIAGNOSTIC PROCEDURES
- The medical assistant may assist with, perform, or schedule these procedures
  1. Fungal, bacterial, and viral cultures
     - Tissue scrapings, purulent material, and exudate sent to the lab to identify pathogenic organisms
  2. KOH (potassium hydroxide) smears
     - Skin scrapings immersed in 20% potassium hydroxide; the sample is examined for fungus
  3. Biopsy
     - a) Excisional: removal of the entire section of tissue for microscopic examination
     - b) Incisional: removal of a portion of the tissue for microscopic examination
     - c) Punch: use of an instrument (dermal punch) to remove only a small amount of tissue for microscopic examination

4. Allergy testing (see Figure 16-3)
   a) Patch test: a small piece of gauze with a small amount of allergen is placed on the skin; a positive reaction occurs if the skin becomes red or blistered after 48 hours
   b) Scratch test: a minute amount of allergen is placed, by scratch, in the skin; a positive reaction occurs if the scratch becomes red and swollen
   c) Intradermal: a small amount of allergen is injected intradermally; a positive reaction is determined by measuring the size of the wheals produced
5. Wood's light examination
   • Examination to detect fluorescent characteristics of certain fungi; the skin is viewed in a darkened room under ultraviolet light that is filtered through Wood's glass
6. Antinuclear antibody titer (ANA)
   • Blood test used to screen for cutaneous lupus erythematosus and similar connective tissue diseases
7. Tuberculin skin testing: test patient for TB antibodies
   a) Mantoux: intradermal injection
   b) Tine: multipuncture method using a small plastic device

C. TREATMENT PROCEDURES
■ The medical assistant may either assist with, perform, or schedule these procedures
1. Cryosurgery
   • Use of extreme cold (liquid nitrogen) to freeze and destroy unwanted tissue

2. Curettage
   • Removal of the surface of the skin or a lesion by scraping with a sharp, spoon-shaped instrument (curette)
3. Dermabrasion
   • Removal of scars or lesions by the use of mechanical or chemical abrasives
4. Electrodesiccation
   • Destruction of growths, warts, or unwanted areas of tissue with electric current (diathermy)
5. Mohs' surgery
   • Removal and microscopic examination of layers of malignant growth

D. MEDICATIONS
1. Anti-acneics
   • Used to treat acne
   • Examples: Accutane, Retin-A, Cleocin, Persagel
2. Antifungals
   • Used to treat fungal infections
   • Examples: Lotrimin, Monistat, Nizocal
3. Antihistamines
   • Used to decrease allergic reactions
   • Examples: Atarax, Benadryl
4. Anti-infectives
   • Used to kill microorganisms
   • Examples: Erythromycin, Keflex, Mycolog, Sumycin
5. Antivirals
   • Inhibit viruses
   • Example: Zovirax
6. Scabicides/pediculocides
   • Used to kill scabies and lice
   • Examples: Lindane, Kwell

Intradermal or "Scratch" test results

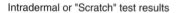
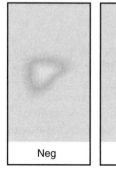
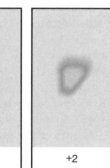
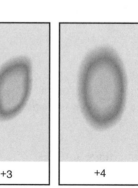

| Neg | ±1 | +2 | +3 | +4 |

Degree of sensitivity measured by area of erythema and a wheal

Neg= no sensitivity or <5mm
  ±1= 5-9mm erythema; further testing needed
  +2= >20mm erythema; with <10mm palpable wheal
  +3= >30mm erythema with <10mm wheal
  +4= >40mm erythema with <15mm wheal

FIGURE 16-3 Allergy testing results. (From Stepp CA, Woods MA: Laboratory procedures for Medical Office Personnel, Philadelphia, 1998, Saunders, p. 352.)

7. Topical steroids
   - Used externally to decrease inflammation
   - Examples: Aristocort, Medrol, Topicort, Kenalog

VIII. Musculoskeletal System (Orthopedics)

■ Deals with disorders of the musculoskeletal systems

■ Specialized physician: orthopedist, orthopod

A. GENERAL EXAMINATION

■ Observes for

1. Decreased range of motion (ROM)
2. Tenderness and swelling
3. Unequal or decreased strength
4. Deformities or growths

B. DIAGNOSTIC PROCEDURES

■ The medical assistant may either assist with, perform, or schedule these procedures

1. Arthrocentesis: removal of joint fluid with a needle for analysis of fluid
2. Arthroscopy: examination of a joint with a viewing scope (arthroscope)
3. Electromyography: recording the strength of muscle contraction as a result of electrical stimulation
4. Muscle biopsy: removal of muscle tissue for examination
5. Bone scan: use of a machine to measure the uptake of a radioactive substance injected intravenously
6. Computerized axial tomography (CAT scan, CT scan): computer-assisted X-ray technique used to distinguish pathological conditions such as tumors or fractures; a noninvasive method of viewing inside the body
7. Magnetic resonance imaging (MRI): production of detailed pictures of internal structures, using magnetism and computers; a noninvasive method of viewing inside the body
8. Skeletal X-ray: plain X-ray of the appropriate body part
9. Erythrocyte sedimentation rate (ESR; sedrate): blood test that can determine whether inflammation is present within the patient's body
10. Latex fixation: test for the presence of rheumatoid factor present in rheumatoid arthritis

C. TREATMENT PROCEDURES

■ The medical assistant may either assist with, perform, or schedule these procedures

1. Wrap/splint: cloth or elastic material or rigid material used to immobilize limbs or joints
2. Cast: application of material (plaster, resin, fiberglass) molded to the affected limb and allowed to harden; holds the affected limb or joint in a fixed position until healing is complete
3. Arthroscopic surgery: surgical procedures performed on joints using an arthroscope
4. Reduction: restoration of a fracture to normal position
   a) Closed reduction: manipulation without an incision
   b) Open reduction: incision is made at the fracture site
5. Physical therapy: use of exercise, heat, cold, and other physical means to reduce pain and swelling, to increase movement and circulation, and to promote healing

D. MEDICATIONS

1. Analgesics
   - Used to reduce pain
   - Examples: aspirin, Tylenol
2. Narcotic analgesics
   - Reduce pain with narcotics
   - Examples: Darvon, Lortab, Percodan
3. Antibiotics
   - Used to kill microorganisms
   - Examples: Cipro, Keflex
4. Nonsteroidal anti-inflammatory agents (NSAIDs)
   - Used to reduce inflammation without the use of steroids
   - Examples: Advil, Motrin, Naprosyn, Indocin, Clinocil
5. Muscle relaxants
   - Used to relax skeletal muscles
   - Examples: Flexeril, Valium

IX. Cardiovascular System (Cardiology)

■ Deals with diseases and disorders of the heart and vessels

■ Specialized physician: cardiologist

A. GENERAL EXAMINATION

■ Listening to the heart with a stethoscope, noting heart sounds, rate, and rhythm

B. DIAGNOSTIC PROCEDURES

■ The medical assistant may either assist with, perform, or schedule these procedures

1. Cardiac catheterization
   - Intensive study of the heart
   - Uses catheters to perform angiocardiography and/or pressure-and-flow measurements
   - Can determine the severity of heart disease and/or vessel blockage
   - Medical assistant would schedule this procedure at the hospital
2. Echocardiogram
   - Graphic recording of ultrasound waves from the heart

3. Electrocardiogram (EKG, ECG) (see details below)
   • Recording of the electrical activity of the heart
4. Holter monitor (see Figure 16-4)
   • Portable ambulatory monitoring system
   • Monitors EKG activity over a 24-hour period
   • Designed so that the patient is able to maintain usual daily activities with minimal inconvenience while being monitored
   • Device is connected to the patient by electrodes placed on the patient's chest and a special portable magnetic tape recorder that continually monitors the heart's activity
   • Recorder is in a protective case that is either worn on a belt around the patient's waist or hung over the shoulder by a strap
   • Patient completes an activity diary; all activities and emotional states are recorded along with any symptoms experienced (chest pain, vertigo, palpitations)
   • Monitor is removed from patient after a 24-hour period, and the tape is evaluated and analyzed
   • Electrodes (floating electrodes) are placed as follows
     1) Right border of the sternum (manubrium)
     2) Left border of the sternum (manubrium)
     3) Right sternal border at the level of the fifth rib
     4) Fifth rib space at the right anterior axillary line
     5) Fifth rib space at the left anterior axillary line

5. Treadmill
   • Motorized machine that allows patient to walk in place; allows evaluation of the patient's heart function while exercising
6. Angiography
   • X-ray of blood vessels after an injection of radiopaque material
7. Arterial blood gases (ABGs)
   • Measures oxygen, carbon dioxide, and metabolic balance in an arterial blood sample
8. Cardiac enzymes
   a) CPK (creatine phosphokinase): enzyme released into the blood when the heart or skeletal muscles are injured
   b) AST (aspartate aminotransferase) (formerly SGOT): found in high concentration in heart muscle and in the liver
   c) LDH (lactic dehydrogenase): enzyme found in heart muscle, skeletal muscles, kidneys, liver, and red blood cells
9. Prothrombin time (PT)
   • Tests coagulation of blood

C. TREATMENT PROCEDURES
   ■ The medical assistant may either assist with, perform, or schedule these procedures
   1. Angioplasty: surgical repair of a blood vessel
   2. Defibrillation (cardioversion): brief charges of electricity applied to the chest to stop cardiac arrhythmia
   3. Coronary artery bypass: open-heart surgery for the purpose of bypassing an obstructed coronary artery
   4. Endarterectomy: removal of the interior portion of an artery and occluding fatty deposits
   5. Phlebotomy: opening into a vein; venipuncture
   6. Vein stripping: removal of a diseased portion of a vein

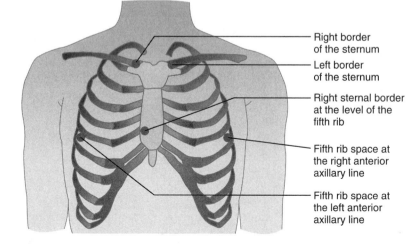

Right border of the sternum

Left border of the sternum

Right sternal border at the level of the fifth rib

Fifth rib space at the right anterior axillary line

Fifth rib space at the left anterior axillary line

FIGURE 16-4 Holter monitor electrode positions. (From Bonewit-West K: Clinical Procedures for Medical Assistants, ed 5, Philadelphia, 2000, Saunders, p. 458.)

D. MEDICATIONS

1. Diuretics
   - Promote urination
   - Examples: Bumex, Dyazide, Lasix, Hydro-Diuril
2. Antihypertensives
   - Decrease blood pressure
   - Examples: Inderal, Lanoxin, Procardia, Tenormin, Minipress
3. Antilipemics
   - Decrease cholesterol levels in blood
   - Examples: Loped, Mivacor

4. Anti-anginals
   - Decrease chest pain
   - Examples: Nitrostat, Transderm-Nitro

E. EKG (See Figure 16-5)

■ Cardiac electrical activity is generated and spreads through the heart and creates an electrical wave
■ This electrical wave is measured as an EKG
   1. Electrical system of the heart
      a) Sinoatrial (SA) node (pacemaker)
      b) Atrioventricular (AV) node
      c) Bundle of His

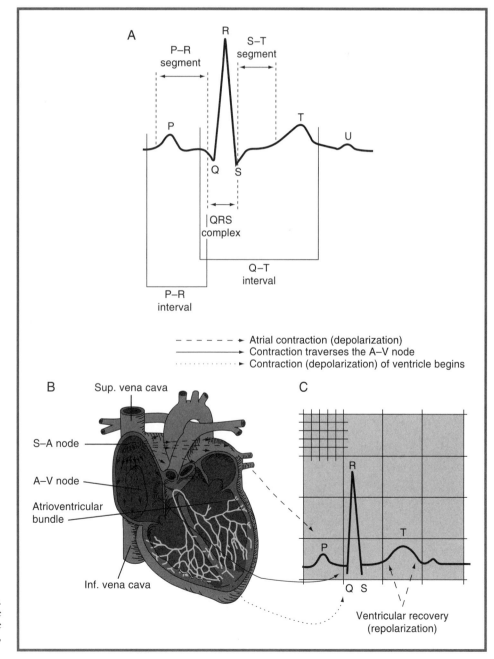

FIGURE 16-5 Cardiac cycle. (From Kinn ME, Woods MA: The Medical Assistant, Administrative and Clinical, ed 8, Philadelphia, 1998, Saunders, p. 509.)

d) Right and left bundle branches
e) Purkinje fibers
2. Electrical states of the heart
   a) Polarization: cardiac muscle cells are resting
   b) Depolarization: cardiac muscle cells contract
   c) Repolarization: cardiac muscle cells transform from active to resting state for recharging
3. Normal EKG—All heartbeats appear as a pattern, consisting of
   a) P-wave: impulse starting in the atria
   b) QRS complex: impulse going through ventricles

c) T-wave: repolarization of ventricles
4. EKG leads (see Figure 16-6)
   • Externally applied electrodes
   • Relative to an axis (a direct line) between two poles
   • Each lead makes up one positive pole, one negative pole, and one ground
   • Leads give an electrical picture of the heart from different angles
   • EKG uses 10 electrodes (4 limb electrodes, and 6 chest electrodes) to give 12 leads
   a) Limb leads
      ■ 6 of the 12 leads
      ■ Electrodes are placed on the patient's ex-

A

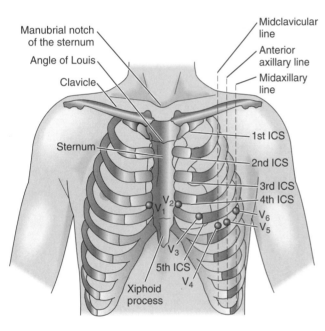

B

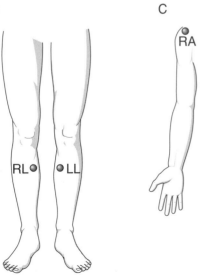

C

FIGURE 16-6 EKG leads. A, Chest lead placement. B, Leg lead placement. C, Arm lead placement. (A from Chester GA: Modern Medical Assisting, Philadelphia, 1998, Saunders, p. 676.)

tremities (upper arms and inside of calves)

1) Bipolar (standard) limb leads (see Figure 16-7)
  > Measures cardiac electrical activity between two extremities (negative and positive pole)
  > Right electrode is used for the ground
    (a) Lead I: measures activity from right arm to left arm (RA to LA)
    (b) Lead II: measures activity from right arm to left leg (RA to LL)
    (c) Lead III: measures activity from left arm to left leg (LA to LL)

2) Unipolar (augmented) limb leads (see Figure 16-8)
  > Measures cardiac electrical activity between the heart and one extremity
    (a) aVR: right side
    (b) aVL: left side
    (c) aVF: left foot

3) Precordial (chest) leads (see Figure 16-8)
  > Provide points of reference across the chest wall
  > Differentiate left- and right-sided heart events
    (a) Lead V1: electrode placed at the fourth intercostal space, to the right of the sternum
    (b) Lead V2: electrode placed at the fourth intercostal space, to the left of the sternum
    (c) Lead V3: electrode placed midway between leads V2 and V4
    (d) Lead V4: electrode placed left-midclavicular line in the fifth intercostal space
    (e) Lead V5: electrode placed at the level of V4 at axillary line
    (f) Lead V6: electrode placed at the level of V5 at the midaxillary line

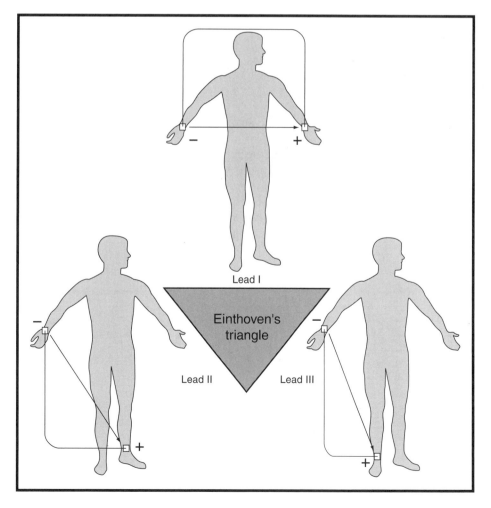

FIGURE 16-7 Bipolar leads and axes. (From Kinn ME, Woods MA: The Medical Assistant, Administrative and Clinical, ed 8, Philadelphia, 1998, Saunders, p. 512.)

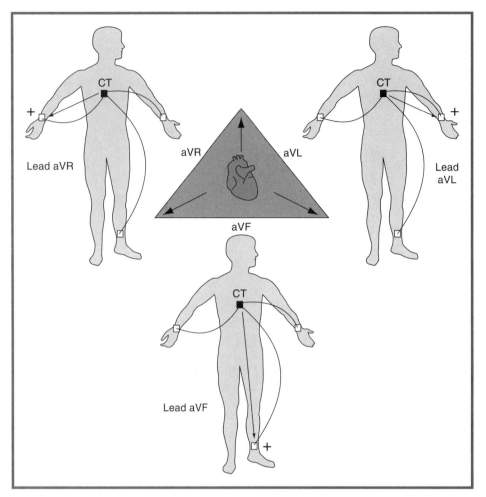

FIGURE 16-8 Augmented leads and precordial leads. (From Kinn ME, Woods MA: The Medical Assistant, Administrative and Clinical, ed 8, Philadelphia, 1998, Saunders, p. 513.)

4) Leads in relation to the anatomy of the heart
    (a) Right side of the heart: V1, aVR
    (b) Left side of the heart: V5, V6, I, aVL
    (c) Transition from right to left sides of the heart: V2, V3, V4
    (d) Inferior heart: II, III, aVF

5. Electrocardiograph
    a) Paper (see Figure 16-9)
      ▪ Records visible record of the heart's electrical activity
      ▪ Paper is heat-sensitive
      ▪ Heated stylus on the machine traces the heart activity onto the paper
      ▪ Composed of 1-millimeter squares: every

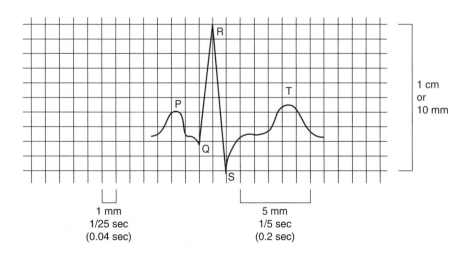

FIGURE 16-9 ECG paper measurement. (From Kinn ME, Woods MA: The Medical Assistant, Administrative and Clinical, ed 8, Philadelphia, 1998, Saunders, p. 511.)

fifth line is darkened, creating large blocks 5 squares wide and 5 squares high
- ■ Cardiac voltage is measured on the vertical scale; time is measured on the horizontal scale
- ■ Horizontally, each large block represents 0.2 second
- ■ Vertically, each large block represents 0.5 millivolt of electricity
- ■ Paper moves continuously through the machine at the rate of 1 inch per second on the standard machine setting

b) Controls
1) Main power switch: turns the machine on and off
2) RUN/STOP: activates (or stops) the amplifier so that the stylus can react to the heartbeat
3) Run-25: moves the paper 25 mm (1 inch) per second (standard speed)
4) Run-50: doubles the paper's speed to 50 mm (2 inches) per second
5) Sensitivity control: regulates the output of the amplifier
6) Standard (STD) button: manually checks the machine's calibration (stylus should deflect 10 millimeters, or 2 large squares)
7) Lead selector: changes leads
8) Marker button: allows manual identification of leads; uses codes of dots or dashes

c) Artifacts: abnormal EKG tracings not caused by heart activity
1) Somatic tremor: caused by the patient's muscle movement
2) Alternating current (AC) interference: caused by nearby operation of electrical equipment
3) Wandering baseline: caused by electrodes applied too loosely or too tightly

X. Blood (Hematology)
- ■ Deals with blood disorders, bone marrow, and coagulation
- ■ Specialized physician: hematologist

A. GENERAL EXAMINATION
- ■ Obtain blood or bone marrow samples for testing
- ■ Palpation of spleen and liver

B. DIAGNOSTIC PROCEDURES
- ■ The medical assistant may either assist with, perform, or schedule these procedures
1. Bone marrow aspiration
   - Insertion of a large needle into the sternum or iliac crest to remove bone marrow for testing

2. Blood cell counts (RBC and WBC)
   - Blood test to determine the number of RBCs and WBCs per cubic millimeter of blood
3. Differential
   - Blood smear on glass slide; stain is applied to the smear; the smear is studied under a microscope to differentiate the types of WBCs
4. Hematocrit (hct)
   - Measures the percentage of RBCs in volume of blood
5. Hemoglobin (hgb)
   - Measures the grams of hemoglobin in volume of blood
6. Platelet count
   - Estimates the number of platelets in volume of blood
7. Prothrombin time (PT)
   - Measures coagulation time of blood

C. MEDICATIONS
1. Anticoagulants
   - Prevent blood from clotting
   - Examples: Coumadin, Heparin
2. Stimulating factors
   - Stimulate production of blood cells
   - Examples: Neupogen, Leukine
3. Thrombolytic agents
   - Dissolve clots
   - Examples: Abbokinase, Streptase
4. Anti-anemics
   - Treat anemias
   - Examples: Epogen, Slow-Fe, Vitamin B12

XI. Respiratory System (Pulmonology)
- ■ Deals with diseases and disorders of the lungs and respiratory system
- ■ Specialized physician: pulmonologist

A. GENERAL EXAMINATION
- ■ Inspection of the nose, face, and throat
- ■ Examination of the mucous membranes
- ■ Inspection and palpation of the sinuses, neck, and lymph nodes
- ■ Auscultation of the lungs

B. DIAGNOSTIC PROCEDURES
- ■ The medical assistant may either assist with, perform, or schedule these procedures
1. Bronchoscopy: visualization of the bronchi through a bronchoscope
2. Spirometry: measurement of the breathing capacity of the lungs
3. Lung biopsy: biopsy of tissue taken from the lungs
4. Pulmonary function test (PFT): evaluates how the patient breathes; determines lung volumes, pulmonary gas exchange, and flow rates
5. Thoracentesis: puncture of the chest wall with a needle to obtain fluid for testing

6. Tracheostomy: emergency or elective procedure that creates an opening through the neck into the trachea
7. Chest X-ray: full view of the lungs from the back (PA) and sides (lat)
8. Sputum culture: collection of a sputum sample and testing it for microorganisms
9. Arterial blood gases (ABGs): measurement of hydrogen, carbon dioxide, pH, and oxygen pressure from an arterial blood sample

C. TREATMENT PROCEDURES
■ The medical assistant may either assist with, perform, or schedule these procedures
1. Endotracheal intubation: a procedure that establishes an airway by inserting a tube through the nose, pharynx, and larynx into the trachea
2. Thoracotomy: surgical insertion of a tube into the chest to drain fluid or air
3. Nebulizer: use of a machine to produce a fine mist of water and medication; the patient receives the medication by inhaling the mist

D. MEDICATIONS
1. Antibiotics
   • Kill microorganisms
   • Examples: Amoxil, Ampicillin, Biaxin, Ceclor, Keflex
2. Antihistamines
   • Counteract the effects of histamine
   • Examples: Benadryl, Phenergan, Seldane
3. Bronchodilators
   • Dilate bronchial tubes
   • Examples: Albuterol, Proventil, Ventolin, Aminophylline
4. Expectorants
   • Produce productive cough
   • Example: Humabid
5. Decongestants
   • Decrease congestion in the nose and nasal passages
   • Examples: Entex, Afrin, Sudafed

XII. Digestive System (Gastroenterology)
■ Treats diseases and disorders of the digestive tract
■ Specialized physician: gastroenterologist

A. GENERAL EXAMINATION
■ Examination of the mouth
■ Palpation of the abdomen and intestines
■ Inspection of the rectum (can be accomplished with a scope)

B. DIAGNOSTIC PROCEDURES
■ The medical assistant may either assist with, perform, or schedule these procedures
1. Colonoscopy: visual examination of the colon using a lighted scope

2. Liver biopsy: removal of a tissue sample from the liver for microscopic examination
3. Proctoscopy (sigmoidoscopy): visual examination of the anus, the rectum, and part of the sigmoid colon
4. Barium enema (BE): infusion of barium into the rectum for visualization by X-ray
5. Cholecystogram: X-ray of the gallbladder
6. Upper gastrointestinal (GI) series: X-ray study of the esophagus, stomach, and duodenum; contrast medium is orally administered
7. Gastric analysis: aspiration of the stomach contents by a tube placed into the stomach, through the nose; contents analyzed
8. Occult blood (Quaiac) test: test for hidden blood in the stool; Hemoccult
9. Ova and parasites (O&P): analysis of a stool sample for the presence of eggs and parasites
10. Liver function tests: tests performed to diagnose liver-related diseases or disorders

C. TREATMENT PROCEDURES
■ The medical assistant may either assist with, perform, or schedule these procedures
1. Appendectomy: removal of the appendix
2. Cholecystectomy: removal of the gallbladder
3. Colostomy: creation of an opening between the colon and the body surface
4. Hemorrhoid ligation: removal of hemorrhoids by using the rubber band technique (ligating)
5. Lithotripsy: crushing of stones
6. Hemorrhoidectomy: excision of hemorrhoids
7. Vagotomy: surgical transaction of the vagus nerve to decrease stomach acid secretion in patients with ulcers

D. MEDICATIONS
1. Antihelmintics
   • Kill helminths (worms)
   • Example: Vermox
2. Antibiotics
   • Kill microorganisms
   • Examples: Sumycin, Flagyl
3. Antispasmodics
   • Decrease spasms of the GI tract
   • Examples: Bentyl, Librax, Donnatal
4. Antidiarrheals
   • Decrease/slow diarrhea
   • Examples: Imodium, Lomotil, Pepto-Bismol
5. H2 antagonists
   • Decrease stomach acids
   • Examples: Tagamet, Zantac, Axid, Pepcid
6. Laxatives
   • Encourage bowel movements
   • Examples: Colace, Dulcolax, Ex-Lax, Milk of Magnesia

XIII. Urinary System (Urology)

■ Treats diseases and disorders of the male and female urinary systems and the male reproductive system
■ Specialized physician: urologist

A. GENERAL EXAMINATION

■ Palpation of the kidneys and bladder
■ Inspection of the external genitalia
■ Palpation of the prostate gland through the rectum

B. DIAGNOSTIC PROCEDURES

■ The medical assistant may either assist with, perform, or schedule these procedures
1. Cystoscopy: visual examination of the bladder with a cystoscope
2. Retrograde pyelogram: X-ray of the kidney after introducing a contrast medium through the ureter
3. Intravenous pyelogram (IVP): study of the kidney using an intravenous contrast medium
4. Renal ultrasound: ultrasound of the kidneys
5. X-ray of the kidney, ureter, and bladder (KUB): X-ray done without injection of air or contrast medium; shows the size and location of the organs
6. Urinalysis (UA): analysis of urine to determine its physical, chemical, and microscopic properties
7. Blood urea nitrogen (BUN): measures the amount of urea in the blood; kidney function test
8. Semen analysis: measures the quantity and motility of sperm
9. Prostate specific antigen (PSA): blood test to check for the presence of prostate cancer

C. TREATMENT PROCEDURES

■ The medical assistant may either assist with, perform, or schedule these procedures
1. Dialysis: artificial means of removing waste products from the blood when the kidneys have failed
2. Lithotripsy: procedure to crush or break up stones in the urinary tract
3. Catheterization: introduction of a flexible tube through the urethra into the urinary bladder
4. Circumcision: removal of the foreskin of the penis
5. Prostatectomy: removal of the prostate
6. Transurethral resection of the prostate (TURP): prostatic tissue removed through an endoscope introduced through the urethra
7. Vasectomy: removal of a segment of the vas deferens; male sterilization technique

D. MEDICATIONS

1. Antibiotics
   • Destroy microorganisms
   • Examples: Bactrim, Furadontin, Gantrisin, Rocephin
2. Analgesics
   • Reduce pain
   • Example: Pyridium
3. Gonadotropins
   • Stimulate gonads
   • Example: Pergonal
4. For impotence
   • Example: Viagra

XIV. Female Reproductive System (Obstetrics/Gynecology)

■ Diagnosis and treatment of diseases and disorders of the female reproductive system and pregnancy
■ Specialized physician: obstetrician (pregnancy and childbirth) and/or gynecologist (female reproductive system)

A. GENERAL EXAMINATION

■ Inspection and palpation of the breasts
■ Inspection of the external genitalia, vagina, and cervix
■ Palpation of the uterus, ovaries, and fallopian tubes
■ Prenatal: includes initial general examination as well as periodic examinations to monitor fetal growth and development

B. DIAGNOSTIC PROCEDURES

■ The medical assistant may either assist with, perform, or schedule these procedures
1. Amniocentesis
   • Puncture of the amniotic sac with a needle to withdraw amniotic fluid for analysis
   • Can detect genetic disorders
2. Cervical biopsy
   • Removal of tissue to evaluate the presence of abnormalities
3. Colposcopy
   • Examination of the cervix with a scope
4. Dilation and curettage (D&C)
   • Expansion of the cervix so that the uterine wall can be scraped
5. Fetal monitoring
   • Recording of the fetal heart rate
6. Laparoscopy
   • Examination of the abdomen by insertion of a laparoscope through the abdominal wall
7. Human chorionic gonadotropin (HCG)
   • Hormone produced by the placenta during pregnancy
   • Basis for pregnancy testing
   • Testing performed on blood or urine

8. Chorionic villi sampling (CVS)
   • Use of ultrasound to guide a needle into the uterine wall to obtain a sample of chorion
   • Can detect chromosomal abnormalities
9. Endovaginal ultrasound
   • Sound probe placed in the vagina for a closer, sharper look within the pelvis
10. Hysterosalpingography
    • X-ray of the uterus and fallopian tubes, using radiopaque material
11. Pelvimetry
    • Measurement of the dimensions of the pelvis
12. Papanicolaou smear (Pap smear)
    • Scrapings from the cervix used to detect tissue changes
    • May indicate cervical cancer

C. TREATMENT PROCEDURES
■ The medical assistant may either assist with, perform, or schedule these procedures
1. Abortion
   • Premature termination of pregnancy
   • May be spontaneous or therapeutic
2. Cauterization
   • Use of heat to destroy abnormal tissue
3. Cesarean section (C-section)
   • Birth of an infant through a surgical incision into uterus
4. Conization
   • Removal of a cone-shaped wedge of tissue from the cervix for examination
5. Cryosurgery
   • Use of cold to destroy abnormal tissue
6. Hysterectomy
   • Surgical removal of the uterus through the abdominal wall or vagina
7. Hysteroscopy
   • Insertion of a scope into the uterus to view the endometrial cavity
8. Kegel exercises
   • Simple exercises to strengthen the pubococcygeal muscles
9. Tubal ligation
   • Tying off the fallopian tubes
   • Female sterilization procedure

D. MEDICATIONS
1. Hormone replacement/hormones
   • Examples: Premaren, Depo-Provera, Ogen
2. Ovulation stimulants
   • Example: Clomid
3. Oral contraceptives
   • Prevent pregnancy
   • Examples: Tri-Phasil, Ovral, Ortho-Novum, Ortho-Tricyclin

4. Supplements
   • Vitamins and iron
   • Examples: Ferro-Sequels, Natalins
5. Antifungals
   • Treat fungal, or yeast, infections
   • Examples: Monistat, Gyne-Lotrimin

XV. Endocrine System (Endocrinology)
■ Diagnose and treats diseases and disorders of the endocrine system
■ Specialized physician: endocrinologist

A. GENERAL EXAMINATION
■ Complete physical examination

B. DIAGNOSTIC PROCEDURES
■ The medical assistant may either assist with, perform, or schedule these procedures
1. Radioactive iodine uptake
   • Measures the uptake of a dose of radioactive iodine by the thyroid gland
2. Thyroid scan
   • Administration of a radioactive compound to visualize the thyroid gland
   • Used to detect tumors and nodules
3. CAT scans
   • Can visualize the endocrine glands
   • Can detect disease processes and masses
4. Ultrasonography
   • Use of sound waves to obtain images
5. Blood tests
   • Used to diagnose and manage disorders
   • Blood tests for
     a) ACTH: from the pituitary
     b) Aldosterone: from the adrenal cortex
     c) Thyroxin: from the thyroid
     d) Calcium: from the parathyroid
     e) Cortisol: from the adrenal cortex
     f) Electrolytes (sodium, potassium, chloride): from the adrenal cortex
     g) Estradial: from the ovaries
     h) FSH: from the pituitary
     i) GH: from the pituitary
     j) Glucose: from the pancreas
     k) Insulin: from the pancreas
     l) LH: from the pituitary
     m) Parathyroid hormone: from the parathyroid
     n) T3 and T4: from the thyroid
     o) Testosterone: from the testes
6. Metabolic rate (BMR)
   • Not an often-ordered test
   • Measures the energy exchange rate of the body in a state of rest
7. Glucose tolerance test (GTT)
   • Blood is tested at specific intervals after the patient ingests a measured amount of glucose

C. TREATMENT PROCEDURES
■ The medical assistant may either assist with, perform, or schedule these procedures
1. Oopherectomy
   • Surgical removal of the ovaries
2. Orchiectomy
   • Surgical removal of the testes
3. Thyroidectomy
   • Total or partial removal of thyroid gland

D. MEDICATIONS
1. Thyroid medications
   • Replace thyroid hormones
   • Examples: Synthroid, Euthroid
2. Corticosteroids
   • Examples: Cortisone, Aristocort, Kenalog, Medrol, Discadron
3. Growth hormones
   • Example: Humatrope
4. Antidiuretic hormones
   • Example: Pitressin
5. Labor inducers
   • Example: Pitocin
6. Oral antidiabetics
   • Examples: Orinase, Glucotrol, Diabinase, Glucophage
7. Insulin
   • Examples: Humulin, Novalin

XVI. Nervous System (Neurology)
■ Diagnosis and treatment of diseases and disorders of the nervous system
■ Specialized physician: neurologist

A. GENERAL EXAMINATION
1. Mental status
   • Includes assessment of intelligence; assessment of memory; orientation to person, place, and time; and general appearance
2. Evaluation of all cranial nerves
3. Motor nerves
   • Includes coordination, strength, Romberg test, walking, finger-to-nose exercise
4. Sensory nervous system
5. Reflexes

B. DIAGNOSTIC PROCEDURES
■ The medical assistant may either assist with, perform, or schedule these procedures
1. Electroencephalography (EEG)
   • Study of the electrical activity of the brain
   • Uses electrodes attached to the scalp
2. Electromyography (EMG)
   • Study of the contraction of a muscle as a result of electrical stimulation
3. Lumbar puncture
   • Procedure for removal of cerebrospinal fluid (CSF) for analysis
4. Brain scan
   • Procedure that uses radioactive chemicals and specialized machines to record the passage through, and absorption into, brain lesions
5. Myelography
   • X-ray of the spinal cord
6. Skull series
   • Standard X-ray views of the skull
7. Cervical, thoracic, and lumbosacral spine
   • Standard X-ray views of specific portions of the spine

C. TREATMENT PROCEDURES
■ The medical assistant may either assist with, perform, or schedule these procedures
1. Craniotomy
   • Surgical opening into the cranium
2. Laminectomy
   • Removal of laminae to decompress pinched spinal nerve roots
3. Halo traction
   • Traction device for neck stability

D. MEDICATIONS
1. Anticonvulsants
   • Decrease seizure activity
   • Examples: Depokote, Delantin, Tegretol
2. Antiemetic (antivertigo)
   • Decrease vomiting, dizziness
   • Examples: Antivert, Compazine, Dramamine
3. Antiparkinson's agents
   • Decrease symptoms of Parkinson's disease
   • Examples: Artane, Cogentin, Sinemet
4. Antidepressants
   • Counteract depression
   • Examples: Paxil, Prozac

XVII. Sensory System (Eyes) (Ophthalmology)
■ Diagnosis and treatment of diseases and disorders of the eye
■ Specialized physician: ophthalmologist

A. GENERAL EXAMINATION
■ Inspection and measurement of the external eye, eyelids, and accessory structures
■ Measurement of eye movements and pupillary distance

B. DIAGNOSTIC PROCEDURES
■ The medical assistant may either assist with, perform, or schedule these procedures
1. Keratometry (K-readings)
   • Measurement of the steepness of the cornea
2. Ophthalmoscopy
   • Visual examination of the interior eye using an ophthalmoscope

3. Visual acuity
   • Determines the amount of myopia, hyperopia, or astigmatism
   • Uses the Snellen Eye Chart
4. Slit lamp examination
   • Examines the cornea, conjunctiva, iris, lens, and vitreous humor using a slit light and biomicroscope
5. Tonometry
   • Measures intraocular tension
   • May indicate the presence of glaucoma
6. Ishihara color vision test
   • Tests color vision

C. TREATMENT PROCEDURES
   ■ The medical assistant may either assist with, perform, or schedule these procedures
   1. Blepharoplasty: surgical repair of the eyelids
   2. Cataract extraction: removal of the lens of the eye
   3. Enucleation: removal of the eye from the socket
   4. Glaucoma operation: procedure that relieves increased intraocular pressure

D. MEDICATIONS
   1. Antibiotic/steroid combinations
      • Example: Tobradex
   2. Antibiotics
      • Examples: Tobrex, Bacitracin Opthalmic
   3. Corticosteroids
      • Examples: Decadron, Opticrom
   4. Glaucoma treatment
      • Examples: Timoptic, Propine, Betagan

XVIII. Ear, Nose, and Throat (Otorhinolaryngology, ENT)
   ■ Diagnosis and treatment of diseases and disorders of the ear, nose, and throat
   ■ Specialized physician: otorhinolaryngologist

A. GENERAL EXAMINATION
   ■ Examination of the ear with an otoscope
   ■ Examination of the nasal structures, throat, and sinuses

B. DIAGNOSTIC PROCEDURES
   ■ The medical assistant may either assist with, perform, or schedule these procedures
   1. Audiometry
      • Use of an audiometer to deliver sound frequencies
      • Determines the patient's hearing threshold
   2. Laryngoscopy
      • Visual examination of the larynx with a laryngoscope
   3. Otoscopy
      • Visual examination of the ear with an otoscope

4. Throat culture
   • Inflamed areas of the throat are swabbed and analyzed for various pathogens
5. Nasal smear
   • Removal of a specimen and analysis for pathogens
6. Skull, mastoid, sinus, and chest X-rays
   • Standard views of specific body parts

C. TREATMENT PROCEDURES
   ■ The medical assistant may either assist with, perform, or schedule these procedures
   1. Adenoidectomy: surgical excision of adenoids
   2. Myringotomy: incision into the eardrum
   3. Myringotomy with tubes: incision into the eardrum with placement of ventilation tubes
   4. Rhinoplasty: reconstruction or plastic surgery of the nose
   5. Tonsillectomy: surgical excision of tonsils
   6. Ear irrigation: irrigation (washing) of external ear canal

D. MEDICATIONS
   1. Antibiotics
      • Examples: Amoxil, Ceclor, Erythromycin, Keflex
   2. Otics
      • Examples: Ceruminex, Cortisporin Otic

XIX. Pediatrics
   ■ Diagnosis and treatment of diseases and disorders associated with childhood and health maintenance for infants, children, and adolescents
   ■ Specialized physician: pediatrician

A. GENERAL EXAMINATION
   ■ Similar to a complete physical examination for an adult
   ■ Examinations fall into two general categories
   1. Well-child (well-baby) visit
      • Evaluates the child's growth and development
      • Physical examination is performed at this time
      • Necessary immunizations are administered
   2. Sick-child (sick-baby) visit
      • Child shows signs and symptoms of a disease process or injury
      • Provider diagnoses and prescribes treatment

B. GROWTH CHART
   ■ Chart used to plot the physical growth pattern of a child
   ■ Includes height, weight, and head circumference
   ■ Identifies the percentile the child's growth falls into, as compared to the measurements listed on the standardized chart
   ■ Should be plotted at each well-baby visit
   ■ Separate charts
   1. Girls, birth to 36 months (see Figure 16-10)
   2. Boys, birth to 36 months (see Figure 16-11)

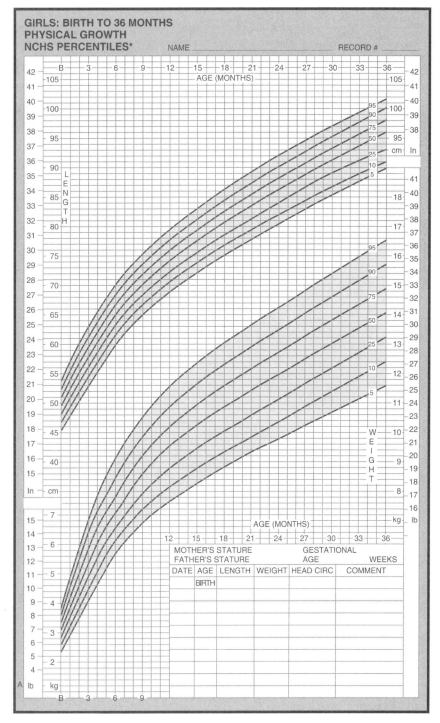

FIGURE 16-10 Growth rate graph: females (0-36 months). (From Kinn ME, Woods MA: The Medical Assistant, Administrative and Clinical, ed 8, Philadelphia, 1998, Saunders, p. 661.)

3. Girls, 2 to 18 years
4. Boys, 2 to 18 years

C. IMMUNIZATIONS

1. Diphtheria tetanus acellular vaccine (DtaP)
   - Total of 5 doses required by law between 2 months and 6 years of age
   - Administer: 0.5 mL IM
2. Adult tetanus vaccine (Td)
   - Given as a booster from age 7 through adult
   - Adults are given one dose each 10 years for life

   - For severe or dirty wounds, a booster is given if the last normal dose was more than 5 years ago
   - For minor or clean wounds, a booster is given if the last normal dose was given 10 or more years ago
3. *Haemophilus influenzae* Type B (HIB)
   - 4 doses administered between 2 months and 18 months of age
   - Administer: 0.5 mL IM
   - Vaccine consists of killed virus grown in chicken embryo tissue

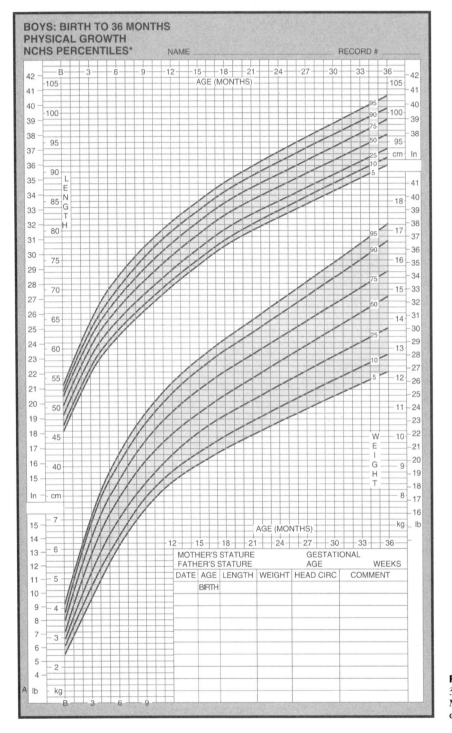

FIGURE 16-11 Growth rate graph: males (0-36 months). (From Kinn ME, Woods MA: The Medical Assistant, Administrative and Clinical, ed 8, Philadelphia, 1998, Saunders, p. 660.)

4. Poliomyelitis vaccine (IPV)
   • 4 doses administered between 2 months and 5 years of age
   • Administer: 0.5 mL IM
5. Hepatitis B vaccine (HepB)
   • 3 doses administered between birth and 18 months of age
   • Administer: 0.5 mL IM
6. Mumps, measles, and rubella (MMR)
   • 2 doses administered between 12 months and 12 years of age
   • Administer: 0.5 mL subq
   • Vaccine consists of attenuated measles, mumps and rubella virus
7. Varicella vaccine (Var; chickenpox)
   • Administered after 12 months of age
   • Administer: 0.5 mL IM
8. Recommended immunization schedule

2 months:	HepB#1, DtaP#1, HIB#1, IPV#1
4 months:	HepB#2, DtaP#2, HIB#2, IPV#2
6 months:	HepB#3, DtaP#3, HIB#3, IPV#3
15 months:	DtaP#4, HIB#4, MMR#1, Var
18 months:	Catch up
4 to 6 years:	DtaP#5, IPV#4, MMR#2
Over 12 years:	HepB series if not vaccinated as an infant, Td every 10 years

XX. Geriatrics

■ Treatment of the aged
■ Specialized physician: gerontologist, internist

A. AGING

■ Complex physiologic, psychologic, and social process
■ Aging is not an illness; it is a normal life process
■ Changes occur in the patient's
   1. Appearance
   2. Abilities
   3. Vision
   4. Hearing
   5. Taste
   6. Smell

B. CARING FOR THE OLDER PATIENT

1. Speak slowly and distinctly if the person is hearing-impaired
2. Use indirect lighting in exam rooms to decrease glare
3. Don't carry on conversations with the patient where there is a large amount of background noise
4. Don't patronize the older patient
5. Touch the older patient as you would any other patient
6. Touch the older patient politely and affectionately, not in a controlling manner
7. Use eye contact when conversing with the older patient
8. Offer assistance to the older patient as needed
9. Treat the older patient as an individual
10. Reinforce treatment instructions by writing them down
11. Never approach a visually impaired person without making your presence known; identify yourself and others in the room

C. PROBLEMS ASSOCIATED WITH AGING

1. Inability to perform personal care, including bathing, dressing, eating, getting out of bed, and using the toilet
2. Inability to live independently, including preparing meals, shopping, managing money, using the phone, and doing housework
3. Functioning such as walking, climbing stairs, lifting, and standing for periods of time

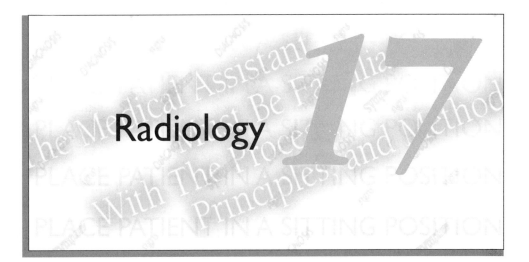

Radiology

A. INTRODUCTION
- High-energy, invisible, electromagnetic waves
- Have the ability to penetrate body structures
- Discovered by Wilhelm Konrad Roentgen in 1895
- Some states limit radiology practices concerning medical assistants (limited radiography license)

B. FUNCTIONS
1. Reveals the presence and position of foreign bodies
2. Reveals the presence of fractures and/or abnormalities of bones
3. Reveals the size and shape of organs
4. Destroys pathological cells

C. EQUIPMENT
1. Table
   - Supports the patient's body
   - Contains grids and Bucky for film placement
2. X-ray tube
   - Glass vacuum tube that produces and transmits the X-rays
3. Collimator
   - Apparatus below the tube that permits the X-ray beam
4. Control panel
   - Allows control of X-ray emissions
   - Regulates the machine
   - Should be located behind lead-lined wall so that the operator is protected from the rays
   a) Main switch: turns machine on and off
   b) Milliamperes (MA) setting: sets the amount of radiation that comes from the tube
   c) Time switch: number of seconds the patient is exposed to the X-rays
   d) Kilovolts peak (KVP) setting: penetrating power of the X-ray beam
   e) Bucky switch: turns on the Bucky
   f) Exposure switch: takes the X-ray
5. Grid
   - Absorbs the scattered radiation
   - Prevents blurring of the film

- Placed between the patient and the film to reduce secondary wave interference
6. Potter-Bucky diaphragm (Bucky)
   - Framelike structure under the table
   - Holds the grid above the film
   - Used when thicker body parts are X-rayed
7. Cassette
   - Device that holds the film
8. Intensifying screen
   - Special plates located within the cassette
   - Reduces the amount of time the patient is exposed to radiation
9. X-ray film
   - Coated with special material that is sensitive to X-rays
   - Creates a visible record
   - Film that receives X-ray appears black and gray; film that does not receive X-ray appears white; the more dense the object, the lighter the image is on the film
   - Use only under safety light in a darkroom to avoid exposure
   - Common sizes are 5×7, 8×10, 10×12, 11×14, 14×17
10. View box
   - Lighted box for viewing the developed X-ray film
11. Caliper
   - Measures the thickness of body parts

D. SAFETY
1. Hazards
   - Radiation has a cumulative effect on the body
   - Exposure damages body cells, especially gametes and the developing fetus
   - Eye exposure can cause cataracts
   - Exposure over a long period of time may cause cancer, sterility, or genetic defects
   - High exposure over a short period of time may cause radiation sickness (nausea, vomiting, diarrhea, hair loss)

2. Precautions
- Appropriate equipment in good condition
- Prevent exposure to gonads by using lead shields or lead aprons
- Always ask women of childbearing age whether there is any chance they are pregnant; if so, the physician must approve the X-ray procedure
- Wear a dosimeter (X-ray badge that contains reactive material that is sensitive to radiation); the badge must be checked periodically to measure the technician's exposure level
- Wear the lead shield or lead apron

E. PATIENT POSITIONING (see Figure 17-1)
- The body part nearest the film gives the greatest detail
  1. AP (anteroposterior): X-ray beam enters the anterior of the surface and exits the posterior of the surface before it hits the film
  2. PA (posteroanterior): X-ray beam enters the posterior of the surface and exits the anterior of the surface before it hits the film
  3. Lateral: X-ray beam passes from one side to the other side before hitting the film; this X-ray order may be right lateral (from the right to the left side) or left lateral
  4. Oblique: X-ray beam passes through the part at an angle

F. PROCEDURE
  1. Select the film and load the cassette in the darkroom
  2. Identify the film
     - Each film is permanently identified
     - Include the patient's name, number, and date of the X-ray
     - Indicate right or left
  3. Position the patient in the center of the film
  4. Measure the body part through the most dense area

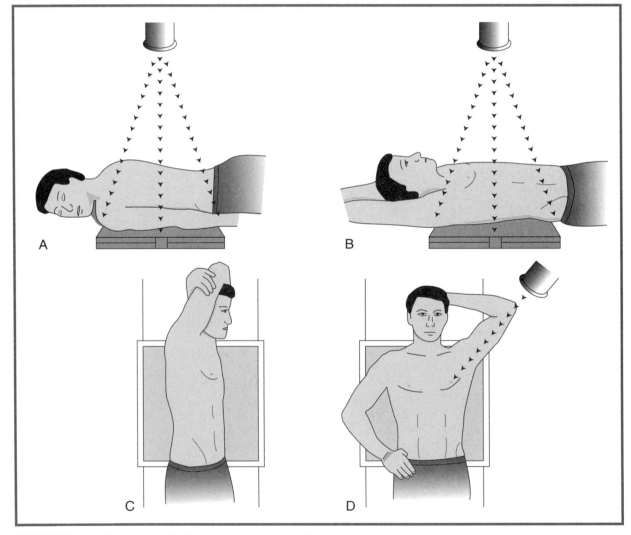

FIGURE 17-1   Positioning the patient for radiological studies. *A,* Posteroanterior view. *B,* Anteroposterior view. *C,* Lateral view. *D,* Oblique view. (From Kinn ME, Woods MA: The Medical Assistant, Administrative and Clinical, ed 8, Philadelphia, 1998, Saunders, p. 819.)

5. Shield the patient with the lead shield or lead apron
6. Place the X-ray film
   - Tabletop: most common use; the film cassette is placed on the table 40 inches from the tube
   - Bucky: the film cassette is placed in the tray under the table
   - Wall mount: the film is placed in the wall stand 72 inches from the tube
7. Position the X-ray tube directly over the body part
8. Adjust the controls
9. Position self behind the lead wall
10. Take the film

G. DARKROOM
- Place where the film is handled and developed
- Lit by a safety light
- Film developer may be manual or automatic
- Development technique includes
  1. Developer
  2. Water bath
  3. Fixer
- Film should be handled by the edges only and be attached to a metal hanger
- After the film is developed and dried, it is placed in a storage envelope or file
- Use a developing timer
- Keep undeveloped film in a lead-lined vault

H. SPECIAL X-RAY STUDIES
1. Angiogram: contrast medium is injected IV; can determine cardiovascular disease
2. Arteriogram: similar to angiogram but specifically studies the arteries
3. Barium enema (Lower GI series): contrast medium is instilled into the colon; test is used to visualize the lower intestines
4. Barium meal (Upper GI series): contrast medium is orally administered; test is used to visualize the esophagus and stomach

5. Bronchogram: contrast medium is administered through the trachea and into the bronchial tree; can detect cancer and other lung disorders
6. Cholecystogram: tablet form of contrast medium is ingested by the patient the night before the procedure; the gallbladder is observed on film
7. Hysterosalpingogram: contrast medium is injected into the fallopian tubes; can detect the patency of the tubes
8. Kidney, ureter, bladder (KUB): basic flat X-ray of the abdominal area
9. Intravenous pyelogram (IVP): contrast medium is injected IV; pathway of the medium (dye) is observed as it is excreted; the outline of the ureters and bladder can be visualized; films are taken at intervals until the dye is completely passed
10. Mammogram: X-ray of the breast; can detect cancer or abnormalities
11. Computed tomography (CT scan, CAT scan): radiographic technique that produces a picture that represents a detailed cross section of tissue structures; more sensitive than X-rays
12. Magnetic resonance imaging (MRI): uses a combination of radio waves and magnetic field to produce images of soft tissues
13. Fluoroscopy: X-ray exam that permits visualization of internal body structures; contrast medium is used; motion of a body part can be observed
14. Ultrasound: not a radiologic procedure; permits visualization of internal structures by the use of high-frequency sound waves; the sound waves echo off the body part and are displayed on a screen; useful for observation of obstetric and soft tissue (brain, eye, breast, reproductive) organs

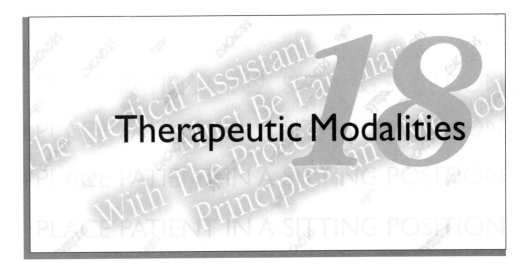

Therapeutic Modalities

■ Use of heat, cold, massage, water, exercise, and/or electricity to restore normal function to injured tissues; physical therapy

■ Objectives include
1. Relief of the patient's pain
2. Increase or improve the patient's circulation
3. Increase or restore the patient's muscle function
4. Improve the patient's strength, range of motion, and joint mobility

■ Physical therapy program may be prescribed by a physician and implemented by a physical therapist

A. HEAT APPLICATION (THERMOTHERAPY)

■ Relieves pain, inflammation, and congestion

■ Promotes muscle relaxation
1. Local effects
   a) Dilation of blood vessels, which results in increased blood supply and tissue metabolism
   b) Increases nutrients and oxygen to area and elimination of waste products
2. Types of heat therapies
   a) Infrared therapy
      ▪ Administered by a heat lamp
      ▪ Lamp placed 2 to 4 feet from the affected area for 15 to 20 minutes
   b) Diathermy
      ▪ Electrical field that produces deep heat penetration
      ▪ Commonly used for muscular injuries and inflammation in joints
      ▪ Can be
        1) Microwave: electromagnetic radiation
        2) Shortwave: high-frequency current
        3) Ultrasound: high-frequency sound waves
   c) Ultrasound
      ▪ High-frequency sound waves used as deep-heating agent
      ▪ Used for strains, sprains, arthritis, edema, and dislocation

      ▪ Coupling agent (oil or gel) is used to increase conductivity
      ▪ Ordered by intensity of sound waves, coupled by time
   d) Paraffin wax
      ▪ Wax is melted and heated to about 125 degrees Fahrenheit
      ▪ Affected part is immersed in the melted wax and lifted out
      ▪ Wax hardens and holds in the heat
      ▪ Used for arthritis, increase of circulation, and reduction of stiffness
   e) Hot water bag
      ▪ Rubber bag filled about one half full with hot water (115 to 125 degrees Fahrenheit)
      ▪ Bag is applied to the affected body part for the prescribed period of time
      ▪ Place some sort of covering (towel, blanket) over the body part before positioning the hot water bag
   f) Hot soaks
      ▪ Basin is filled with a warmed solution (105 to 110 degrees Fahrenheit)
      ▪ Body part is immersed in the basin for the prescribed period of time
      ▪ As the solution cools, replace it with more warmed solution
   g) Hot compress
      ▪ Immerse cloth or gauze squares in warm solution (105 to 110 degrees Fahrenheit)
      ▪ Wring out excess fluid and place the material over the affected body part
      ▪ Replace the hot compress every 2 to 3 minutes for the prescribed time

B. COLD APPLICATION (CRYOTHERAPY)

■ Prevents edema by constricting vessels

■ Applied immediately after the trauma

■ Relieves pain by numbing
1. Local effects: vascular constriction, which leads to decreased blood supply to the area, decreased tissue metabolism, and decreased accumulation of wastes

2. Types of cold therapies
   a) Ice bag
      - Ice bag is filled one half to two thirds full of ice
      - Applied to the affected area for the prescribed time
      - Place some sort of covering (towel, blanket) over the body part before positioning the ice bag
      - Check for pallor, numbness, or cyanosis and report any immediately
   b) Cold compress
      - Immerse cloth or gauze squares in a basin filled with cold water and ice
      - Wring out excess fluid and place the material over the affected body part
      - Replace the cold compress every 2 to 3 minutes for the prescribed time

C. HYDROTHERAPY
   - Use of external water applications for therapeutic purposes
   - Used for
     1. Relaxation
     2. Increased circulation
     3. Improved mobility
   - Modalities
     1. Whirlpool: moist heat with massage action
     2. Contrast baths: patient moves affected part from hot, to cold, to hot baths
     3. Underwater exercise: buoyant effect of water facilitates exercise

D. ULTRAVIOLET THERAPY (UV)
   - Produced by the sun and sunlamps
   - Capable of killing bacteria
   - Activates the formation of Vitamin D in skin
   - Used to treat acne, psoriasis, wound applications, and pressure sores
   - Cover eyes when using UV therapy

E. EXERCISE THERAPY
   - Use of body motion to help the patient regain function
   - Dosage must be constantly adjusted for the patient to benefit
   - Types include
     1. Active: patient performs the exercise
     2. Passive: exercises are performed on the patient by someone else
     3. Aided: active exercise helped by a physical aid (such as a pool)
     4. Active resistance: counterpressure is applied
     5. Range of motion: active or passive joint mobility

F. MASSAGE
   - Manipulation of external body tissues to promote healing

- Patient must be relaxed to receive benefit
- Lubricating oil or cream should be used
- Approaches
  1. Stroking: systematic movement of the hand across the patient's skin
  2. Compression: squeezing, kneading, or pressing the patient's soft tissues
  3. Percussion: thumping or striking the patient's skin with the hand

G. DEVICES TO ASSIST PATIENT MOBILITY
   1. Crutches
      - Wood or aluminum devices that serve as aids for walking
      - Patient's weight is transferred from the legs to the arms
      - Types
        a) Axillary crutches
           - Crutch that extends from the patient's axillary region to the ground
           - Used for temporary assistance
           - Measured to fit for each individual patient
        b) Lofstrand crutches
           - Cuff and handgrip that extend from the patient's forearm to the ground
           - Used by patients who require permanent walking assistance
      - Crutch gaits
        a) Four-point gait
           - Patient must be able to bear own weight on both legs
           - Used for muscle weakness
           - Right crutch moves forward, left foot moves to the level of the left crutch; left crutch moves forward and right foot moves to the level of the right crutch
        b) Three-point gait
           - Used when the patient cannot bear own weight on one leg
           - Move both crutches and weak leg forward, then move the strong leg forward while balancing on both crutches
        c) Two-point gait
           - Similar to four-point gait
           - Move the right crutch and left foot forward simultaneously, then move the left crutch and right foot forward simultaneously
        d) Swing gait
           - Used by patients with lower extremity paralysis
           - Patient moves both crutches forward simultaneously, then swings both legs through

2. Cane
- Wood or aluminum pole with a handle or handgrip
- Provides a balance point and/or support to the patient with leg weakness on one side
- Used on the side of the strong leg
- Measured so that the handle is level with the greater trochanter; the elbow should be flexed at 25 to 30 degrees
- Types
  1) Standard cane: the least amount of support; used by patients who require slight assistance
  2) Tripod cane: three legs and a bent shaft; provides greater stability because of wider support base
  3) quad cane: four legs and a bent shaft; provides the same support as a tripod

- Gait
  - Cane is held on the strong side; move the cane forward 12 inches, move the weak leg to the level of the cane, move the strong leg ahead of the weak leg and the cane
  - Patient needs to stand erect and not lean on the cane to ensure good balance and support

3. Walker
- Aluminum frame consisting of handgrips for both of the patient's hands and four squarely placed legs
- Provides optimum balance for patients with balance problems
- Gait
  - Pick up the walker and move it forward 6 inches, move the right foot, then the left foot forward into the walker, then move the walker again

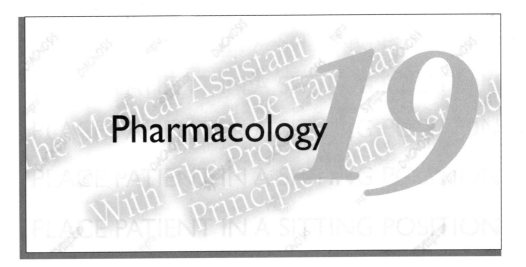

Pharmacology 19

■ Pharmacology: science that deals with the study of drugs and their actions, uses, properties, and origins

I. Drugs

■ Any substances that cause a change in body functions and/or structure

A. USES
1. Therapeutic
   - Treats diseases
   - Relieves symptoms
   - Replaces a necessary body substance
2. Prophylactic
   - Prevents disease
3. Diagnostic
   - Helps to diagnose diseases and disorders

B. SOURCES
1. Plant
   - Naturally occurring substance from plants
   - Parts used includes roots, leaves, fruits
2. Animal
   - Substances obtained from animals
   - Includes glands, organs, and tissues
3. Mineral
   - Naturally occurring substances obtained from the earth or soil
4. Synthetic
   - Artificially prepared substances
   - Prepared using chemicals and techniques in a laboratory

C. NAMES
1. Chemical name
   - Drug's chemical formula that identifies its molecular structure
2. Generic name
   - Official name of the drug
   - Not capitalized
3. Trade name
   - Brand name
   - Name owned by the manufacturer
   - Always capitalized

D. DRUG REFERENCES
1. Physician's Desk Reference (PDR)
   - Common reference book
   - Provides information on uses, precautions, indications, and dosages for a variety of drugs
   - Organized in color-coded sections
     a) Section 1 (white)
        ■ Manufacturer's Index
        ■ Lists manufacturers who have given product information for use in the book
     b) Section 2 (pink)
        ■ Product Name Index
        ■ Gives trade and generic names alphabetically
     c) Section 3 (blue)
        ■ Product Category Index
        ■ Drugs are listed according to their classification
     d) Section 4 (yellow)
        ■ Generic and Chemical Name Index
        ■ Lists drugs alphabetically according to main ingredient
     e) Section 5 (noncolored pages)
        ■ Product Identification
        ■ Color photographs of the drugs on plain-color pages
     f) Section 6 (white)
        ■ Product Information
        ■ Detailed descriptions of the drugs
2. Product insert
   - Folded sheet of paper within the drug container or box
   - Contains information similar to the information on the drug contained in the PDR
3. United States Pharmacopoeia/National Formulary (USP/NF)
   - Published every 5 years
   - All drugs listed have met federal governmental standards
4. PDR for Nonprescription Drugs
   - Similar to PDR but for over-the-counter medications

E. DRUG FORMS

1. Syrup
   - Drug is dissolved in water, mixed with sugar and flavoring
2. Solution
   - Liquid preparation containing one or more solutes dissolved in a solvent
3. Suspension
   - Drug that does not dissolve evenly in a liquid; must be shaken to mix before administration
4. Emulsion
   - Mixture of water and oil; must be shaken to mix before administration
5. Tincture
   - Drug is dissolved in alcohol
6. Elixir
   - Drug is dissolved in a mixture of water, alcohol, and sugar
7. Lotion
   - Topical preparation that is nongreasy
   - Contains suspended particles of the drug mixed in an aqueous solution
8. Liniment
   - Drug is mixed with soap, oil, or water
   - Applied topically to produce a feeling of heat and warmth
9. Aerosol
   - Drug is suspended in a liquid and administered in a spray/aerosol form
10. Capsule
    - Powdered or liquid drug within a gelatin capsule
11. Gelcap
    - Drug contained within gelatin-coated capsule
12. Spansule
    - Granulated drug is enclosed within a capsule
    - Designed to release the drug at various times after ingestion
13. Tablet
    - Powdered medication is compressed into a disk shape
    - May be scored for breaking into halves or quarters
    - May be enteric-coated for dissolution in intestines instead of stomach
14. Caplet
    - Capsule-shaped tablet
15. Geltab
    - Gelatin-coated tablet
16. Suppository
    - Drug is mixed with a base of fat or wax
    - Shaped into a cone or cylinder
    - Made to be inserted into the rectum, vagina, or urethra
    - Suppository dissolves at body temperature
17. Ointment
    - Semisolid preparation
    - Drug is combined with oil or fat; topically applied
18. Lozenge (troche)
    - Medicine is mixed within a candylike base made to be dissolved within the mouth

F. TRANSACTIONS

1. Prescribe: an order for a medication by a practitioner
2. Administer: to give a medication that has been prescribed
3. Dispense: to prepare and give out to a patient
4. All practitioners who prescribe, administer, or dispense controlled substances MUST register with the Drug Enforcement Agency (DEA)
   - Practitioner receives a DEA registration number that is valid for 3 years
   - All controlled substances MUST be stored separately apart from other medications within the office; MUST be kept locked
   - Separate records MUST be kept of all controlled substances
   - Controlled substance inventory MUST be counted and recorded daily
   - Discarded liquid controlled substances must be poured down the sink drains
   - Discarded solid controlled substances must be crushed and flushed down the toilet

G. DRUG REGULATIONS AND CONTROLS

1. Controlled Substances Act of 1970
   - Federal legislation designed to control dispensing of drugs that have a high potential for abuse
   - Five schedules, based on medical usefulness and potential for abuse
   a) Schedule I
      - Drugs with a high potential for abuse and no acceptable medical use
      - Examples: heroin, LSD
   b) Schedule II
      - Drugs with some accepted medical use but high potential for abuse
      - Examples: morphine, cocaine
   c) Schedule III
      - Drugs with moderate abuse potential; require prescription with refills limited to 5 within 6 months
      - Example: Tylenol with codeine
   d) Schedule IV
      - Drugs with low abuse potential; prescription is limited to 5 refills within 6 months
      - Example: Valium

e) Schedule V
- Low abuse potential, may be purchased over the counter, depending on the state's laws
- Examples: Contac, Drixoral

2. Federal Food, Drug and Cosmetic Act
   - Allows FDA (Food and Drug Administration) to protect the public by requiring rigid standards for drug development
3. Drug Enforcement Agency
   - Responsible for controlling narcotics abuse and illegal sales of drugs

H. PHARMACOKINETICS

- Study of how drugs are used within the body
- Process includes

1. Absorption
   - How a drug enters the body
   - Depends on how the drug is administered
2. Distribution
   - How a drug is transported from the site of administration to the site(s) of action
3. Action
   - Changes that the drug causes when it reaches the site(s) of action
4. Biotransformation
   - How the drug is inactivated
   - Usually occurs within the liver
5. Elimination
   - Route by which the drug is eliminated from the body

II. Prescriptions (see Figure 19-1)

- An order written by the practitioner for the compounding, dispensing, and administration of a particular drug for a particular patient
- A prescription is a legal document
- It is acceptable to use common/accepted abbreviations when writing a prescription

A. PARTS OF A PRESCRIPTION

1. Preprinted physician's name, address, phone number, and DEA number
2. Date the prescription was written
3. Patient's name, address, phone number, and age (if a child)
4. Superscription
   - Symbol "Rx" which means "take thou"
5. Inscription
   - Name, form, and strength of drug prescribed
6. Subscription
   - Practitioner's instructions to the pharmacist
   - Includes the number of doses prescribed and special preparations
7. Signature
   - "Sig" (label)
   - Patient instructions for taking the drug

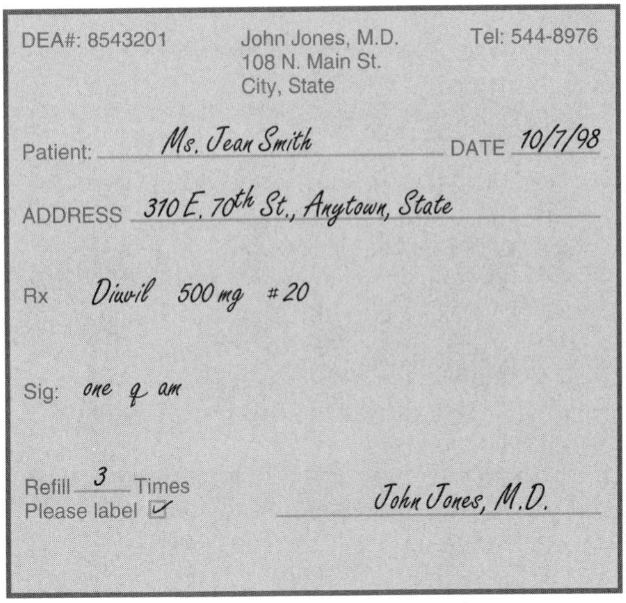
DEA#: 8543201
John Jones, M.D.
108 N. Main St.
City, State
Tel: 544-8976

Patient: Ms. Jean Smith DATE 10/7/98

ADDRESS 310 E. 70th St., Anytown, State

Rx Diuril 500 mg #20

Sig: one q am

Refill 3 Times
Please label ☑
John Jones, M.D.

FIGURE 19-1 A sample prescription. (From Kinn ME, Woods MA: The Medical Assistant, Administrative and Clinical, ed 8, Philadelphia, 1998, Saunders, p. 1000.)

8. Refill information:
   - Number of refills allowed for the prescription, if any
9. Practitioner's handwritten signature

B. PRESCRIPTION PADS

- Kept locked up except when being used
- NEVER presign blank prescription forms
- NEVER use blank prescription forms for scratch paper
- NEVER leave blank pads in examination rooms

III. Drug Classifications

A. ANTI-INFECTIVES: TREAT, PREVENT INFECTIONS

1. Antibiotic: destroys or inhibits the growth of microorganisms
2. Antifungal: kills or prevents the growth of fungi and yeast
3. Antiviral: prevents or treats viral infections
4. Antiparasitic: prevents or treats parasitic infections

B. DERMATOLOGY AGENTS

1. Antiacneic: treats acne vulgaris
2. Antiseptic: kills or inhibits the growth of microorganisms
3. Anesthetic: causes loss of sensation, local numbing
4. Emollient: soothes skin and mucous membranes
5. Keratolytic: causes sloughing of hardened skin

C. MUSCULOSKELETAL AGENTS

1. Antiarthritic: treats arthritis
2. Antigout: treats gout (gouty arthritis)

3. Anti-inflammatory: decreases inflammation
4. Muscle relaxant: aids in the relaxation of skeletal muscles

D. CARDIOVASCULAR AGENTS
1. Angiotensin-converting enzyme (ACE) inhibitor: decreases blood pressure
2. Antianginal: reduces chest pain
3. Antiarrhythmic: regulates the heart rhythm and rate
4. Anticoagulant: prevents or delays blood clotting
5. Antihypertensive: decreases blood pressure
6. Calcium channel blocker: decreases blood pressure
7. Cardiotonic: increases heart muscle strength
8. Hematenic: increases blood iron levels
9. Hemostatic: controls or stops bleeding
10. Vasoconstrictor: constricts blood vessels, raises blood pressure
11. Vasodilator: dilates blood vessels, lowers blood pressure

E. ENDOCRINE AGENTS
1. Contraceptive: prevents conception/pregnancy
2. Hypoglycemic: lowers blood glucose levels
3. Thyroid: replaces thyroid hormones
4. Hormone replacement therapy (HRT): replaces hormones lost through surgery, disease processes, aging, and so on

F. NERVOUS SYSTEM AGENTS
1. CNS stimulant: increases brain and body activity
2. CNS depressant: decreases brain and body activity
3. Analgesic: relieves pain
   a) Narcotic agents: highly addictive
   b) Non-narcotic agents
4. Antipyretic: reduces fever
5. Anticonvulsant: controls seizure activity
6. Antidepressant: relieves depression
7. Tranquilizer: reduces anxiety; calms the patient
8. Sedative: produces relaxation
9. Hypnotic: induces sleep

G. RESPIRATORY AGENTS
1. Antihistamine: relieves allergic symptoms; reduces secretions
2. Antitussive: suppresses cough
3. Bronchodilator: opens air passages (bronchi)
4. Decongestant: relieves congestion in respiratory tract
5. Expectorant: liquifies mucus; helps to expel secretions

H. GASTROINTESTINAL AGENTS
1. Antacid: neutralizes stomach acid
2. Antiemetic: prevents nausea and vomiting
3. Antidiarrheal: controls or stops diarrhea
4. Cathartic/laxative: relieves constipation
5. Emetic: induces vomiting
6. Antispasmotic: prevents, controls, spasms of the GI tract
7. Antiulcer: treats gastric or duodenal ulcers

I. URINARY AGENTS
1. Diuretic: promotes or increases urination

J. CANCER AGENTS
1. Antineoplastic: inhibits growth of malignant cells

IV. 50 Most-Prescribed Drugs of 1999

1. Premarin
   • Generic: estrogen
   • Classification: hormone replacement
   • Treatment: hormone replacement
2. Synthroid
   • Generic: levothyroxine
   • Classification: hormone replacement
   • Treatment: hypothyroidism
3. Lipitor
   • Generic: atorvastatin
   • Classification: antilipemic
   • Treatment: high cholesterol
4. Prilosic
   • Generic: omeprazole
   • Classification: antiulcer
   • Treatment: ulcers, acid reflux
5. Hydrocodone with APAP
   • Generic: same
   • Classification: analgesic
   • Treatment: pain
6. Albuterol
   • Generic: salbetamol
   • Classification: bronchodilator
   • Treatment: asthma
7. Norvasc
   • Generic: amlodipine
   • Classification: antianginal
   • Treatment: angina
8. Claritin
   • Generic: loratadine
   • Classification: antihistamine
   • Treatment: seasonal allergies
9. Trimox
   • Generic: amoxicillin
   • Classification: anti-infective
   • Treatment: infection, UTI
10. Prozac
   • Generic: fluoxetine
   • Classification: antidepressant
   • Treatment: depression
11. Zoloft
   • Generic: sertraline
   • Classification: antidepressant
   • Treatment: depression

12. Glucophage
    - Generic: metformin
    - Classification: antidiabetic
    - Treatment: diabetes
13. Lenoxin
    - Generic: digoxin
    - Classification: cardiotonic
    - Treatment: arrhythmia, CHF
14. Prempro
    - Generic: estrogen and progesterone
    - Classification: hormone replacement
    - Treatment: hormone replacement, menopause
15. Paxil
    - Generic: paroxitine
    - Classification: antidepressant
    - Treatment: depression
16. Zithromax Z-pak
    - Generic: azithromycin
    - Classification: anti-infective
    - Treatment: infections
17. Zestril
    - Generic: lisinopril
    - Classification: antihypertensive
    - Treatment: hypertension
18. Zocor
    - Generic: simvastatin
    - Classification: antilipemic
    - Treatment: high cholesterol
19. Prevacid
    - Generic: lansoprazole
    - Classification: antiulcer
    - Treatment: ulcers
20. Augmentin
    - Generic: amoxicillin/clavulanate
    - Classification: anti-infective
    - Treatment: respiratory and ear infections
21. Celebrex
    - Generic: celecoxib
    - Classification: anti-inflammatory
    - Treatment: arthritis
22. Coumadin
    - Generic: warfarin sodium
    - Classification: anticoagulant
    - Treatment: embolism, MI
23. Vasotic
    - Generic: enalapril
    - Classification: antihypertensive
    - Treatment: hypertension
24. Amoxicillin trihydrate
    - Generic: amoxicillin trihydrate
    - Classification: anti-infective
    - Treatment: systemic infections
25. Furosemide (Lasix)
    - Generic: furosemide
    - Classification: diuretic
    - Treatment: edema, HTN
26. Levoxyl
    - Generic: levothyraxine sodium
    - Classification: hormone replacement
    - Treatment: thyroid replacement
27. Cipro
    - Generic: ciprofloracin
    - Classification: anti-infective
    - Treatment: infections
28. Cephalexin
    - Generic: cephalexin monohydrate
    - Classification: anti-infective
    - Treatment: infections
29. K-Dur
    - Generic: potassium chloride
    - Classification: hormone replacement
    - Treatment: hormone replacement
30. Prednisone
    - Generic: prednisone
    - Classification: anti-inflammatory
    - Treatment: severe inflammation, immunosuppression
31. Pravachol
    - Generic: pravastatin sodium
    - Classification: antilipemic
    - Treatment: high blood lipid levels
32. Amoxil
    - Generic: amoxicillin
    - Classification: anti-infective
    - Treatment: URI, UTI
33. Trimethoprim/sulfate
    - Generic: same
    - Classification: anti-infective
    - Treatment: UTI
34. Biaxin
    - Generic: clarithromycin
    - Classification: anti-infective
    - Treatment: infection, URI
35. Ortho-Tri-Cyclen 28
    - Generic: ethinyl estradiol and norethindrone
    - Classification: contraceptive (triphasic)
    - Treatment: birth control
36. Acetaminophen with codeine
    - Generic: same
    - Classification: narcotic analgesic
    - Treatment: pain
37. Tenormin
    - Generic: atenolol
    - Classification: antihypertensive
    - Treatment: hypertension
38. Zyrtec
    - Generic: cetirizine
    - Classification: antihistamine
    - Treatment: seasonal allergies
39. Ambien
    - Generic: imidazopyridine
    - Classification: hypnotic
    - Treatment: insomnia

40. Darvon
    - Generic: propoxyphine-N
    - Classification: narcotic analgesic
    - Treatment: pain
41. Xanax
    - Generic: alprazolam
    - Classification: anti-anxiety
    - Treatment: anxiety
42. Ultram
    - Generic: tramadol
    - Classification: non-narcotic analgesic
    - Treatment: pain
43. Accupril
    - Generic: quinapril
    - Classification: antihypertensive
    - Treatment: hypertension
44. Prinivil
    - Generic: lisinopril
    - Classification: antihypertensive
    - Treatment: hypertension
45. Cardizem CD
    - Generic: diltiazem
    - Classification: antianginal
    - Treatment: angina
46. Glucotrol XL
    - Generic: glipizide
    - Classification: antidiabetic
    - Treatment: diabetes
47. Allegra
    - Generic: fixofinadine
    - Classification: antihistamine
    - Treatment: allergies
48. Toprol-XL
    - Generic: metoprolol
    - Classification: antihypertensive
    - Treatment: hypertension
49. HCTZ (hydrochlorothiazide)
    - Generic: same
    - Classification: diuretic
    - Treatment: edema and hypertension
50. Flonase
    - Generic: fluticasone
    - Classification: antihistamine
    - Treatment: allergic rhinitis

V. Calculation of Dosages

A. METRIC SYSTEM
- Based on multiples of 10
- Used to weigh and measure
    1. Basic units of measure
        a) Gram (g): used to measure solids
        b) Liter (L): used to measure liquids (volume)
        c) Meter (m): used to measure length
    2. Basic metric prefixes
        a) Micro-: one millionth (0.000001)
        b) Milli-: one thousandth (0.001)
        c) Centi-: one hundreth (0.01)
        d) Deci-: one tenth (0.1)
        e) Unit (g, m, L): "one" (1.0)
        f) Deka-: ten (10.0)
        g) Hecto-: one hundred (100.0)
        h) Kilo-: one thousand (1000.0)
        i) Mega-: one million (1000000.0)
    3. Metric conversion
        a) Changing from larger unit to smaller unit
            1) Multiply by the number of smaller units that are in the larger unit
            2) Move the decimal point to the right the number of places equal to the number of zeros found in the smaller unit
        b) Changing from smaller unit to larger unit
            1) Divide by the number of smaller units that are in the larger unit
            2) Move the decimal point to the left the number of places equal to the number of zeros in the smaller unit

B. ADULT DOSAGE CALCULATION
- Dosage given is dosage ordered divided by the available strength times the dosage form
$$\frac{\text{dosage ordered}}{\text{available}} \times \text{form} = \text{dosage given}$$
    1. Dosage given: amount administered to the patient to fill the practitioner's order
    2. Dosage ordered: amount of drug the practitioner orders be given to the patient
    3. Available strength: concentration of medicine on hand
    4. Dosage form: number of tablets (or capsules) or amount of liquid that contains the available strength
- Example: practitioner orders 500 mg Amoxicillin; 250 mg/cap Amoxicillin is available
$$\frac{500 \text{ mg}}{250 \text{ mg}} \times 1 = 2 - 250 \text{ mg caps administered}$$

C. PEDIATRIC DOSAGE CALCULATION
    1. Young's rule
        - Used for children under 12, based on age
        - Formula: child's age, divided by (child's age + 12), multiplied by average adult dose, gives the amount administered to the child
    2. Fried's rule
        - Used for infants and children under age 2, based on age in months
        - Formula: infant's age in months, divided by 150, multiplied by the average adult dose, gives the amount administered to the child
    3. Clark's rule
        - Used for children under 12, based on weight in pounds
        - Formula: (child's weight in pounds divided by 150) multiplied by the average adult dose, gives the amount administered to the child

VI. Administration of Medications

A. ROUTES OF ADMINISTRATION

1. Buccal: medication is placed between cheek and gum and dissolves
2. Oral: medication is administered by mouth and swallowed
3. Sublingual: medication is placed under the tongue and dissolves
4. Inhalation: medication is delivered to lungs by means of a nebulizer (inhaler unit)
5. Topical: medication is externally applied to skin, eyes, ears, nose, or mucous membranes
6. Vaginal: medication is inserted into, or applied to, the vagina
7. Rectal: medication is inserted into the rectum and absorbed
8. Parenteral: medication is administered by a needle

B. SEVEN "RIGHTS" OF ADMINISTRATION

1. The right patient
2. The right drug
3. The right dose
4. The right route
5. The right time
6. The right technique
7. The right documentation

C. SAFETY

1. Three "befores": read the drug label 3 times when preparing the medication
   - Before removing the medication from storage
   - Before preparing the medication for administration
   - Before replacing the medication back in storage
2. Be familiar with the drug; use references
3. Prepare medication in a clean, quiet, well-lit area, away from distractions
4. Do NOT use a medication that does not appear normal (changes in color, odor, or appearance of sediment in the medication)
5. Check the expiration date; NEVER administer a date-expired medication
6. Verify the patient's identity before administering (call by name; ask patient their name)
7. Always check for allergies
8. Correctly chart the procedure: include date, time, medication, dose, route, patient reactions, medical assistant's initials

D. CONSIDERATIONS

1. Age: children and the elderly require smaller doses
2. Sex: women require smaller doses than men
3. Weight: smaller patients require smaller doses
4. Tolerance: a patient who has taken this medication over a long period of time may require a larger dose for required results
5. Condition of the patient: physical and psychological conditions
6. Route: parenteral medications are absorbed more quickly than oral medications
7. Timing: medications are absorbed more quickly on an empty stomach

E. ALLERGIC REACTIONS

1. Mild reaction: rash, pruritis, rhinitis
2. Severe reaction: pruritis, edema, dyspnea, cyanosis, shock; untreated, this can lead to coma and/or death
3. Prevention
   a) Monitor the patient after administration of the drug
   b) Observe the patient for signs and symptoms
   c) Notify the practitioner immediately of any reaction
   d) Be prepared to provide emergency assistance

VII. Parenteral Administration

A. EQUIPMENT

1. Syringe (see Figure 19-2)
   - Parts include
   a) Barrel: holds medication; calibrated for measuring (cc/mL and minims)
   b) Flange: rim at the end of the barrel; place to put the fingers while depressing the plunger and keeps the syringe from rolling off a flat surface

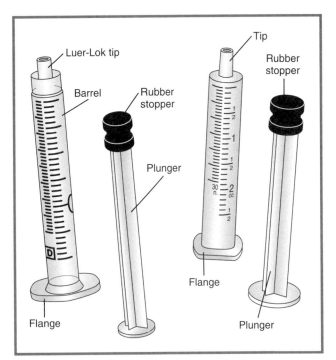

FIGURE 19-2 Parts of a syringe. (From Kinn ME, Woods MA: The Medical Assistant, Administrative and Clinical, ed 8, Philadelphia, 1998, Saunders, p. 1038.)

c) Plunger: fits inside the barrel; brings the medication into and out of the barrel
d) Tip: end of the barrel where the needle attaches
• Types include (see Figure 19-3)
    a) Regular hypodermic
        ▪ Most commonly calibrated in 2 cc, 3 cc, 5 cc, or 10 cc
        ▪ May be disposable (plastic) or nondisposable (glass)
        ▪ May come with needle attached or without needle
    b) Tuberculin (TB)
        ▪ Small syringe calibrated in 0.1 cc
        ▪ Holds up to a total volume of 1.0 cc
    c) Insulin
        ▪ Calibrated in units (U40, U80, U100)
        ▪ Used for insulin injections
        ▪ Syringe must correspond to the type of insulin prescribed
    d) Tubex, carpuject
        ▪ Closed injection system
        ▪ Disposable medication cartridge/needle unit fits into a reusable plastic or metal holder

2. Needle (see Figure 19-4)
    • Parts include
        a) Hub: the part of the needle that connects to the syringe
        b) Shaft: length of the needle; inserted into the body
        c) Point: sharpened end of the shaft
        d) Lumen: inside opening of the shaft
        e) Bevel: slant of the point
    • Measured by
        a) Gauge: size of the lumen
            ▪ The smaller the gauge, the larger the needle
            ▪ 13G to 27G
        b) Length
            ▪ Varies according to use
            ▪ 1/4 inch to 6 inch
B. ADMINISTRATION
    1. Intradermal (ID)
        a) Needle and syringe size
            ▪ Syringes: TB (1 cc)
            ▪ Needle gauge: 26G to 27G
            ▪ Needle length: 3/8 inch to 1/2 inch
        b) Sites
            ▪ Anterior forearm
            ▪ Midback

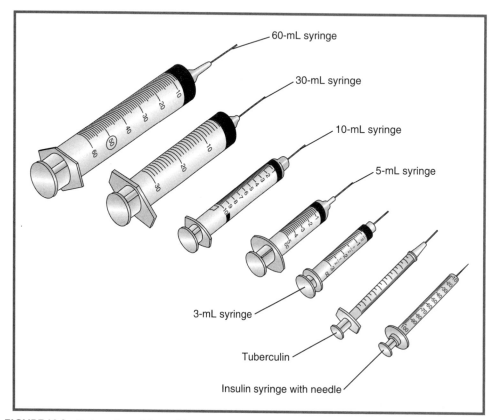

FIGURE 19-3   Various sizes of disposable syringes. (From Kinn ME, Woods MA: The Medical Assistant, Administrative and Clinical, ed 8, Philadelphia, 1998, Saunders, p. 1039.)

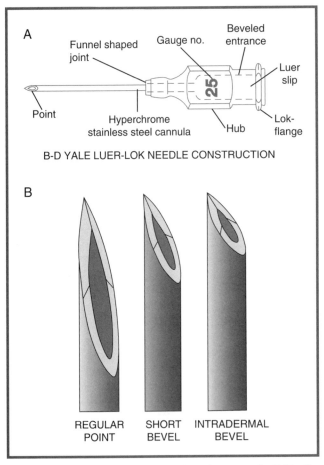

FIGURE 19-4 *A,* The construction of a hypodermic needle. *B,* Needle points. (From Kinn ME, Woods MA: The Medical Assistant, Administrative and Clinical, ed 8, Philadelphia, 1998, Saunders, p. 1038.)

c) Uses of route
- Allergy skin testing
- TB skin testing medication (Mantoux/ PPD)

d) Injection angle: 10 to 15 degrees (with bevel facing up)

e) Goal of injection: formation of a wheal

f) Amount given: 0.01 to 0.02 cc

2. Intramuscular (IM)

a) Needle and syringe size
- Syringe: 1 cc to 2 cc (depending on the amount administered)
- Needle gauge: 22G to 25G (depending on the area of the body and the consistency of the medication)
- Needle length: 5/8 inch to 2 inches (depending on the size of the patient and the consistency of the medication)

b) Sites
- Deltoid (not for infant or small child)
- Dorsogluteal (not for infant or small child)
- Vastus lateralis (used for infants and small children)

c) Uses of route
- Adult and childhood immunizations (deltoid and vastus)
- Thick or oil-based medications (gluteal)

d) Injection angle: 90 degrees

e) Goal of injection: to deliver medication into muscle tissue

f) Amount given
- less than 2 cc (deltoid and vastus)
- 2 to 5 cc (gluteal)

3. Subcutaneous (SQ, subq, SC)

a) Needle and syringe size
- Syringe: insulin, TB, or 2 to 3 cc syringe
- Needle gauge: 25G to 27G
- Needle length: 3/8 inch to 5/8 inch

b) Sites
- Upper arm (under deltoid, back of arm)
- Thigh
- Back
- Abdomen
- Any area where there is fat

c) Uses of route
- Insulin
- Allergy injections
- MMR immunization
- Epinephrine

d) Injection angle: 45 degrees

e) Goal of injection: delivery of medication into subcutaneous (fatty) tissue

f) Amount given: less than 2 cc

Clinical Lab 20

I. Orientation to the Lab

A. LAB DEPARTMENTS

1. Blood bank
   - Analyzes blood and blood components for transfusions
   - Examples: type and cross-match
2. Chemistry
   - Analyzes blood and body fluids for presence and quantity of chemical substances
   - Examples: glucose, cholesterol, electrolytes
3. Cytology/Histology
   - Examines cells and tissues to diagnose diseases
   - Examples: Pap smear, biopsy
4. Hematology
   - Performs tests on blood and blood components
   - Examples: CBC, sed rate, coagulation studies
5. Microbiology
   - Identification and study of pathogenic microorganisms
   - Includes bacteriology (bacteria), parasitology (parasites), and virology (viruses)
6. Serology
   - Examination of blood to detect diseases through antigen/antibody reactions
   - Examples: rubella titer, mononucleosis testing

B. LAB PERSONNEL

1. Pathologist: physician in charge of the lab
2. Medical technologist: bachelor's degree-prepared lab technician
3. Medical lab technician: lab technician who has completed 1 to 2 years of training
4. Phlebotomist: obtains blood samples from patients

C. OSHA STANDARDS

1. Hazard communication standard
   a) Employer must provide information and training to employees who are exposed to hazardous agents (chemicals, noise, radiation, infectious agents)
   b) Standards must be in writing and include
      1) Training outline
      2) List of hazards and MSDS forms
      3) Warning and labeling system
      4) Method of informing employees
   c) MSDS (Material Safety Data Sheets)
      - Must be kept for each hazardous substance on-site
      - Prepared by manufacturer
      - Describe chemical and physical properties, hazards, precautions, and first aid
      - Signs posted in lab
   d) All hazardous agents must be labeled
      1) Name of hazardous substance
      2) Specific product warnings
      3) Name and address of manufacturer
2. Blood-borne pathogen standard
   a) Disease-causing microorganisms transmitted through blood and body fluids
   b) OSHA requires employers to ensure the safety of employees and provide training about exposure
   c) Blood-borne pathogens transmitted when contaminated blood or body fluids come into contact with nonintact skin or mucous membranes of another person
   d) Prevention includes
      - Engineering controls: structural/mechanical devices that minimize exposure (sharps containers, eyewash stations)
      - Work practice controls: promotion of behaviors necessary to use the engineering controls properly
      - Personal protective equipment (PPE): equipment that decreases exposure (gloves, masks, lab aprons)
      - Standard precautions: concept that all bodily secretions should be treated as if they are contaminated
      - Body secretions include
         1) Blood and body fluids containing blood
         2) Semen

3) Cerebrospinal fluid
4) Saliva
5) Sputum
6) Vaginal secretions
7) Feces
8) Urine
9) Sweat and tears
10) Vomitus
11) Unidentifiable body fluids

D. LAB SAFETY
1. Post evacuation routes
2. Post emergency phone numbers (fire, police, poison control)
3. First aid kit accessible and up to date
4. Safety equipment accessible, and in working order
   • Eyewash station
   • Shower
   • Fire extinguisher
5. Lab coats or aprons worn at all times; remove before leaving the lab
6. Hair is pulled back; only minimal jewelry is allowed; fingernails are short
7. Dispose of sharps and broken glass immediately in a puncture-resistant container
8. Observe hazard identification labels
9. Work under the hood in a well-ventilated area when working with chemicals
10. NEVER pipette by mouth
11. Close all reagent containers when not in use
12. Label all reagent containers with name, expiration date, date of preparation, and preparer's initials
13. Pour acids into water when preparing solutions
14. Properly ground all electrical equipment
15. Wash hands after handling specimens and before leaving the lab
16. Do not eat, drink, smoke, apply makeup, or handle contact lenses in the lab
17. Do not store food in the lab refrigerator
18. Do not recap, break, or bend contaminated needles
19. Cap all tubes before centrifuging
20. Dispose of all contaminated nonsharps in labeled biohazard containers (red trash can or red trash bag)

E. CLINICAL LABORATORY IMPROVEMENT ACT OF 1988 (CLIA '88)
   ■ Legislation developed to regulate testing of specimens to diagnose, prevent, and treat diseases and disorders
   ■ Enforced by CDC and HCFA
   ■ Lab must be in compliance with CLIA to receive Medicare/Medicaid reimbursement

■ 3 main standards
1. Personnel standards
   • Identify qualifications of persons directing or performing testing
   • Qualifications depend on the complexity levels of the testing
2. Testing standards
   • Identify the tests that fall into one of three levels of complexity
      a) Waived tests
         ▪ Not subject to personnel or quality assurance requirements
         ▪ Common in medical office (POL)
      b) Moderately complex tests
      c) Highly complex tests
3. Quality assurance standards
   • Identify quality assurance requirements for qualified labs
   • Apply only to labs that perform moderately and highly complex testing
   • Standards include
      a) Written policies and standards
      b) Personnel training
      c) Procedure manual
      d) Maintenance, and documentation of the maintenance, of instruments
      e) Quality control documentation
      f) Proficiency testing

II. Collection of Specimens

A. URINE
   ■ Sterile liquid waste product
   ■ Should be analyzed within 30 minutes of collection but may be refrigerated for up to 8 hours
   ■ Specimen types include
   1. First-morning specimen
      • Specimen of choice
      • Most concentrated
   2. Random specimen
      • Specimen collected at any time of the day
   3. Midstream specimen
      • Used for routine urinalysis
      • Patient is instructed to retract foreskin or labia, void the first portion of the urine stream into the toilet, collect the midportion of the stream into a sterile container, and void the remaining portion of the stream into the toilet
      • Properly label the container
   4. Clean-catch specimen
      • Used for culture
      • Patient is instructed to thoroughly cleanse the glans penis or urethral meatus with an antiseptic solution, continue with the midstream specimen collection technique, and collect in a sterile container

5. Twenty-four-hour specimen
   • Used to measure volume
   • Used for quantitative analysis (amount) of chemicals
   • Specimen requires a preservative and refrigeration (specimen container usually provided by lab)
   • Patient is instructed to void first morning urine into the toilet; collect all urine into the same container for the next 24 hours, including the first morning specimen of the next day; bring the entire specimen in the container to the lab

B. BLOOD
■ Consists of liquid and cellular components
■ Sample can be separated into components by centrifuging or settling
   a) Plasma
      ■ Liquid component of circulating blood; if whole blood is allowed to clot, the liquid portion is called serum; serum contains no clotting factors (formed clot)
      ■ Appears clear and light yellow
   b) Buffy coat
      ■ Consists of WBCs and platelets
   c) Red blood cells
1. Blood collection tubes
   • Vacuum tubes with color-coded stoppers
   • Tube utilized depends on the test to be performed on the sample
      a) Yellow stopper
         ■ Used for serum collection
         ■ Has no additive
         ■ Tube is sterile and used for bacteriological testing
      b) Red stopper
         ■ Used for serum collection
         ■ Contains no additives
         ■ Tube must sit for 15 minutes to allow a clot to form, then centrifuge
         ■ Used for samples for chemistry and serology
      c) Tiger/speckled/SST (serum separator tube)
         ■ Red-and-black mottled stopper
         ■ Used to collect serum
         ■ Tube contains a silicon gel that creates a barrier between the serum and the clotted cells when centrifuged
         ■ Tube must sit for 15 minutes to allow a clot to form, then centrifuge
         ■ Used for the same purpose as red stopper
      d) Lavender stopper
         ■ Used to collect plasma
         ■ Tube contains anticoagulant (EDTA) (ethylene diamine tetraacetic acid)

         ■ Used for hematology
         ■ Tube must be gently mixed after collection
      e) Blue stopper
         ■ Used to collect plasma
         ■ Contains anticoagulant sodium citrate
         ■ Used to perform coagulation testing
      f) Green stopper
         ■ Used to collect plasma
         ■ Contains anticoagulant sodium heparin
         ■ Used in chemistry for stat testing
      g) Gray stopper
         ■ Contains anticoagulant sodium fluoride
         ■ Used in chemistry for glucose testing and alcohol testing
2. Order of collection: when multiple tubes are to be collected, collect in the following order
      a) Yellow stopper
      b) Red/SST stopper
      c) Blue stopper
      d) Lavender stopper
      e) Green stopper
      f) Gray stopper
3. Venipuncture (phlebotomy) (see Figures 20-1, 20-2)
   • Puncture of vein to withdraw blood sample
   • Usually performed on the median cubital vein in the antecubital area
      a) Apply tourniquet about 3 to 4 inches above site; palpate/observe for the vein; release the tourniquet (do not leave the tourniquet on for more than 60 seconds)
      b) Assemble all equipment
      c) Reapply the tourniquet

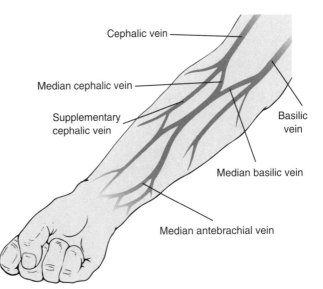

FIGURE 20-1 Veins of the arm commonly used for venipuncture sites. (From Stepp CA, Woods MA: Laboratory procedures for Medical Office Personnel, Philadelphia, 1998, Saunders, p. 116.)

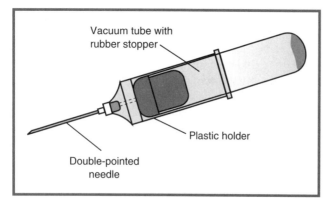

FIGURE 20-2 Evacuated tube system used for venipuncture. (From Kinn ME, Woods MA: The Medical Assistant, Administrative and Clinical, ed 8, Philadelphia, 1998, Saunders, p. 880.)

   d) Glove; cleanse the site with an alcohol wipe and allow it to dry
   e) Anchor the vein; insert the needle at approximately 15 degrees, bevel up
   f) Fill the syringe by slowly pulling back on the plunger or by inserting the vacuum tube onto the needle in the holder
   g) As the blood fills, release the tourniquet
   h) After collection is complete, place a clean cotton ball or gauze over the site and quickly withdraw the needle; instruct the patient to apply pressure to the site; apply a pressure dressing to the site
   i) Label the specimen; dispose of the needle into a sharps container
 4. Capillary puncture (see Figure 20-3)
   • Used to collect small amounts of blood
   • Sites used include
     ■ Middle or ring finger of the nondominant hand
     ■ Earlobe
     ■ Heel or big toe on an infant
   a) Cleanse the site with alcohol and allow it to dry
   b) Quickly puncture the skin with a lancet; wipe away the first drop of blood
   c) Collect a sample in the appropriate container

C. CEREBRAL SPINAL FLUID (CSF)
 ■ Fluid that surrounds the brain and spinal cord
 ■ Normal CSF is clear and colorless
 ■ Collected by lumbar puncture procedure between L3, L4, or L5
 ■ Fluid may be cultured for bacteria, analyzed for chemical components (glucose and protein), or tested for the presence of blood cells

D. SEROUS FLUIDS
 ■ Includes pericardial, plural, and peritoneal fluids
 ■ Normal fluids appear clear and light yellow
 ■ May be tested for chemical components, cultured and smeared for bacteria, or tested for cell counts

E. SYNOVIAL FLUID
 ■ Fluid that lines and lubricates joints
 ■ Normal fluid appears yellow and viscous
 ■ Collected through joint puncture
 ■ May be cultured, analyzed for cells and crystals, tested for glucose and protein

F. FECES
 ■ Collected in a clean container
 ■ Avoid contamination from water or urine
 ■ Tests include
   1. Occult blood
     • Detects hidden blood
     • Helps diagnosis of cancer or bleeding
     • Hemoccult

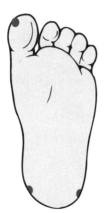
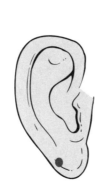

Infant's heel/great toe   Earlobe   Ring/great finger

FIGURE 20-3 Skin puncture sites for microcapillary blood collection. (From Stepp CA, Woods MA: Laboratory procedures for Medical Office Personnel, Philadelphia, 1998, Saunders, p. 131.)

2. Ova and parasites (O&P)
   • Detects eggs and parasites in the intestinal tract
3. Culture
   • Detects microorganisms

G. SPUTUM
■ Secretions of trachea and bronchi
■ Avoid contamination with saliva and nasal secretions
■ Patient is instructed to cough deeply into the container for the culture

H. OTHER SECRETIONS
■ Collected with sterile swabs for cultures, includes
   1. Wound secretions
   2. Throat secretions
   3. Genital secretions

III. Microscope
■ Precision magnifying instrument
■ Total magnification equals objective magnification times ocular magnification
■ Consists of two lenses
   • Objective
   • Ocular

A. PARTS OF THE MICROSCOPE (see Figure 20-4)
1. Base: portion that supports the microscope
2. Arm: supports lenses and focus knobs
3. Stage: platform that holds the objects being observed; contains clips for holding the objects on the stage
4. Light source: lightbulb in base that illuminates the objects; knob controls the intensity of the light
5. Condenser: lens over the light source that directs and focuses the light on the object
6. Iris diaphragm: shutter mechanism on the bottom of condenser; regulates the amount of light passing through the object
7. Ocular: one or two eyepieces; contains a lens that magnifies the image
8. Objectives: lenses mounted on a revolving nosepiece; microscope usually contains 3 lenses on the objective
   a) Low power: usually 10X; used for initial focusing
   b) High/dry power: usually 40X; used for cellular specimens, wet preps, and urine sediment
   c) Oil immersion: usually 100X; requires the use of immersion oil to prevent refraction; used to study cell detail and bacteria

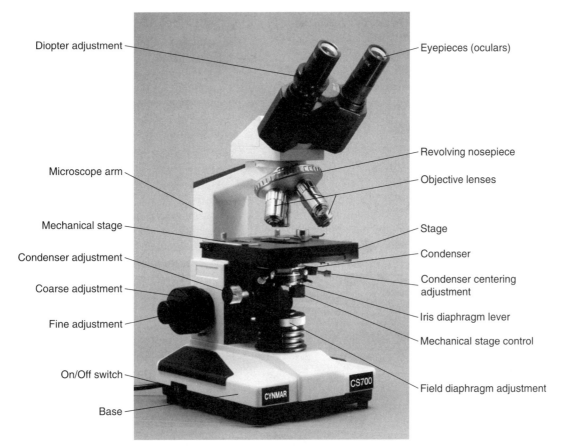

FIGURE 20-4 Parts of a microscope. (Courtesy of CARLSAN Inc., Carlinville, Illinois.)

9. Coarse adjustment: large focusing knob; moves the stage up or down for rough focus

10. Fine adjustment: small focusing knob; allows for precise focusing

B. CARE

1. Transport with one hand under the base, the other on the arm

2. Wipe immersion oil off the objective immediately after use

3. Store with 10X objective over the stage; bring the stage to the lowest level and cover

4. Lenses should be cleaned only with lens paper to decrease the possibility of scratches

IV. Urinalysis

■ Physical, chemical, and microscopic examination of urine

■ Provides information about the conditions of the kidneys and urinary tract

■ Can help in the diagnosis of metabolic and systemic disorders

A. PHYSICAL EXAMINATION

1. Color
   a) Normal: yellow; color is due to urochrome pigment
   b) Pale (straw): dilute urine
   c) Dark yellow (amber): concentrated urine; may be seen in fever or dehydration
   d) Yellow-brown or green/brown: presence of bilirubin; will foam when shaken
   e) Bright orange: seen in patients taking Pyridium; will interfere with reagent strips
   f) Red: clear red may indicate hemoglobin; cloudy red indicates the presence of RBCs (hematuria)
   g) Dark brown/black: presence of melanin
   h) Pink, green, or blue: results from foods, dyes, chemicals, or vitamins

2. Clarity
   a) Normal: clear, but becomes cloudy on standing
   b) Hazy: solid particles make urine appear hazy; print is not distorted when viewed through the sample
   c) Cloudy: solid particles make print difficult to see through the sample
   d) Turbid: solid particles make print impossible to see through the sample
   e) Normal cloudiness may be caused by
      1) Mucus
      2) Certain crystals
      3) Epithelial cells
      4) Sperm cells
   f) Abnormal cloudiness may be caused by
      1) Certain crystals
      2) WBCs and RBCs

   3) Pus
   4) Epithelial cells
   5) Casts
   6) Fats

3. Specific gravity (SG)
   • Measures the amount of dissolved solids in urine
   • Compares weight to an equal amount of distilled water
      a) Normal SG is 1.005 to 1.035
         ■ SG inverses with volume
            > Low volume has high specific gravity (concentrated urine)
            > High volume has low specific gravity (dilute urine)
      b) Methods of measuring SG
         ■ Reagent strip
         ■ Urinometer
         ■ Refractometer

4. Odor
   • May be noted if abnormal
      a) Normal: faintly aromatic; not unpleasant
      b) Ketones: sweet or fruity odor
      c) Ammonia: due to bacterial growth that breaks down urea
      d) Strong food ingestion may cause odor

B. CHEMICAL EXAMINATION

■ Chemical components are measured by use of a reagent strip

■ Presence of a chemical causes a color change on the reagent pad on the strip

■ Tests are qualitative

■ Specimen should be well mixed before testing

■ Completely immerse the strip into the sample

■ Remove the strip and keep it in a horizontal position (avoids cross-contamination of pads)

■ Compare the color of the reagent pad to the color on the bottle or chart at the time specified

■ Testing includes

1. pH: measures acidity/alkalinity of urine; normal is 5 to 7

2. Protein: significant for renal disease; normal is "negative"

3. Blood: significant for kidney disease or hemorrhage in the urinary tract; normal is "negative"

4. Nitrite: significant for UTI (some bacteria convert nitrate to nitrite); normal is "negative"

5. Leukocytes: significant for UTI; normal is "negative"

6. Glucose: significant for diabetes mellitus; normal is "negative"

7. Ketones: end product of metabolism; significant for diabetes mellitus and starvation; normal is "negative"

8. Bilirubin: by-product of RBC destruction; significant for liver disease or bile duct obstruction; normal is "negative"

9. Urobilinogen: result of breakdown of bilirubin in the intestine; significant for anemias and malaria; normal is "small amount"

C. MICROSCOPIC EXAMINATION

- Examined under low power (10X)
- Examined under high power (40X) for cells and bacteria
- Examination includes
  1. RBCs: normal is 0 to 2 per HPF; cells appear small, round, and clear
  2. WBCs: normal is 0 to 5 per HPF; cells appear 2 to 3 times the size of RBCs and round with a grainy appearance
  3. Epithelial cells
     a) Squamous epithelial cells: normal: not significant unless a large quantity per HPF; appear about the same size as WBCs
     b) Renal epithelial cells: normal is 0 per HPF; presence indicates renal tubule destruction; appear round and grainy, about twice the size of WBCs
  4. Bacteria: normal are a few per HPF; more indicates UTI; appear as tiny grains
  5. Yeast: normal are a few per HPF; more indicates yeast infection (*Candida albicans*); they appear as round, clear bodies; some have buds (hyphae); may be confused with RBCs
  6. Mucus threads: wavy, threadlike structures
  7. Spermatozoa: appear as small oval bodies, with tail; normal in males, contamination in females
  8. Casts: structures formed in nephron tubules; material solidifies in tubules and may contain cells, fat, and bacteria; normal is 0 to 2 per LPF; appear as cylindrical bodies, longer than wide
     - Types include
     a) Hyaline: colorless and semitransparent
     b) Fatty cast: contains fat globules
     c) RBC cast: orange-yellow in color
     d) WBC cast: contains WBCs
     e) Granular cast: sandlike granules
     f) Waxy cast: yellowish, wide cast with irregular edges
  9. Crystals
     a) Normal crystals found in acidic urine
        1) Uric acid: appears lemon-shaped
        2) Calcium oxalate: square shape with an "x"
     b) Normal crystals found in alkaline urine
        1) Triple phosphate: coffin-lid-shaped
        2) Calcium phosphate: flat plates
     c) Abnormal crystals found in acidic urine
        1) Cystine: hexagonal plates
        2) Tyrosine: fine needles
        3) Leucine: yellow spheres
        4) Sulfonamides: large needles in rosettes

5) Cholesterol: large, flat, hexagonal plates with notched corners

V. Serology

- Tests done on serum to evaluate antigen-antibody reaction
- Helps detect disease or amount of antibodies present (titer)
- Some tests available in kit and/or "rapid" forms
- Reactions include
  - Precipitation: antigen-antibody complex visibly settles out of solution
  - Agglutination: type of precipitation method that creates visible clumping
- Tests include

A. INFECTIOUS MONONUCLEOSIS

- Disease caused by Epstein-Barr virus
- Body produces heterophil antibodies in response
- Tests (Monospot) are designed to detect heterophil antibody

B. STREPTOCOCCUS

- Group A beta hemolytic streptococcus causes strep throat, rheumatic fever, impetigo
- Tests detect antibody antistreptolysin-O (ASO)

C. RHEUMATOID FACTOR

- Group of proteins (autoantibodies)
- Causes rheumatoid arthritis
- Test detects antibodies against factor

D. HUMAN CHORIONIC GONADOTROPIN (HCG)

- Hormone produced by the placenta
- Test for hormone in blood and urine
- Basis of pregnancy testing

E. BLOOD GROUPS

- Blood cells are mixed with antisera; agglutination indicates the presence of antigens on RBCs
- Can detect ABO group (A, B, AB, or O)
- Can detect Rh (Rh+, or Rh−)

F. SYPHILIS

- Antibody test for *Treponema pallidum*
- Tests include
  - RPR: rapid plasma reagin
  - VDRL: venereal disease research lab

G. SYSTEMIC LUPUS ERYTHEMATOSUS

- Testing to detect ANA (antinuclear antibodies)

VI. Chemistry

A. LIPIDS

- Before lipid testing, the patient should fast for 12 to 14 hours; no alcohol for 24 hours before the test; reduce fat intake for 2 weeks before the test
- These tests can assess the risk of coronary and vascular disease

■ Lipid profile is made up of the following tests
  1. Cholesterol
     • Fatty compound
     • Necessary for production of sex hormones and bile
     • Helps in formation of cell membranes
     • Normal value: <200 mg/dL
  2. High-density lipoproteins (HDL)
     • "Good cholesterol"
     • Removes excess cholesterol from cells and carries it back to the liver for excretions
     • Normal value for female: 55 mg/dL
     • Normal value for male: 45 mg/dL
  3. Low-density lipoproteins (LDL)
     • "Bad cholesterol"
     • Picks up fat from liver and carries it in the blood
     • Normal value: 60 to 180 mg/dL
  4. Triglycerides
     • Form fat in the bloodstream
     • Transported in blood by LDLs
     • Make up most of the fat in the body
     • Normal value for female: 35 to 135 mg/dL
     • Normal value for male: 40 to 160 mg/dL

B. GLUCOSE
  ■ Simple sugar from the breakdown of carbohydrates
  ■ Provides energy for cells and tissues
  ■ Excess is stored as glycogen in the liver
  ■ Blood levels regulated by hormones produced by pancreas
     • Glucagon: converts glycogen to glucose (increased blood levels)
     • Insulin: transports glucose into cells (decreased blood levels)
  ■ Tests include
  1. Fasting blood sugar (FBS)
     • Testing done on blood sample of patient after fasting for 8 to 12 hours (water permitted)
     • Test is commonly used in the diagnosis or evaluation of diabetes mellitus
     • Normal value: 70 to 105 mg/dL
  2. Postprandial glucose (2-hour PPBS)
     • Measures the amount of glucose in the patient's blood after a meal is ingested
     • Blood level should return to the premeal range within 2 hours
     • Normal value: 70 to 105 mg/dL
  3. Glucose tolerance test (GTT)
     • Assists in the diagnosis of diabetes mellitus
     • Patient's blood glucose levels are evaluated at fasting, then 30, 60, 120, and 180 minutes after ingestion of a standard oral glucose solution
     • Urine samples are evaluated at the same times

     • Patient is to fast 12 hours before the test
     • Fasting blood sugar is drawn
     • Patient drinks 75 g of glucose
     • Collect blood samples and urine samples 30, 60, 120, and 180 minutes (or any combination of these times) after the patient takes the glucose solution
     • Patient may drink water during the test, but NO coffee, tea, or tobacco
     • Normal glucose values
        ■ Fasting: 70 to 105 mg/dL
        ■ 30 min: 200 mg/dL
        ■ 1 hour: 200 mg/dL
        ■ 2 hours: 140 mg/dL
        ■ 3 hours: 70 to 115 mg/dL

C. ELECTROLYTES
  ■ Charged particles of the body
  ■ Includes
     • Cation: positively charged ions
     • Anion: negatively charged ions
  ■ Found in extracellular fluids
  ■ Body strives for neutrality (balance of anions and cations); if balance is not achieved, could be dangerous or fatal for the patient
  ■ Lungs and kidneys control the electrolyte balance
  1. Functions of electrolytes
     a) Maintain water balance in the body
     b) Maintain pH of the body
     c) Help with blood coagulation
     d) Control neuromuscular excitability
  2. Sodium (Na)
     • Major extracellular cation
     • Helps maintain osmotic pressure
     • Low sodium level: hyponatremia
     • High sodium level: hypernatremia
     • Normal value: 136 to 146 mEq/L
  3. Potassium (K)
     • Major intracellular cation
     • Influences muscle activity of heart
     • Works with sodium for acid-base balance
     • Low potassium level: hypokalemia
     • High potassium level: hyperkalemia
     • Normal value: 3.5 to 5.0 mEq/L
  4. Chloride (Cl)
     • Major extracellular anion
     • Counterbalances sodium for neutrality in body fluids
     • Helps maintain osmotic pressure (water distribution between cells), plasma, and interstitial fluid
     • Helps maintain acid-base balance
     • Normal value: 98 to 106 mEq/L
  5. Bicarbonate (HCO_3)
     • Major anion
     • Measured by blood carbon dioxide levels
     • Works with chloride
     • Normal value: 21 to 31 mEq/L

D. BILIRUBIN
- Yellow pigment in bile
- Comes from heme portion of hemoglobin (heme released when RBCs break down)
- Two types
  - Unconjugated (indirect): transported by albumin to the liver
  - Conjugated (direct): becomes water soluble in the liver and enters the bile; transported to the small intestine, where it is converted into urobilinogens
- Increased levels may indicate
  - Destruction of RBCs
  - Impaired liver function
  - Obstruction of flow of bile
- Exposure to UV lights results in oxidation of bilirubin
- Normal values: 0.1 to 1.0 mg/dL

E. PROTEINS
- Make up muscles, enzymes, hormones, hemoglobin, and other important functional and structural substances in the body
  1. Albumin
     - Principal plasma protein
     - Found in liver
     - Functions
       - Maintenance of osmotic pressure
       - Transportation of drugs, hormones, and enzymes
     - Can be a measure of nutritional status
     - Normal values: 3.5 to 5.0 g/dL
  2. Globulin
     - Building block of antibodies, lipids, and clotting factors
     - Transport mechanism
     - Can be measure of nutritional status
     - Normal values: 2.3 to 3.4 g/dL
  3. Total protein
     - Albumin plus globulin
     - Component of osmotic pressure (keeps fluids within vascular system)
     - Normal values: 6.0 to 8.5 g/dL

F. NITROGENOUS COMPOUNDS
- Forms of nitrogen in the body
- Waste product of metabolism
  1. Blood urea nitrogen (BUN)
     - Main indicator of kidney function
     - Urea is main nonprotein nitrogen in blood
     - Urea is formed in the liver and is the waste product of the breakdown of protein
     - Normal value: 7 to 18 mg/dL
  2. Creatinine
     - End product of creatine metabolism in muscles
     - Constantly being formed; the amount has a direct relationship to muscle mass
     - Filtered by the kidneys and excreted in urine
     - Reliable screening test for renal function
     - Normal value: 0.7 to 1.5 mg/dL
  3. Uric acid
     - By-product of protein metabolism
     - Blood levels from food metabolism (high-protein diet) and muscle tissue breakdown
     - Normal value: 4 to 6 mg/dL

G. ENZYMES
- Substances that speed up chemical reactions but remain unchanged themselves
- Values expressed in IU (International Units)
- Always end with the suffix "-ase"
- Can originate in cells, specific organs, or tissues
- Release may be due to damage or disease of tissues
  1. Aspartate aminotransferase (AST)
     - Formerly SGOT
     - Found in highly metabolic tissues (heart muscle, liver, skeletal muscles)
     - Levels increase post MI (indication of MI)
     - Normal value: 8 to 20 IU/L
  2. Creatine phosphokinase (CPK, CK)
     - Enzyme found in mitochondria of cells
     - High concentration in the heart, skeletal muscles, and brain
     - Useful in diagnosis of MI and muscle disease
     - Normal value: 25 to 130 IU/L
  3. Alkaline phosphatase
     - High concentration in bone and liver
     - Bone growth or liver disease can cause levels to rise
     - Normal value: 30 to 85 IU/L
  4. Acid phosphatase
     - Largest source is the prostate gland
     - Elevated in prostate cancer
     - Normal value: 0 to 0.8 IU/L

H. MINERALS
  1. Calcium (Ca)
     - Found in bone tissue
     - Required for
       - Bone development
       - Cardiac function
       - Blood clotting
       - Transmission of nerve impulses
       - Muscle contractions
     - Normal values: 9 to 11 mg/dL
  2. Phosphorus (P)
     - Required for metabolism of protein, calcium, and glucose
     - Combines with calcium
     - Normal values: 3.0 to 4.5 mg/dL
  3. Magnesium (Mg)
     - Found in bone
     - Binds with ATP molecule for energy
     - Required for

- Muscle action
- Nerve impulse transmission
- Calcium regulation
- Enzyme activity
  - Normal values: 1.2 to 2.0 mEq/L

I. THYROID
  1. Triiodothyronine (T_3)
     - Evaluates thyroid function (hyperthyroidism, hypothyroidism)
     - Monitors thyroid replacement and suppressive therapy
     - Normal values: 70 to 205 ng/dL
  2. Thyroxine (T_4)
     - Initial test done for assessing thyroid function
     - Used to diagnose thyroid function
     - Used to monitor replacement and suppressive therapy
     - Normal values for female: 5 to 12 mcg/dL
     - Normal values for male: 4 to 12 mcg/dL

VII. Hematology
  ■ Study of blood and blood components

A. BLOOD COMPONENTS
  ■ Part of the circulatory system
  ■ Functions as transport mechanism for nutrients, waste, and defense agents to tissues and cells
  ■ Specimens collected by venipuncture (anticoagulated specimens) or capillary puncture
  1. Plasma
     - Liquid portion of circulating/unclotted blood
     - 55% of total blood volume made up of
       - 90% water
       - 10% solutes (proteins, hormones, vitamins, carbohydrates, enzymes, lipids, and salts)
  2. Formed elements
     - Blood cells
     - 45% of total blood volume made up of
       - Erythrocytes: red blood cells (RBCs)
       - Leukocytes: white blood cells (WBCs)
       - Thrombocytes: platelets (plt)

B. ERYTHROCYTES
  ■ Mature cells are anuclear biconcave discs
  ■ Contain hemoglobin (hgb)
     - Heme (iron-containing portion) plus globin (protein-containing portion)
     - Transports oxygen
  1. Color
     - Normally appear pinkish-red (depends on hgb concentration)
     - Anisochromia: variations in color (depends on hgb concentration)
  2. Size
     - Normally 6 to 8 micrometers
     - Anisocytosis: variation in size

3. Shape
   - Normally appear round
   - Poikilocytosis: variation in shape
4. Diseases and disorders
   a) Anemia: caused by
      - Blood loss
      - Increase in plasma volume (overhydration, pregnancy)
      - Iron deficiency caused by hgb decrease
   b) Polycythemia
      - Increase in RBC numbers
5. Lab testing
   a) Hemoglobin (hgb test)
      - Measures the total amount of hgb in the blood
      - Rapid indirect measurement of RBC count
      - Evaluates anemic patients
      - Routine portion of CBC
      - Blood sample is diluted with Drabkin solution; lyses RBCs and releases hgb into the solution; chemicals in the reagent react with released hgb and forms the pigment cyanmethemoglobin, which can be measured by photometer
      - Normal hgb values
        > Newborn: 14 to 24 g/dL
        > Infant: 9.5 to 14 g/dL
        > Child: 9.5 to 15.5 g/dL
        > Adult male: 14 to 18 g/dL
        > Adult female: 12 to 16 g/dL
   b) Hematocrit (hct, microhematocrit, crit)
      - Direct measurement of percentage of RBCs in total blood volume
      - Indirect measurement of RBC number and volume
      - Rapid measurement of RBC count
      - Routine portion of CBC
      - Height of RBC column is measured after the blood sample is centrifuged; compared to the height of the column of whole blood (height of the column of whole blood is 100%)
      - After centrifuging, blood separates into 3 layers
        1) Plasma (top) layer
        2) Buffy coat: thin middle layer made up of WBCs and platelets
        3) RBCs (bottom) layer
      - Hgb value multiplied by 3 gives the hct value (± 3)
      - Procedure
        1) 2 tubes needed (for comparison; to balance centrifuge; if one breaks)
        2) Fill two capillary tubes 3/4 full with blood from capillary puncture or

lavender-stoppered tube from veni-puncture

3) Wipe the ends to remove blood from the outside of the tubes and seal with clay (Critoseal)

4) Place in a hematocrit centrifuge with the sealed ends facing outward; spin for 5 minutes

5) Read tubes by comparing them to the printed reading device

6) To be valid, the tubes should read within 2% of each other; report the average reading; repeat the test if not within 2%

7) Normal hct values
> Newborn: 44% to 64%
> Infant: 29% to 43%
> Child: 30% to 40%
> Adult female: 37% to 47%
> Adult male: 42% to 52%

c) RBC count (see Figures 20-5, 20-6, 20-7, 20-8)
■ Counts the number of circulating RBCs in 1 cu. mm of peripheral venous blood
■ Routine portion of CBC
■ Closely related to hgb and hct values
■ Procedure (for manual count)
1) Fill RBC unopette
2) Let sit for 10 minutes; expel a few drops
3) Charge the hemocytometer; let stand for 5 minutes
4) Under 40X magnification, observe the center square

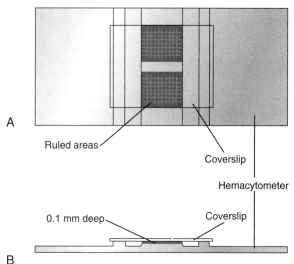

A

Ruled areas   Coverslip

Hemacytometer

0.1 mm deep   Coverslip

B

FIGURE 20-6 Hemacytometer: top (*A*) and side (*B*) views. The blood sample should fill the shaded areas when the chamber is properly filled. (From Kinn ME, Woods MA: The Medical Assistant, Administrative and Clinical, ed 8, Philadelphia, 1998, Saunders, p. 913.)

5) Count the cells within the smaller center and four squares on both sides; do not count cells that sit on bottom or left lines

6) Counts from both sides should be within 10% of each other; if not, repeat

7) Average the sides count and multiply by 10,000

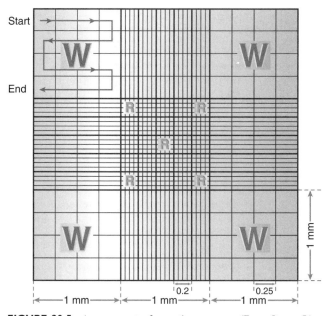

FIGURE 20-5 Arrangement of counting squares. (From Stepp CA, Woods MA: Laboratory procedures for Medical Office Personnel, Philadelphia, 1998, Saunders, p. 141.)

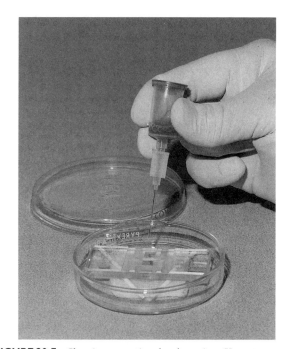

FIGURE 20-7 Charging a counting chamber using a Unopette system. (From Stepp CA, Woods MA: Laboratory procedures for Medical Office Personnel, Philadelphia, 1998, Saunders, p. 142.)

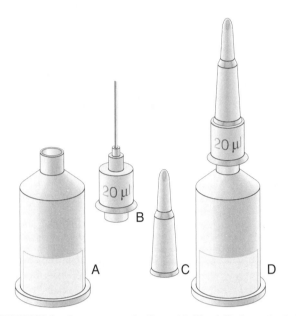

FIGURE 20-8 Components of a disposable blood-diluting unit. *A*, A pre-filled reservoir, containing pre-measured diluting fluid, is sealed with a diaphragm. *B*, A capillary pipette with overflow chamber and capacity marking. *C*, A pipette shield. *D*, Assembled unit. (From Stepp CA, Woods MA: Laboratory procedures for Medical Office Personnel, Philadelphia, 1998, Saunders, p. 141.)

8) Count can also be performed by automation (Coulter, etc.); follow the manufacturer's directions
9) Automated counts are faster, are more accurate, and decrease the chances of contamination by sample
10) Normal RBC values (million per cu. mm)
> Newborn: 4.8 to 7.1
> Infant: 3.5 to 5.2
> Child: 4.0 to 5.5
> Adult female: 4.0 to 5.0
> Adult male: 4.5 to 6.0

d) Indices
■ Provide information about RBC size, weight, and hgb concentration
■ Part of automated CBC
■ Results of RBC count, hct, and hgb necessary to calculate indices
1) Mean corpuscular volume (MCV)
> Measure of average size/volume of an RBC
> Used to classify anemias

hct (%) $\times$ 10 MCV = RBC (million per cu. mm)

> Normal values
Newborn: 95 to 96
Child/adult: 80 to 95
2) Mean corpuscular hemoglobin (MCH)
> Measures amount/weight of hgb within an RBC

hgb (g/dL) $\times$ 10 MCH = RBC (million per cu. mm)

> Normal values
Newborn: 32 to 34 pg
Child/adult: 27 to 31 pg
3) Mean corpuscular hemoglobin concentration (MCHC)
> Measure of average concentration/percentage of hgb in a single RBC

hgb (g/dL) $\times$ 100 MCHC = hct (%)

> Normal values
Newborn: 32% to 33%
Child/adult: 32% to 36%

e) Reticulocyte count
■ Reticulocytes are immature RBCs
■ Indication of ability of bone marrow to respond to anemia and make RBCs
■ Used to classify and monitor anemia therapy
■ Count is percentage of total number of RBCs
■ Procedure
1) Mix a drop of blood and a drop of Wright's or Giemsa stain
2) Prepare smear
3) Examine under 100X magnification
4) Appear as RBCs with small dark granules
5) Count the number of cells in 10 fields
6) Total the number of cells and divide by 10

> Normal values
Newborn: 0.5% to 2% of total RBCs
Infant: 0.5% to 3.1% of total RBCs
Child/adult: 0.5% to 2% of total RBCs

f) Erythrocyte sedimentation rate (ESR, sed rate)
■ Nonspecific test used to detect illnesses associated with acute and chronic infection, inflammation, and neoplasms
■ Measures the rate at which RBCs settle in plasma over a specified time period (1 hour)
■ Methods include
1) Wintrobe
2) Westergren
3) Landau-Adams
■ All methods are based on the same principle, although they vary in the amount of blood needed, the tube size, and calibration
■ Procedure
1) Fill the tube according to manufacturer's directions
2) Place the tube perfectly upright in the rack; let the tube sit for 1 hour without being disturbed

3) After 1 hour, note how many millimeters cells fall (settle)
> Normal values
Newborn: 0 to 2 mm/hr
Child: 0 to 10 mm/hr
Adult female: 0 to 15 mm/hr
Adult male: 0 to 20 mm/hr

C. LEUKOCYTES
■ Mature cells vary in morphology depending on type
1. Neutrophil (segmented neutrophil, seg, poly, PMN): most numerous of granulocytes
   a) Size: 10 to 15 micrometers
   b) Nucleus: contains 2 to 5 lobes with constrictions (as sausage links): stains deep reddish-purple
   c) Cytoplasm: abundant; stains light to medium pink, with many small granules
   d) Distribution: 35% to 70% of circulating WBCs
   e) Increased number: shift to the right
2. Bands (stabs): immature form of seg
   a) Size: 10 to 15 micrometers
   b) Nucleus: peanut-, band-, or rod-shaped; no lobes or constrictions
   c) Cytoplasm: same as seg
   d) Distribution: 1% to 5% of circulating WBCs
   e) Increased number: shift to the left
3. Eosinophil (eos): granulocyte
   a) Size: 11 to 16 micrometers
   b) Nucleus: not significant; stains dark pinkish-red
   c) Cytoplasm: stains pink; contains large, reddish-orange granules
   d) Distribution: 1% to 5% of circulating WBCs; increase seen in allergic reactions, parasite infestation, and inflammation
4. Basophil (baso): granulocyte
   a) Size: 10 to 15 micrometers
   b) Nucleus: indistinct; usually occludes by granules
   c) Cytoplasm: small amount; stains purplish-blue; contains large, dark-purple-to-black granules; granules contain histamine and heparin
   d) Distribution: 0% to 1% of circulating WBCs; increase seen in allergic reactions, radiation exposure, and post splenectomy
5. Monocytes (mono): agranulocyte
   a) Size: 15 to 20 micrometers
   b) Nucleus: large, foamy, and round; stains reddish-purple to medium purple
   c) Cytoplasm: large amount; may appear foamy; stains sky-blue to blue-gray
   d) Distribution: 3% to 5% of circulating WBCs

6. Lymphocyte (lymph): agranulocyte
   ■ Smallest in size of all WBCs
   a) Size: 6 to 10 micrometers
   b) Nucleus: round; fills most of the cell; stains dark purple
   c) Cytoplasm: small amount; encircles the nucleus; stains sky-blue to medium blue
   d) Distribution: 30% to 40% of circulating WBCs; infants and children normally have more than adults; increase seen in acute and chronic infections
7. Lab testing (see Figures 20-5, 20-6, 20-7, 20-8)
   a) WBC count
      ■ Measurement of total number of WBCs
      ■ Routine part of CBC
      ■ Helps evaluate/diagnose infection, allergy, neoplasm, or immunosuppression
      ■ Procedure (manual count)
      1) Fill WBC unopette and let stand for 10 minutes
      2) After standing, expel a few drops
      3) Charge the hemocytometer; let stand for 5 minutes
      4) Locate four large corner squares under 10X power; count all 16 smaller squares in a zigzag pattern, moving from left to right; do not count the cells sitting on the bottom or left lines
      5) Repeat for other side; counts should be within 10% of each other
      6) Average the two sides; multiply by 50
      ■ Normal values
      Newborn: 9,000 to 30,000 per cu. mm
      Child: 6,200 to 17,000 per cu. mm
      Adult: 5,000 to 10,000 per cu. mm
      ■ Can also be performed by automation (read and follow manufacturer's directions)
   b) Differential (diff)
      ■ Measurement of different WBCs in a smear
      ■ Smear is stained with polychromatic stain (Wright's)
      ■ Preparation of smear
      1) Small drop of blood is placed about 1/2 inch from the end of the slide
      2) Spreader slide is held at a 35 to 40 degree angle and moved back into the drop of blood slide; blood should be completely spread across the edge of the spreader's edge; push the spreader smoothly from the blood across the slide
      3) Allow to air-dry; a smooth feather-edge should be seen
      4) Stain the smear following the manufacturer's directions and completely air-dry
      ■ Procedure for differential
      1) Place the prepared slide under 100X magnification using immersion oil

2) Classify the first 100 cells seen; use the differential counter; record the result

3) Also note RBC morphology and estimation of platelets (adequate platelets are 7 to 20 cells seen in 10 fields)

- ■ Normal values
  segs: 35 to 70
  bands: 1 to 5
  lymphs: 30 to 40
  monos: 3 to 5
  eos: 1 to 5
  basos: 0 to 1

D. THROMBOCYTES

1. Platelet count test is the actual count of the number of platelets in a cubic millimeter of blood
   - Used to monitor the course of disease/ therapy for thrombocytopenia and bone marrow failure
   - Small round or oval bodies; have no nucleus
   - Stain dark blue on a different smear
   - Procedure
     a) Fill a platelet unopette following the manufacturer's directions
     b) Let sit 10 minutes and then expel a few drops
     c) Charge the hemocytometer, then allow to sit 5 minutes
     d) Find the large center square; count under 40X magnification all 25 smaller squares within the center square; do not count cells that sit on the bottom or left lines
     e) Count both sides; counts should be within 10% of each other
     f) Average both sides and multiply by the factor determined by the manufacturer
   - Normal values
     Newborn: 150,000 to 300,000 cu. mm
     Infant: 200,000 to 415,000 cu. mm
     Child/adult: 150,000 to 400,000 cu. mm
2. Bleeding time
   - Measures platelet function by noting the length of time it takes for bleeding to stop
   - 2 methods
     a) Ivy method: small incision in the patient's arm
     b) Duke method: small incision in the patient's earlobe (not commonly performed)
   - Ivy procedure
     a) Place the sphygmomanometer on the patient's upper arm; inflate to 40 mmHg; maintain this pressure for the entire procedure

b) Cleanse the area on the patient's forearm

c) Use an automatic lancet device to make a puncture/incision

d) Activate a stopwatch when the first drop of blood appears

e) Every 30 seconds, blot away the blood using the edge of the filter paper; do not touch the puncture with the filter paper

f) Note the time the bleeding stops

g) Normal value is 1 to 9 minutes for bleeding to stop

3. Prothrombin time (PT, pro-time)
   - Used to evaluate clotting mechanism
   - Used to monitor Coumadin therapy
   - Normal value is from 11 to 12.5 seconds
4. Partial thromboplastin time (PTT)
   - Used to evaluate the pathway to clot formation
   - Used to monitor heparin therapy
   - Normal value is from 60 to 70 seconds

VIII. Microbiology

- ■ Study of microorganisms
- ■ Includes
  - Bacteria
  - Fungi
  - Viruses
  - Rickettsiae
  - Mycobacteria
  - Parasites
- ■ Main objective is to identify the organism so that the practitioner can properly treat

A. CLASSIFICATION OF ORGANISMS

- ■ Scientific study of classification process is taxonomy
- ■ Simple, orderly method
- ■ Places organisms into categories according to similar morphological and biochemical properties
  1. Species: basic unit; based on reproduction (members of the same species can mate successfully)
  2. Genus: share biological likenesses
  3. Family: similar genera
  4. Order: related families
  5. Class: related orders
  6. Phylum: classes with common characteristics
- ■ Organisms in lab setting have two separate names
  1. Genus: name is capitalized; often abbreviated, using the first initial
  2. Species: name in lowercase
- ■ Both names are underlined or italicized when written

B. BACTERIA (BACTERIOLOGY)
1. Characteristics: help with identification of organisms in the lab (see Figure 20-9)
   a) Shape
      1) Cocci: round (singular: coccus)
      2) Bacilli: rod-shaped (singular: bacillus)
      3) Vibrio: comma-shaped
      4) Spirilla: spiral-shaped (singular: spirillum)
   b) Arrangement
      1) Diplo: arranged in pairs
      2) Strepto: arranged in chains
      3) Staphylo: arranged in grapelike clusters
      4) Tetra: four cocci together in capsule
   c) Staining properties
      1) Gram stain
         > Gram-positive: stain blue or dark purple
         > Gram-negative: stain pink or red
      2) Acid-fast stain
         > Type of stain used on bacteria that are difficult to stain with other stains
   d) Oxygen requirements
      1) Aerobic: requires oxygen to survive
      2) Anaerobic: requires no oxygen to survive
      3) Facultative: can survive in either environment
   e) Colony growth
      1) Size
      2) Color
      3) Shape
      4) Elevation
      5) Texture
      6) Margins
      7) Hemolysis (present or absent)
   f) Chemical reactions: bacteria respond differently to chemical reagents
2. Gram-stain procedure
   a) Apply the specimen in a thin layer to the slide; allow to air-dry
   b) Fix the smear by passing the slide over a flame; allow to cool
   c) Flood the slide with crystal violet; let stand 60 seconds (this stains the specimen purple)

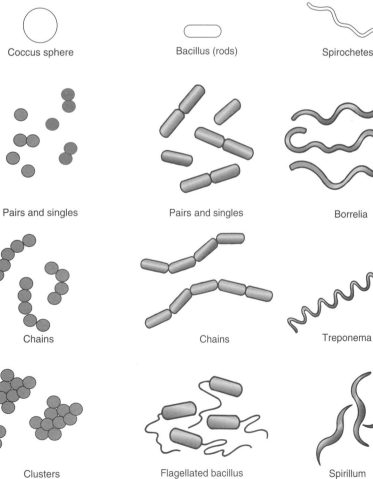

Coccus sphere Bacillus (rods) Spirochetes

Pairs and singles Pairs and singles Borrelia

Chains Chains Treponema

Clusters Flagellated bacillus Spirillum

FIGURE 20-9 The three basic shapes of bacteria. (From Stepp CA, Woods MA: Laboratory procedures for Medical Office Personnel, Philadelphia, 1998, Saunders, p. 325.)

d) Rinse gently with water

e) Flood the slide with iodine solution; let stand 60 seconds (iodine is a mordant that fixes the crystal violet to the cell)

f) Rinse gently with water

g) Apply decolorizer (alcohol-acetone solution) until the purple color no longer runs off the slide

h) Rinse gently with water

i) Flood the slide with safranin stain; let stand 60 seconds (turns bacteria that lost the purple stain during decolorization red or pink)

j) Rinse gently with water

k) Allow to dry; view under 100X using immersion oil

3. Common pathogenic bacteria

   a) Gram-positive cocci

      1) Staphylococcus (appears in clusters, dark purple)

         (a) *S. aureus:* skin infections, impetigo

         (b) *S. epidermis:* normal flora of the skin

         (c) *S. saprophyticus:* UTI

      2) Streptococcus (appears in chains, dark purple)

         (a) *S. pyogenes:* URI, rheumatic fever

         (b) *S. pneumoniae:* otitis media, pneumonia, meningitis

         (c) *S. viridans:* gum disease, endocarditis

   b) Gram-negative cocci

      1) Neisseria (appears as diplococci, pink)

         (a) *N. gonorrhoeae:* gonorrhea

         (b) *N. meningitidis:* meningitis

   c) Gram-negative bacilli

      1) *Escherichia coli* (*E. coli*): normal flora of the colon; UTI

      2) Salmonella

         (a) *S. typhi:* constipation

         (b) *S. enteritidis:* gastroenteritis

      3) Shigella

         (a) *S. dysenteriae:* severe dysentery

      4) *Klebsiella pneumoniae*

         (a) Normal flora of the colon and respiratory tract

         (b) UTI, wound infections, pneumonia

      5) *Proteus vulgaris:* normal flora of the GI tract; UTI, wound infections

      6) *Pseudomonas aeruginosa:* UTI, wound and burn infection

      7) *Haemophilus influenzae:* severe meningitis, otitis media (HIB vaccination)

   d) Gram-negative vibrio and spirochetes

      1) *Treponema pallidum* (spirochete): syphilis

      2) *Borrelia burgdorferi* (spirochete): Lyme disease

      3) *Vibrio cholerae* (vibrio): cholera

   e) Gram-positive bacilli

      1) *Corynebacterium diphtheriae:* diphtheria

      2) *Mycobacterium tuberculosis:* TB

      3) *Mycobacterium leprae:* leprosy

4. Rickettsia

  • Extremely small, Gram-negative bacteria

  • Parasites; require living cells to live

  • Transmitted by the bite of fleas, ticks, lice, and mites

  • *Rickettsia rickettsii:* Rocky Mountain spotted fever

5. Chlamydia

  • Gram-negative cocci

  • Parasites; depend on host for food and energy source

   a) *C. psittaci:* parrot fever

   b) *C. trachomatis:* conjunctivitis

6. Mycoplasma

  • Simplest form of bacteria

  • Normal flora of the respiratory system and genitalia

C. CULTURE MEDIA

■ Contains known amount of substances for optimal growth and diagnostic properties of bacteria

■ May contain

  • Sugar

  • Vitamins and minerals

  • Proteins

  • Dyes for diagnostics

1. Forms

   a) Semisolid/solid

     ■ Usually made of agar (from seaweed)

     ■ Allows for general growth

     ■ Allows for identification of colony size, color, and shape

   b) Liquid

     ■ Broth

     ■ Allows for general growth

     ■ Allows for study of gas production or patient changes

2. Bacterial growth requirements

   a) Nutrients: differ among species

   b) Temperature: usually thrive at normal body temperature (98.6 degrees Fahrenheit, 37 degrees Celsius)

   c) Oxygen: differs among species (aerobic or anaerobic)

   d) pH: human pathogens thrive at 7 (neutral); blood, milk, seawater are neutral

e) Sterile: medium must be sterile and non-contaminated for use

f) Moisture: most bacteria require some level of moisture

3. Classification of media

a) Differential: contains substances (dyes) that give organisms easily identifiable characteristics

b) Selective: inhibits growth of some species

c) Supportive: allows most organisms to grow equally

4. Common media

a) Blood agar
  ▪ Used for primary plating
  ▪ Contains sheep's blood
  ▪ Demonstrates hemolysis (staph and strep cultures)

b) Chocolate agar
  ▪ Contains denatured blood
  ▪ Used for organisms that require a rich food source and moisture

c) Mueller-Hinton: selective for Neisseria; used for sensitivity testing

d) Thayer-Martin (TM): selective for *N. gonorrhoeae* and *N. meningitidis*

D. PROCEDURE FOR STREAKING CULTURE PLATES (PLATING) (see Figure 20-10)

■ Used to culture bacteria and isolate colonies for identification

1. Collect a specimen with a sterile swab; may use a sterile inoculating loop if already plated

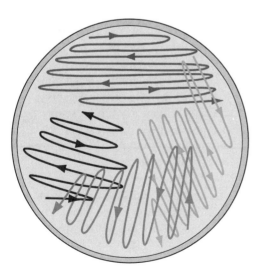

　First quadrant (swab)
　Second quadrant (loop)
　Third quadrant (loop)
　Fourth quadrant (loop)

FIGURE 20-10　Basic streaking pattern. (From Stepp CA, Woods MA: Laboratory procedures for Medical Office Personnel, Philadelphia, 1998, Saunders, p. 338.)

2. Primary streak
  • Streak a swab (or loop) over one fourth of the plate using a back-and-forth motion; do not gorge or break the agar

3. Secondary streak
  • Sterilize (or flame) the loop and let it cool
  • Turn the plate counterclockwise 45 degrees
  • Touch the primary streak with the loop and draw a new streak to cover one fourth of the plate (carry the material from the primary streak into a secondary streak)

4. Tertiary streak
  • Sterilize (or flame) the loop and let it cool
  • Repeat the secondary procedure for this streak

5. Quaternary streak
  • Repeat the above process
  • Carry the last streak into the center part of the plate that had not been streaked

6. Sterilize (or flame) the loop

7. Incubate the plate
  • Place into the incubator face down
  • Identify the plat on the plate, not the lid

E. COLLECTION OF MOST COMMON SPECIMENS

1. Throat culture
  • Use a sterile swab and swab the back of throat in a "rainbow" pattern
  • Collect any material in the area
  • Transport/send the specimen to the lab using a transport medium or streak immediately

2. Urine culture
  • Collect a clean-catch specimen in a sterile container
  • Use a sterile loop to streak the plate

3. Genitourinary culture
  • Collect a specimen using a sterile swab
  • Roll the swab over the plate in a "Z" or "W" pattern
  • Streak across the Z or W, using a sterile loop

4. Blood culture
  • Collect a specimen in a yellow-stoppered tube
  • Cleanse the skin with betadine before venipuncture
  • Inject approximately 10 mL of the specimen into 2 separate blood culture bottles

5. Wound culture
  • Collect a specimen with a sterile swab
  • Streak the plate using the "Z" or "W" method

6. Fecal culture
  • Collect a specimen in a clean container
  • Streak the plate with a sterile loop

F. CULTURE AND SENSITIVITY (C&S): DETERMINES AN ORGANISM'S SUSCEPTIBILITY TO SELECTED ANTIBIOTICS

1. Streak the plate with culture; cover the entire plate, rotating 45 degrees between each streak
2. Apply antibody disks using a dispenser or sterile forceps; make sure the disk is in contact with the medium
3. Incubate; check after 24 hours
4. Measure the zones of inhibition around each disk; compare to the chart provided by the manufacturer
5. Report the results

G. MYCOLOGY

■ Study of fungus
■ Medical mycology fungal forms
   • Molds
      ■ Multicellular organisms made up of hyphae
      ■ Produce powdery, fuzzy, or fluffy colonies on media
   • Yeasts
      ■ Single-cell organisms
      ■ Multiply by budding
      ■ Produce moist, creamy colonies on media

1. Common pathogenic fungi
   a) Trichophyton: causes various forms of tinea infections
   b) Microsporum: transmitted by animals and humans; causes ringworm
   c) *Candida albicans:* yeast; normal flora of bowel and skin; causes thrush and vaginal yeast infections
   d) *Aspergillus fumigatus:* affects respiratory tract and ears
   e) *Penicillium notatum:* used to make penicillin; causes pulmonary infections, UTI
   f) *Phycomycites mucor:* causes opportunistic infections in poorly managed patients with diabetes

2. Identification methods
   a) KOH prep
      ■ Place the specimen on a slide
      ■ Mix potassium hydroxide (KOH) with the specimen and allow to sit for 15 to 20 minutes
      ■ Observe under low power
   b) India ink
      ■ Helps identify capsules
      ■ Mix bodily fluid with ink on the slide
      ■ Observe under low power
      ■ Cells will appear to have halo around them

H. VIROLOGY

■ Study of viruses
■ Intracellular parasites that require a host to carry out their functions
■ Do not have cellular structure (nucleic acid and protein layer)
1. Reproductive by replication
2. Common viruses
   a) Adenovirus: conjunctivitis
   b) Arbovirus: yellow fever, encephalitis (carried by insects)
   c) Coxsackie: herpangina
   d) Echovirus: meningitis, encephalitis
   e) Hepatitis B virus (HBV): hepatitis B
   f) Herpes virus: herpes simplex, varicella (chickenpox), varicella zoster (shingles), Epstein-Barr
   g) Human immunodeficiency virus (HIV): AIDS
   h) Myxovirus: influenza
   i) Paramyxovirus: mumps, rubeola (measles)
   j) Papovirus: verruca (warts)
   k) Poliomyelitis: polio
   l) Rhabdovirus: rabies
   m) Rhinovirus: common cold

I. PARASITOLOGY: STUDY OF PARASITES; UNICELLULAR ORGANISMS THAT REQUIRE A HOST

1. Relationships
   a) Commensalism: neither organism harmed; one benefits
   b) Mutualism: both organisms benefit
   c) Parasitism: one organism benefits at the expense of the other
   d) Symbiosis: dependant relationship between two dissimilar organisms
2. Infection: invasion of microscopic parasites causing disease
3. Infestation: external or internal invasion of animal-like parasites
4. Classifications
   a) Protozoa: unicellular organisms
      1) Transmission
         > Ingestion of cysts in fecally contaminated water or food
         > Become adults after infection; they multiply in the intestine and are passed in feces
      2) Amoeba
         > Move by means of pseudopods ("false foot")
         > *Entamoeba hystolyica:* amebic dysentery

3) Flagellates
> Move by flagella
> *Trichomonas vaginalis:* vaginal flagellate; vaginitis
4) Ciliates
> Move by cilia
> *Balantidium coli:* largest protozoan; causes dysentery
5) Sporozoans
> Have sexual and asexual reproductive cycles
> Plasmodium: malaria
> *Pneumocystis carinii:* pneumonia in AIDS patients
b) Helminths: parasitic worms
1) Nematodes: roundworms
> *Ascaris lumbricoides:* intestinal roundworms
> *Enterobius vermicularis:* pinworms
> *Necator americanus:* hookworms
> *Trichuris trichiura:* whipworms
> *Strongyloides stercoralis:* threadworms
2) Cestodes: tapeworms
> *Diphyllobothrium latum:* broad tapeworms
> *Taenia saginata:* beef tapeworms
> *Taenia solium:* pork tapeworm
3) Trematodes (flukes)
> Schistosoma: blood fluke
c) Arthropods: organisms with exoskeletons and jointed appendages; can serve as vector or as intermediate host

1) Insects
> Pediculosis species: head and body lice
2) Fleas
3) Mosquitoes
> Anopheles species: malaria
4) Arachnids
> *Sarcoptes scabiei:* scabies (itch mite)
2. Diagnostic procedures
a) Ova and parasites (O&P)
■ Examination of feces for parasites and/or eggs
> Collect a sample in a clean, dry container; do not allow the specimen to touch water or urine
> Scoop out an amount of specimen and place in prepared specimen containers as directed by the manufacturer
b) Scotch-tape test
■ Pinworm diagnosis
■ Adult female lays eggs in area around anus
1) Affix tape onto the end of a slide and drape over the slide so that the adhesive side faces outward
2) Gently touch the anal area with the adhesive side of the tape
3) Undrape the tape and stick it to the slide
4) Send the slide with tape on it to the lab

the medical

al identifi-

ENTS

ved or

on under

dressings

issues

fascia

adhesive
r)

nder su-

dard)

■ Different sizes and shapes (#15 is standard)

B. GRASPING AND CLAMPING INSTRUMENTS (see Figures 21-3, 21-4, 21-5, 21-6, 21-7)
■ Used to retract, clamp, hold, or manipulate tissue, other instruments, or sterilized materials
1. Hemostat forceps (hemostats)
   • Jaws may or may not be serrated
   • Used to clamp small vessels or hold tissue
     a) Kelly hemostats
     b) Mosquito hemostats
2. Needle holders (needle pushers)
   • Jaws shorter and look stronger than hemostat
   • Used to grasp suture needles
3. Splinter forceps
   • Fine tip for foreign body retrieval or removal
   • Various designs and construction
4. Thumb forceps (dressing forceps)
   • Serrated jaws with teeth
   • Used to insert packing into a wound or to remove objects from cavities
5. Allis tissue forceps
   • Blunt teeth
   • Used to grasp tissue, muscle, or skin, surrounding a wound
6. Adson thumb forceps (tissue forceps)
   • Have teeth for grasping tissue
   • Used to grasp tissue and in suturing
7. Bayonet forceps
   • Smooth-tipped
   • Used to insert or remove objects from nose and ear
8. Towel clamps (forceps)
   • Have very sharp hooks
   • Various lengths
   • Used to hold drapes in place during surgery
9. Transfer forceps
   • Many sizes and lengths
   • Sterile forceps used to arrange objects on sterile field

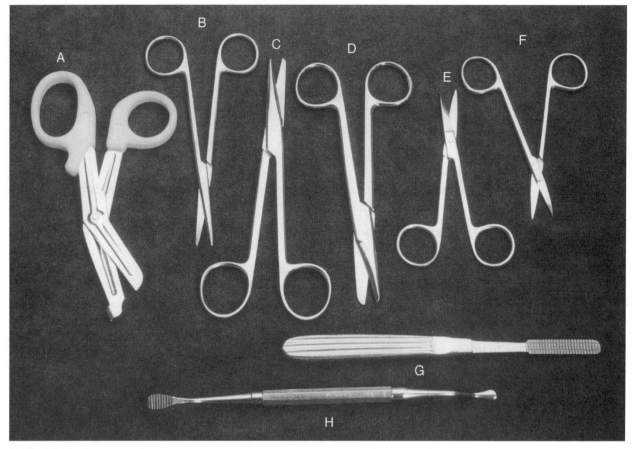

FIGURE 21-1 Operating scissors. *A,* Bandage scissors. *B,* Metzenbaum ("Metz") scissors. *C,* Curved Mayo scissors. *D,* Straight Mayo scissors. *E,* Straight ins scissors. *F,* Curved ins scissors. *G,* Bone rasp, single ended. *H,* Bone rasp, double ended. (From Kinn ME, Woods MA: The Medical Assistant, Administrative and Clinical, ed 8, Philadelphia, 1998, Saunders, p. 1069.)

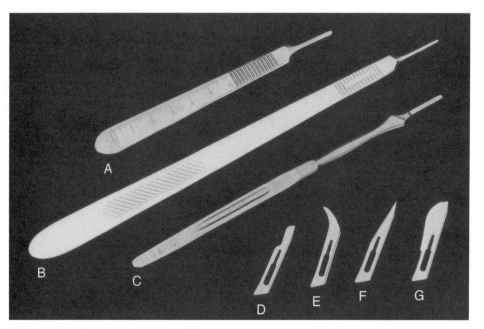

FIGURE 21-2 Scalpels. *A,* No. 3 scalpel blade. *B,* No. 3 long scalpel handle. *C,* No. 7 scalpel handle. *D,* No. 15 blade. *E,* No. 12 blade. *F,* No. 11 blade. *G,* No. 10 blade. (From Kinn ME, Woods MA: The Medical Assistant, Administrative and Clinical, ed 8, Philadelphia, 1998, Saunders, p. 1070.)

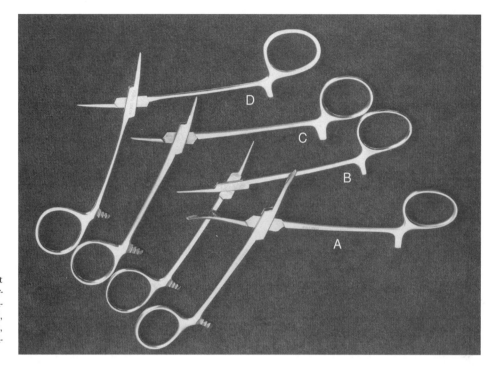

FIGURE 21-3 *A,* Kelly hemostat forceps. *B,* Mosquito hemostat forceps. *C,* Needle holder. *D,* Smooth-tip needle holder. (From Kinn ME, Woods MA: The Medical Assistant, Administrative and Clinical, ed 8, Philadelphia, 1998, Saunders, p. 1070.)

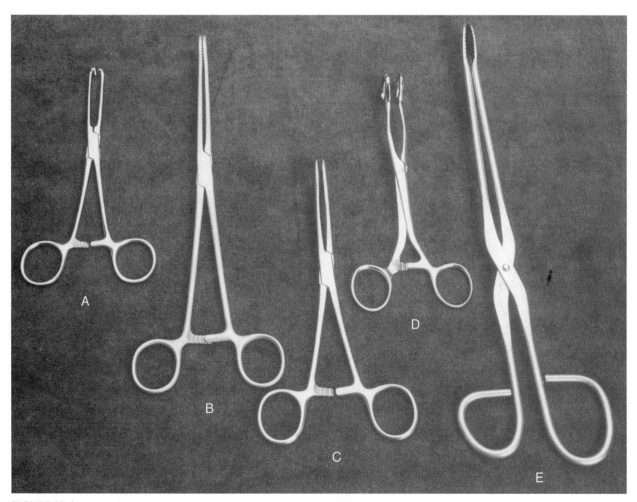

FIGURE 21-4 *A,* Allis forceps. *B,* Foerster sponge forceps. *C,* Straight transfer forceps. *D,* Short transfer forceps. *E.* Long transfer forceps. (From Kinn ME, Woods MA: The Medical Assistant, Administrative and Clinical, ed 8, Philadelphia, 1998, Saunders, p. 1072.)

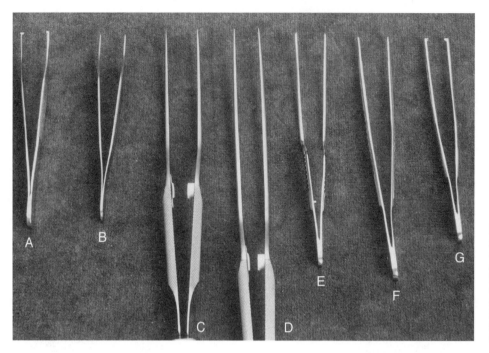

FIGURE 21-5 *A,* Toothed Adson forceps. *B,* Smooth Adson forceps. *C,* Medium long bayonet forceps. *D,* Long bayonet forceps. *E,* Short bayonet forceps. *F,* Plain-tip tissue forceps. *G,* Toothed tissue forceps. (From Kinn ME, Woods MA: The Medical Assistant, Administrative and Clinical, ed 8, Philadelphia, 1998, Saunders, p. 1072.)

C. RETRACTING INSTRUMENTS (see Figure 21-8)
  ■ Holds tissue away from surgical incision
    1. Rake retractor
      • Has pronged end
    2. Senn retractor
      • Pronged end may be sharp or dull
      • Flat end is blunt retractor
    3. Skin hook
      • Sharp point is used to retract small incisions or to secure skin edge for suturing

    4. Ribbon retractor (Crile Malleable Retractor)
      • Used to hold back tissues and organs in large wounds
D. PROBING AND DILATING INSTRUMENTS (see Figures 21-9, 21-10)
  ■ Used for surgery and exams
  ■ Probes search a cavity or wound
  ■ Dilators used to stretch a cavity or opening
    1. Specula
      • Most common dilator used
      • Valves spread apart and dilate the opening
      • Includes vaginal, nasal, rectal, and ear specula
    2. Trocars and obturators
      • Consist of sharply pointed instrument (trocar) contained within an outer tube
      • Used to withdraw fluids from cavities or for draining and irrigating with a catheter
    3. Probes
      • Different lengths (from 4 inches to 12 inches)
      • Used to enter body cavities
    4. Sound
      • Long, slender probe
E. SPECIALTY INSTRUMENTS
  ■ Fall into 4 main categories
  ■ Specific for particular exams in a specialty
    1. Gynecology (see Figure 21-11)
      a) Sponge forceps
        ■ Used like dressing forceps
      b) Uterine dressing forceps
        ■ Can reach the cervix and vagina
        ■ Used to swab the area or to apply medications

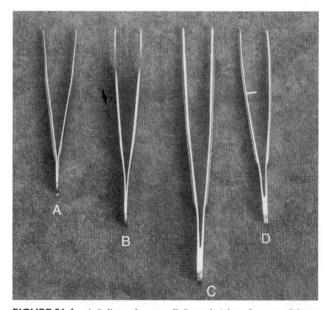

FIGURE 21-6 *A,* Splinter forceps, *B,* Smooth Adson forceps. *C,* Long plain-tip forceps. *D,* Short plain-tip tissue forceps. (From Kinn ME, Woods MA: The Medical Assistant, Administrative and Clinical, ed 8, Philadelphia, 1998, Saunders, p. 1071.)

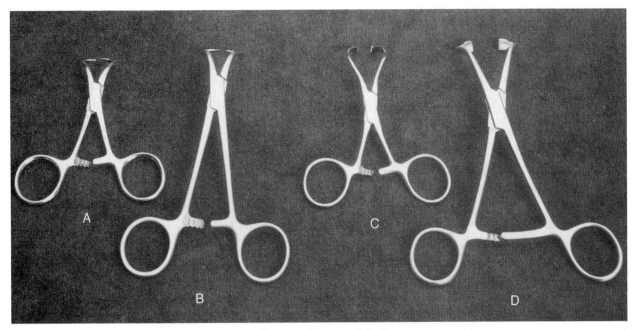

FIGURE 21-7 *A,* Small sharp towel forceps. *B,* Large sharp towel forceps. *C,* Small atraumatic towel forceps. *D,* Large atraumatic towel forceps. (From Kinn ME, Woods MA: The Medical Assistant, Administrative and Clinical, ed 8, Philadelphia, 1998, Saunders, p. 1071.)

c) Curettes (endocervical and uterine Sims)
 ■ Hollow and spoon-shaped
 ■ Used to remove polyps, secretions, and tissue
d) Schroder tenaculum forceps
 ■ Sharp, pointed tips
 ■ Used to hold tissue or cervix while obtaining specimen
e) Hegar uterine dilators
 ■ Used to dilate the cervix for dilation and curettage (D&C)

2. Ophthalmology and otolaryngology (see Figure 21-12)
 a) Krause nasal snare
 ■ Wire loop on tip
 ■ Used to remove polyps
 b) "Alligator ear" forceps
 ■ Used to remove foreign bodies
 c) Laryngeal mirror
 ■ Various sizes
 ■ Used to examine larynx and postnasal area

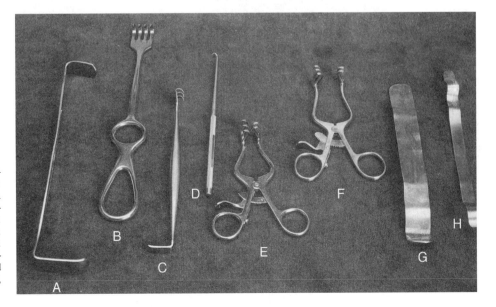

FIGURE 21-8 *A,* Army-Navy retractor. *B,* Four-prong rake retractor. *C,* Senn retractor. *D,* Single skin hook. *E,* Sharp 3/2 Weitlaner retractor. *F,* Dull 3/2 Weitlaner retractor. *G,* Wide Crile (ribbon) retractor. (H, Narrow Crile (ribbon) retractor. (From Kinn ME, Woods MA: The Medical Assistant, Administrative and Clinical, ed 8, Philadelphia, 1998, Saunders, p. 1073.)

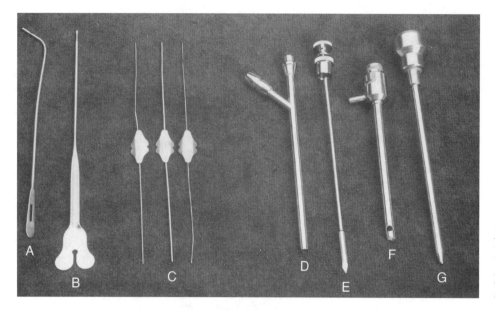

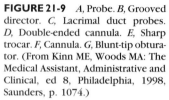

FIGURE 21-9 *A,* Probe. *B,* Grooved director. *C,* Lacrimal duct probes. *D,* Double-ended cannula. *E,* Sharp trocar. *F,* Cannula. *G,* Blunt-tip obturator. (From Kinn ME, Woods MA: The Medical Assistant, Administrative and Clinical, ed 8, Philadelphia, 1998, Saunders, p. 1074.)

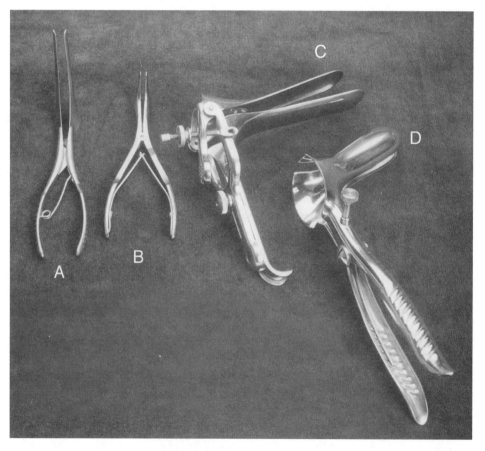

FIGURE 21-10 *A,* Long nasal speculum. *B,* Short nasal speculum. *C,* Graves vaginal speculum. *D,* Anal speculum, self-retaining. (From Kinn ME, Woods MA: The Medical Assistant, Administrative and Clinical, ed 8, Philadelphia, 1998, Saunders, p. 1074.)

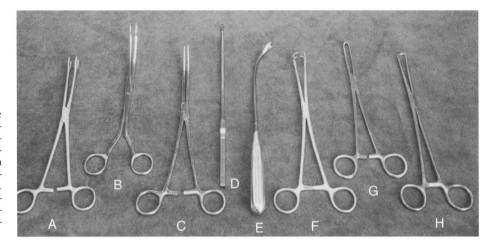

FIGURE 21-11 *A,* Foerster sponge forceps. *B,* Placenta forceps. *C,* Bozeman uterine dressing forceps. *D,* Endocervical curette. *E,* Sims uterine curette. *F,* Schroeder uterine vulsellum forceps. *G,* Long Allis forceps. *H,* Schroeder uterine tenaculum forceps. (From Kinn ME, Woods MA: The Medical Assistant, Administrative and Clinical, ed 8, Philadelphia, 1998, Saunders, p. 1075.)

d) Buck ear curette
  ■ Sharp or blunt scraper end
  ■ Used to remove foreign matter from ear canals
3. Biopsy
  a) Cervical biopsy forceps
    ■ Used to obtain specimens
  b) Punch biopsy
    ■ Used to remove tissue specimens
  c) Biopsy needle
    ■ Works on the same principle as obturator
  d) Abscess needle
    ■ Used to withdraw fluids or pus from cyst or abscess
    ■ Usually disposable

4. Genitourinary
  • Foley catheter
    ■ Manufactured in sizes 8 to 32 (French)
    ■ Used as an indwelling catheter
5. Endoscopes
  • Hollow, cylindrical instruments
  • Used to visualize the interior of a cavity or opening
    a) Sigmoidoscope: used to visualize the sigmoid colon
    b) Proctoscope: used to visualize the rectum
    c) Anoscope: used to visualize the superficial rectum
    d) Bronchoscope: used to visualize the larynx, trachea, and bronchi

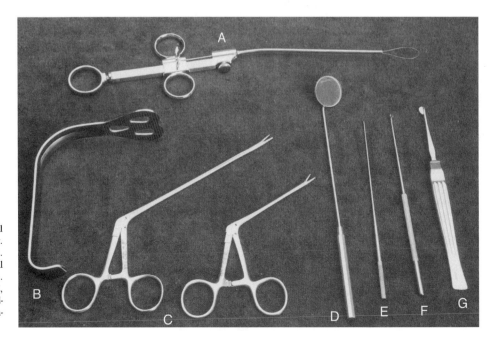

FIGURE 21-12 *A,* Krause nasal snare. *B,* Metal tongue depressor. *C,* Long and short alligator forceps. *D,* Laryngeal mirror. *E,* Ivan metal applicator. *F,* "Buck" ear curette. *G,* Sharp ear dissector. (From Kinn ME, Woods MA: The Medical Assistant, Administrative and Clinical, ed 8, Philadelphia, 1998, Saunders, p. 1076.)

e) Otoscope: used to visualize the external and middle ear

f) Cytoscope: used to visualize the urinary bladder

g) Laparoscope: used to visualize the peritoneal and abdominal cavities

II. Sutures and Needles

■ Suture: act of stitching or sewing together

■ Material used to stitch or sew

■ May also be used to ligate (tie off)

A. TYPES

1. Absorbable
   • Dissolves and is absorbed by body's enzymes
   • Includes
     a) Surgical catgut (surgical gut)
        ▪ Used in tissues that heal rapidly
        ▪ Obtained from sheep, cattle, pig intestines
        ▪ Packaged in alcohol to keep it pliable
     b) Chromic
        ▪ Catgut coated with chromic salts
        ▪ Delayed absorption of up to 80 days
     c) Vicryl
        ▪ Synthetic suture made of polyglactin
        ▪ Takes up to 11 weeks to absorb

2. Nonabsorbable
   • Left in the body, where it embeds in scar tissue or must be removed when healing is complete
   • Used frequently in office minor surgeries
     a) Silk
        ▪ Strong
        ▪ Easy to tie and remove
     b) Cotton
        ▪ Not used much (polyester more common)
     c) Polyester fiber
        ▪ Strongest of all suture material
     d) Stainless steel
        ▪ Surgical staples
        ▪ Used on skin, nerves, blood vessels
        ▪ Applied with a skin stapler

B. SIZING

■ Diameter of strand determines the size

■ Sized from 6-0 (smallest) to 6 (largest)

■ Length of strands are precut (into 18-, 24-, 54-, and 60-inch lengths)

■ 2-0 to 6-0 most common

C. SUTURE REMOVAL

■ Physician determines the length of time sutures remain in place

■ Must always be left in place long enough for proper healing to take place

■ In general

• Skin sutures in head and neck: remove in 3 to 5 days

• Skin sutures in other areas: 7 to 10 days

D. NEEDLES

■ Chosen according to area used

■ Classified by
   1. Shape
      • Straight
      • Curved (more easily manipulated)
   2. Type of point
      • Tapered (for delicate tissue)
      • Cutting (for skin)
   3. Eye
      • Eyelet (have to thread the needle)
      • Eyeless (suture material attached to the needle; atraumatic)

E. ADHESIVE SKIN CLOSURES

■ Sterile, nonallergenic tape

■ Available in a variety of widths and lengths

■ Used when not much tension exists on the skin edges

■ Applied transversely across the incision line

■ Eliminate the need for sutures and anesthetic

■ Easily applied and removed

■ Less scarring

■ Example: Steri-Strips

III. Drapes

■ Sterile paper or cloth material placed over or around the operative site

■ Used to maintain sterility

■ Types
   1. Plain
   2. Fenestrated
      • Contains a precut opening
      • Opening is placed over the operative site
   3. Incisional
      • Adhesive-backed plastic
      • Drape adheres directly to skin
      • Incision is made through the drape

IV. Anesthesia

■ Injected into the surgical site to prevent the sensation of pain

■ Medications used for anesthesia end in the suffix "-cain(e)"

■ Example of anesthesia medication: Xylocaine, lidocaine, Novocaine

■ May contain epinephrine
   • Enhances the effect of the anesthesia
   • Minimizes bleeding at the operative site

■ Takes effect in from 5 to 15 minutes; will be effective for 1 to 3 hours

■ Types of local anesthesia
   1. Infiltration: solution is injected under the skin to anesthetize nerve endings

2. Nerve block: solution is injected into an accessible main nerve
3. Topical: solution is painted (or sprayed) directly onto the skin or mucous membrane

V. Surgical Asepsis (see Table 21-1)

■ Destruction of organisms before they enter the body
■ Used any time skin or mucous membrane is punctured, pierced, or incised

A. BASIC RULES

1. Clean with clean
2. Dirty with dirty
3. Sterile with sterile
4. When in doubt, throw it out

B. SURGICAL SCRUB

1. Hands and forearms scrubbed for 3 to 10 minutes
2. Use surgical soap with a brush
3. Clean under the fingernails
4. Hands held up; rinsed from fingertips to elbows
5. Dry with sterile towels
6. Glove immediately

C. STERILE GLOVES

■ Used whenever the patient needs to be protected from microorganisms (all surgical procedures)
■ Used when handling sterile instruments or sterile supplies
1. Select the proper glove size
2. Open the package
3. With the nondominant hand, lift the glove for the dominant hand by the folded edge of the cuff
4. Put on the glove, keeping it above your waist
5. Pick up the second glove by placing the gloved fingers under the cuff; insert the hand; adjust the cuffs and fingers
6. Always keep gloved hands above your waist and away from your body

D. STERILE FIELD

■ Any surface on which sterile items are placed
■ Created by draping sterile towels over a Mayo stand
■ Sterile field is also a draped surgical site after the patient's skin is prepped and draped
■ Any item placed below the waist is considered contaminated
■ The 1-inch edge around the entire sterile field is considered nonsterile
■ Edges of all wrappers, packs, and towels are nonsterile
■ Sides of containers are nonsterile
■ Moisture carries bacteria from nonsterile to sterile surfaces

E. HANDLING INSTRUMENTS AND SUPPLIES

■ Sterile forceps are used to handle sterile instruments or sterile supplies when sterile gloves are not being worn
1. Lift forceps out of the container without touching the sides of the container
2. Touch the tips of the forceps to sterile gauze to dry
3. Always keep forceps tips facing down
■ Lids removed from containers are placed face up on surfaces; hold face down if not placed on surfaces
■ Pour solutions to avoid splashing; avoid touching the rim of a sterile receptacle with the bottle
■ Do not reach over the sterile field
■ Cover the setup with a sterile towel if it is not to be used immediately

Table 21-1. How to Distinguish Between Medical and Surgical Asepsis

	Medical Asepsis	Surgical Asepsis
Definition	Destruction of organisms *after* they leave the body	Destruction of organisms *before* they enter the body
Purpose	Prevent reinfection of the patient. Avoid cross-infection from one person to another	Care for open wounds. Use in surgery
Technique	Universal blood and body-fluid precautions Isolation techniques	Sterile technique
Procedure	Clean objects are kept from contamination	Objects must be sterile
	Clean gloves and clean barriers used	Sterile gloves and articles used
	Objects disinfected as soon as possible after contact with the patient	Objects must be sterilized before contact with the patient
When used	For examinations that do not involve open wounds or breaks in the skin or mucous membranes but do involve patient blood or body fluids. Isolating infected persons from others	Surgery, biopsy, wound treatment, insertion of instruments into sterile body cavities
Handwashing technique	Hands and wrists washed for 1 to 2 minutes; soap, water, and plenty of friction used to remove oil and microorganisms from fingers	Hand and forearms scrubbed for 3 to 10 minutes; surgical soap, running water, friction, and sterile brush used; fingernails must be cleaned
	Hands held downward, running water allowed to drain off fingertips; hands dried with paper towels	Hands held up, under running water, to drain off elbows; hands dried with sterile towels

From Kinn ME, Woods MA: The Medical Assistant: Administrative and Clinical, 8th ed., Philadelphia, 1999 WB Saunders, p. 1087.

F. SKIN PREPARATION

- Skin cannot be sterilized
- Resident and transient bacteria must be completely removed
- Skin prep is performed by a gloved assistant
- Make sure that the patient is not allergic to the surgical scrub solution used (examples: Betadine, iodine)
- Area is cleansed in a circular motion from the inside of the circle out; repeat the cleansing with a new sponge; dry with sterile, dry sponges

VI. Wounds

- Interruption in continuity of internal or external body tissues

A. TYPES OF WOUNDS

1. Closed wound
   - Nonpenetrating
   - No outward opening
   - Underlying tissue is damaged

2. Open wound
   - Skin is broken
   - Underlying tissue is exposed
   - Classified according to the appearance of the opening
     a) Laceration: jagged, irregular, breaking or tearing of tissues
     b) Puncture: skin is pierced by a pointed object (e.g., pin, nail, splinter)
     c) Abrasion: superficial wound; scraping of the skin
     d) Avulsion: tissue is torn away or separated
     e) Surgical incision: neat, clean-cut
     f) Contusion: closed, nonpenetrating wound; blood from broken vessels accumulates in tissues

B. WOUND HEALING (see Figure 21-13)

- All wounds go through healing (repair)
- Three phases

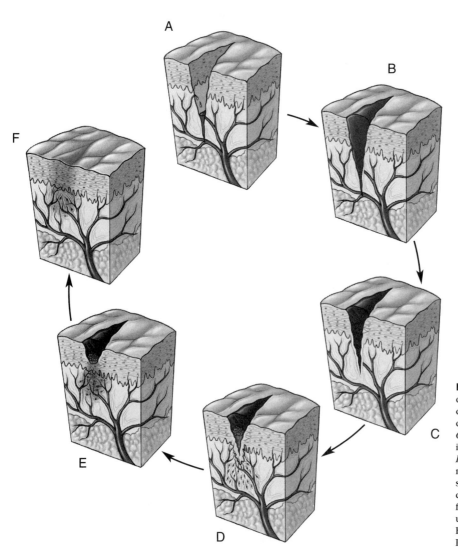

FIGURE 21-13 Steps in tissue repair. *A,* A deep wound to the skin severs blood vessels, causing blood to fill the wound. *B,* A blood clot forms, and as it dries, it forms a scab. *C* and *D,* The process of tissue repair begins. Scar tissue forms in the deep layers. *E,* At the same time, surface epithelial cells multiply and fill the area between the scar tissue and the scab. *F,* When the epithelium is complete, the scab detaches. The result is a fully regenerated layer of epithelium over an underlying area of scar tissue. (From Herlihy B, Maebius N: The Human Body in Health and Illness, Philadelphia, 1999, Saunders, p. 86.)

1. Lag phase
   - Blood vessels contract to control bleeding
   - Platelets form a plug
   - Fibrin is released to begin clotting (dried clot becomes the scab)
   - WBCs arrive at the site to clear away debris
   - Within 1 to 4 days, fibrin threads contract and pull the edges of the wound together under the scab
2. Proliferation phase
   - Lasts from 5 to 20 days
   - Tissues repair themselves
   - Wound continues to contract and seal
3. Remodeling phase
   - Day 21 on
   - Scar tissue forms
   - Scar tissue is not true skin; very strong and nonelastic
   - Scar tissue is connective tissue without blood or nerve supply

C. CLASSIFICATION OF WOUND REPAIR
1. First intention
   - Minimal tissue damage and scarring
   - Wound may be sutured closed
2. Second intention
   - Wound edges are not sutured or approximated
   - Heals slowly from bottom up
   - Large amount of scarring
3. Third intention
   - Infected wound requires reopening

VII. Dressings and Bandages

A. DRESSINGS: STERILE COVERING PLACED OVER WOUND
1. Protect wound from injury and/or contamination

2. Maintain constant pressure on the wound
3. Help hold wound edges together
4. Control bleeding
5. Absorbs drainage and secretions
6. Hide temporary disfigurement
7. May need to be removed periodically so that the wound can be checked for healing or suture removal
8. Always note drainage in chart
   a) Sanguineous: contains mostly blood
   b) Purulent: contains pus
   c) Serosanguineous: contains blood and serous fluid
   d) Serous: contains no blood
   e) May note color and odor

B. BANDAGES
■ Nonsterile material used to hold dressings in place
1. Splints and protects injured tissue
2. Maintains pressure on the wound
3. Aids in circulation
■ Made up of different materials and different sizes
1. Gauze roller bandage
2. Kling (self-adhering)
3. Elastic cloth (Ace)
4. Adhesive bandage (Band-Aid)
5. Seamless tubular gauze (Tube-gauze)

VIII. Patient Education

■ Instruct the patient to contact the practitioner immediately to report
1. Excessive bleeding at the wound site
2. Fever
3. Redness, swelling, or streaking around the wound site

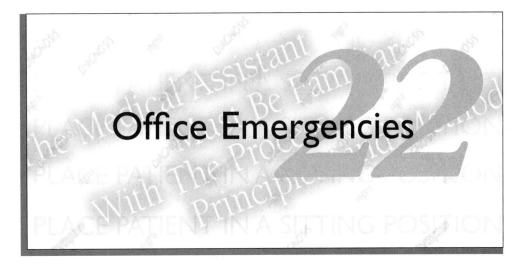

Office Emergencies

■ First aid: immediate care given to a person who has been injured or suddenly taken ill

I. Rules for Emergencies

A. STAY CALM; REASSURE THE PATIENT AND MAKE THE PATIENT AS COMFORTABLE AS POSSIBLE

B. SURVEY THE SITUATION AND DECIDE WHETHER THE NEED IS EMERGENT

C. EXAMINE THE SCENE

D. AIRWAY IS FIRST PRIORITY

E. IF THE PATIENT IS CONSCIOUS, MUST GET CONSENT; IF THE PATIENT IS UNCONSCIOUS, CONSENT IS IMPLIED

F. CARE FOR LIFE-THREATENING CONDITIONS FIRST

G. AFTER THE EMERGENCY IS UNDER CONTROL, ACCURATELY DOCUMENT THE EVENTS AND MEDICATIONS USED

H. FOLLOW STANDARD PRECAUTIONS AT ALL TIMES

II. Common Emergencies

A. FAINTING (SYNCOPE)
1. Lay the patient with the patient's head lower than the heart
2. Loosen the patient's tight clothing
3. Maintain an open airway
4. Apply a cool cloth to the patient's head
5. Pass aromatic spirits of ammonia under the patient's nose
6. Keep the patient supine for 10 minutes after consciousness is regained

B. CHOKING
1. Do not interfere if the patient can speak, cough, or breathe
2. Use the Heimlich maneuver if the victim cannot speak, cough, or breathe
3. If the patient becomes unconscious, position the patient on his/her back; call for help
4. Begin CPR after removing the foreign body

C. CHEST PAIN
1. Sit the patient down
2. Keep the patient quiet and warm
3. Loosen the patient's tight clothing
4. Take the apical and radial pulse
5. Administer oxygen if the practitioner so orders
6. Bring the emergency ("crash") cart into the room
7. If cardiac arrest occurs, perform CPR

D. CEREBROVASCULAR ACCIDENT (CVA)
1. Protect the patient against injury
2. Keep the patient lying down
3. Maintain an open airway
4. Do not give food or water

E. POISONING
1. Ask what was taken, how much was taken, how long ago, and whether or not vomiting has occurred
2. Call the poison control center
3. Induce vomiting (unless a corrosive had been ingested) or dilute with 1 to 2 cups of water or milk; give 1 tablespoon of syrup of ipecac (or follow specific directions given by the poison control center)

F. ANIMAL BITES
1. Thoroughly wash the wound with soap and water
2. Report the bite to the authorities

G. INSECT BITES AND STINGS
1. Remove the stinger by brushing it off or using tweezers
2. Apply ice to the bite area
3. Be aware of patient allergy to insect bites or stings; if the patient is allergic, this is a true emergency

H. SHOCK
1. Ensure and maintain an open airway
2. Place the patient on his/her back with legs elevated above the heart
3. Loosen the patient's tight clothing
4. Cover the patient with a blanket to maintain warmth

I. ASTHMA ATTACK
1. Assist the patient with an inhaler
2. Assist the patient to relax
3. Patient may breathe into a paper bag if hyperventilating

J. SEIZURES
1. Lay the patient on his/her back
2. Loosen the patient's tight clothing
3. Do not restrain the patient
4. Protect the patient's head from injury
5. Give the patient nothing by mouth
6. Let the patient rest after the seizure subsides

K. SPRAIN
1. Elevate the sprained area
2. Apply mild compression
3. Apply ice

L. FRACTURES
1. Make the patient as comfortable as possible
2. Prevent movement of the injured area
3. Apply ice
4. Control bleeding if applicable

M. BURNS
1. Remove the patient's clothing from the burned area
2. Stay with the patient; assist the practitioner

N. LACERATIONS
1. Keep the patient as quiet as possible
2. Cover the area with a sterile dressing
3. Apply direct pressure to the wound to control bleeding
4. Elevate the injured area above the level of the patient's heart
5. Ask the patient about when the last tetanus injection was given
6. Cleanse the wound if it is not bleeding severely

O. NOSEBLEEDS (EPISTAXIS)
1. Keep the patient quiet and in a sitting position
2. Apply direct pressure to the affected nostril by pinching

P. HEMORRHAGE
1. Apply direct pressure over the area; do not remove the original pad when it becomes saturated; add additional pads
2. Elevate the injured part above the patient's heart
3. Apply pressure over the area's pressure point
4. As a last resort, apply a tourniquet

Q. HEAD INJURIES
1. Lay the patient flat
2. Do not move the patient if a neck injury is suspected
3. Do not administer the patient anything by mouth
4. Keep the patient warm and quiet
5. Watch the patient's pupils for changes

R. DIABETIC EMERGENCIES
1. For hypoglycemia (insulin shock): give juice, candy, or soda (a sugar source)
2. For hyperglycemia (diabetic coma): if the patient is conscious, administer fluids; if you are uncertain whether this is insulin shock or diabetic coma, give the patient a sugar source

S. FOREIGN BODY IN THE EYE
1. Place the patient in a darkened room
2. Apply a cool, wet compress to the affected eye; do not apply pressure

■ Caregiver is covered by the good Samaritan laws at the scene of an accident
■ Keep emergency phone numbers near phones
■ Keep your CPR and first aid cards current
■ Do not provide care beyond your scope of training or beyond your abilities

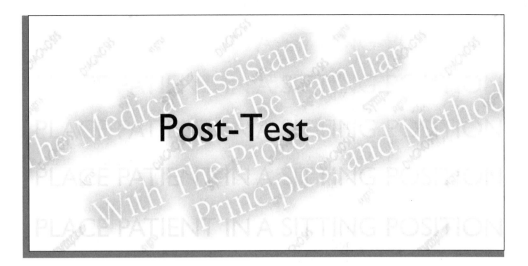

Post-Test

Directions: Each of the following questions is followed by five possible responses. Select the *best* response by completely filling in the corresponding circle on your answer sheet. Answer sheets are located at the back of the book.

1. An abnormal decrease in the size of a muscle is
   A. Myopathy
   B. Atrophy
   C. Dystrophy
   D. Hypertrophy
   E. Myotrophy

2. The cell from which a muscle develops is
   A. A myeloblast
   B. An osteoblast
   C. A myoblast
   D. A myoclast
   E. An erythroblast

3. The abbreviation for "right ear" is
   A. AD
   B. AS
   C. AU
   D. OD
   E. OS

4. An otoscope is used to
   A. Inspect the nasal cavity
   B. Inspect the exterior ear canal
   C. Measure eyeball pressure
   D. Inspect the oral cavity
   E. Measure O_2 levels

5. The procedure that is used to puncture the chest to remove fluid is called
   A. Spirometry
   B. Bronchoscopy
   C. Intubation
   D. Thoracentesis
   E. Tracheostomy

6. Which of the following lab tests would be abnormal for a patient with anemia?
   A. Differential
   B. Hematocrit/hemoglobin
   C. Blood glucose
   D. Total cholesterol
   E. WBC count

7. Hyperparathyroidism may be treated by which medical specialist?
   A. Cardiologist
   B. EMT
   C. Endocrinologist
   D. Hematologist
   E. Obstetrician

8. An abnormal increase in total number of WBCs is
   A. Anemia
   B. Leukopenia
   C. Leukosis
   D. Leukocytosis
   E. Polycythemia

9. Extremely rapid breathing is called
   A. Hyperpnea
   B. Hypopnea
   C. Dyspnea
   D. Apnea
   E. Hypertension

10. Which of the following suffixes refers to pain?
    A. -phagea
    B. -desis
    C. -pnea
    D. -algia
    E. -lysis

11. A suffix used to denote a surgical repair is
    A. -pexy
    B. -desis
    C. -plasty
    D. -lysis
    E. -centesis

12. A mammogram is a radiograph of the
    A. Chest
    B. Bladder
    C. Breast
    D. Lymph nodes
    E. Axilla

13. The term alopecia is synonymous with
    A. Excessive hair growth
    B. Itching
    C. Myopia
    D. Baldness
    E. Whitish pigmentation of the skin

14. Another term for chewing is
    A. Mastication
    B. Obstipation
    C. Deglutition
    D. Peristalsis
    E. Regurgitation

15. A nevus in the antecubital area is a
    A. Mass on the shoulder
    B. Polyp on the lower back
    C. Wart on the ankle
    D. Scar on the knee
    E. Mole on the inside of the elbow

16. An inflammation of a joint is
    A. Arthrodesis
    B. Arthrodynia
    C. Arthroclasis
    D. Arthritis
    E. Arthrocentesis

17. Fat makes up
    A. The epidermis
    B. Adipose tissue
    C. Muscle tissue
    D. Tendons
    E. Lymphatic tissue

18. The cause of disease is referred to as
    A. Biology
    B. Epidemiology
    C. Pathology
    D. Etiology
    E. Physiology

19. The function of the olfactory nerve is
    A. Touching
    B. Tasting
    C. Smelling
    D. Seeing
    E. Hearing

20. An oophorectomy is a surgical procedure of the
    A. Uterus
    B. Ovaries
    C. Knee
    D. Vagina
    E. Ear

21. The study of diseases and treatment of the male and female urinary systems is
    A. Nephrology
    B. Oncology
    C. Urology
    D. Proctology
    E. Gynecology

22. A diagnostic procedure that allows for visualization of the urinary bladder is
    A. Urethral dilation
    B. IVP
    C. Cystography
    D. Cystoscopy
    E. TURP

23. A patient with hives most likely will report that he or she has
    A. Urticaria
    B. Verruca
    C. A nevus
    D. Shingles
    E. Alopecia

24. The membrane that surrounds the heart is the
    A. Endocardium
    B. Endometrium
    C. Pericardium
    D. Perineum
    E. Myocardium

25. A mucous membrane
    A. Lines closed cavities of the body
    B. Covers the lungs
    C. Lines the abdominal cavity
    D. Lines body cavities that open to the outside
    E. Surrounds the heart

26. The ventral region of the body is described as
    A. Superior
    B. Lateral
    C. Medial
    D. Anterior
    E. Posterior

27. The body cavity that contains the intestines is the
    A. Thoracic
    B. Spinal
    C. Abdominal
    D. Pleural
    E. Peritoneal

28. Movement of a body part toward the midline of the body is
    A. Supination
    B. Pronation
    C. Adduction
    D. Abduction
    E. Rotation

29. The plane that divides the body into front and back halves is
    A. Frontal
    B. Horizontal
    C. Median
    D. Oblique
    E. Transverse

30. Reye's syndrome
    A. Can follow a viral illness in children
    B. Is caused by high fever
    C. Is a symptom of AIDS
    D. Causes muscular dystrophy
    E. Is the common cold

31. The vertebrae of the lower back are the
    A. Cervical
    B. Thoracic
    C. Lumbar
    D. Sacral
    E. Coccyx

32. An acute infectious skin disease caused by strep or staph is
    A. Impetigo
    B. Psoriasis
    C. Athlete's foot
    D. Melanoma
    E. Eczema

33. The bone located in the posterior of the skull is the
    A. Frontal
    B. Ethmoid
    C. Temporal
    D. Occipital
    E. Mandible

34. The type of bone fracture in which the bone is bent and partially broken is a
    A. Simple fracture
    B. Compound fracture
    C. Greenstick fracture
    D. Comminuted fracture
    E. Complete fracture

35. The peripheral nervous system is composed of how many pairs of spinal nerves?
    A. 2
    B. 5
    C. 12
    D. 20
    E. 31

36. The pons and medulla make up the
    A. Brain stem
    B. Cerebellum
    C. Cerebrum
    D. Thalamus
    E. Right hemisphere

37. A failure of bone marrow to produce red blood cells results in which type of anemia?
    A. Aplastic
    B. Hemolytic
    C. Pernicious
    D. Microcytic
    E. Leukemia

38. Protrusion of a part of the stomach through the esophageal opening in the diaphragm is a(n)
    A. Esophageal aneurysm
    B. Esophageal varices
    C. Hiatal hernia
    D. Pyloric stenosis
    E. GERD

39. The tympanic membrane is the
    A. Ossicle
    B. Cochlea
    C. Auricle
    D. Eardrum
    E. Organ of Corti

40. The largest artery in the body is the
    A. Brachial artery
    B. Temporal artery
    C. Radial artery
    D. Aorta
    E. Femoral artery

41. The SA node
    A. Stimulates the diaphragm
    B. Is the same as the AV node
    C. Is the pacemaker of the heart
    D. Divides the heart into right and left
    E. Regulates blood flow to the brain

42. An X-ray taken to confirm a fracture of the distal forearm includes the
    A. Tibia and fibula
    B. Radius and ulna
    C. Femur and trochanter
    D. Calcaneus and malleolus
    E. Humerus and scapula

43. Which of the following demonstrates an involuntary muscle action?
    A. Heartbeat
    B. Breathing
    C. Peristalsis
    D. Pupil dilation
    E. All of the above

44. Which of the following organs are located in the RUQ?
    A. Liver
    B. Right ovary
    C. Appendix
    D. Uterus
    E. Stomach

45. The diaphragm is stimulated by which nerve?
    A. Trochlear
    B. Accessory
    C. Sciatic
    D. Phrenic
    E. Vagus

46. An abnormal lateral curvature of the spine is known as
    A. Spondylosis
    B. Kyphosis
    C. Scoliosis
    D. Ankylosis
    E. Lordosis

47. The alpha cells in the pancreas are responsible for the production of
    A. Insulin
    B. Glucagon
    C. HCL
    D. Pepsin
    E. Gastrin

48. The surgical removal of the gallbladder is a
    A. Cholectomy
    B. Colostomy
    C. Cholecystectomy
    D. Laparoscopy
    E. Gastrectomy

49. The cranial nerve involved in blindness is the
    A. Abducens
    B. Oculomotor
    C. Trigeminal
    D. Olfactory
    E. Optic

50. The number of permanent teeth is
    A. 20
    B. 24
    C. 28
    D. 32
    E. 36

51. Legally, a physician
    A. May not refuse treatment in an emergency situation
    B. May refuse to provide follow-up care after initial treatment
    C. Must provide a diagnosis to a patient's employer if requested
    D. Must provide a medical history to the patient's insurance company if the insurance company requests it
    E. May refuse to accept a patient if he or she chooses

52. An itinerary
    A. Is a yearly schedule
    B. Is a travel guide
    C. Contains tickets
    D. Is a detailed outline of a trip
    E. Makes travel arrangements

53. Professionalism may best be displayed by
    A. Keeping emotions to one's self
    B. Staying calm when dealing with angry patients
    C. Showing no consideration for other members of the team
    D. Referring all problems to the physician
    E. Arriving late or leaving early

54. The ability to imagine taking the place of the patient and accepting the patient's behavior is
    A. Objectivity
    B. Empathy
    C. Sympathy
    D. Industry
    E. Subjectivity

55. The patient's medical record belongs to
    A. The patient's spouse
    B. The physician
    C. The patient
    D. The patient's attorney
    E. The state medical board

56. A breast mass is found in a woman whose mother and sister have died from breast cancer. She cancels her next three follow-up appointments. Which defense mechanism is she using?
    A. Denial
    B. Anxiety
    C. Acceptance
    D. Isolation
    E. Suppression

57. Personality differences are due to
    A. Age
    B. Experience

C. Heredity
D. Environment
E. All of the above

58. Which is *not* a characteristic desirable in a medical assistant?
   A. Appreciation
   B. Impatience
   C. Flexibility
   D. Friendliness
   E. Concern

59. Which is *not* an example of stereotyping?
   A. Similar people have similar needs
   B. Elderly patients have hearing deficits
   C. Medicaid patients are lazy
   D. Educated patients have no fear of illness
   E. Young children react differently to stressful situations

60. To release medical information,
   A. The physician must sign a waiver
   B. The insurance company must make the request in writing
   C. The patient must sign a release form
   D. A certified record technician must be employed by the office
   E. The patient must deliver the records in person to the requester

61. Which of the following should be reported to the health department?
   A. Otitis media
   B. Strep throat
   C. Flu
   D. Vaginal yeast infection
   E. HIV

62. Which of the following is objective data?
   A. Family history
   B. Vital signs
   C. Past surgical history
   D. LMP
   E. Insurance information

63. Which of the following phone calls should be given immediately to the physician?
   A. Another physician
   B. An angry patient
   C. A patient's family member
   D. A salesperson
   E. An insurance company

64. In Maslow's hierarchy of needs, the need to be loved and free from loneliness is a
   A. Physiological need
   B. Safety need

C. Social need
D. Self-esteem need
E. Self-actualization need

65. If a patient refuses to consent to treatment, the medical assistant should
   A. Schedule the patient for another appointment
   B. Force treatment on the patient
   C. Force the patient to consent
   D. Delay treatment and inform/consult the physician
   E. Terminate the patient

66. An enforceable contract contains
   A. An offer
   B. An acceptance
   C. A consideration
   D. A capacity
   E. All of the above

67. The opposite of anterior is
   A. Distal
   B. Medial
   C. Proximal
   D. Posterior
   E. Lateral

68. Informed consent should include which of the following elements?
   A. Benefits and risks of the treatment
   B. Purpose of treatment
   C. Nature of the patient's condition
   D. Assessment of the patient's understanding of the treatment
   E. All of the above

69. All of the following are reasons for revoking a physician's license *except*
   A. Mental incapacity
   B. Physical incapacity
   C. Conviction of a crime
   D. Unprofessional conduct
   E. Providing atypical care

70. The control center of a cell is
   A. DNA
   B. Organelles
   C. Nucleus
   D. Ribosomes
   E. Cell membrane

71. Subcutaneous tissue
   A. Is found under the skin
   B. Contains fat
   C. Is an injection site
   D. Connects the dermis to the muscle surface
   E. All of the above

72. Which is *not* a bone of the lower extremity?
    A. Femur
    B. Humerus
    C. Tibia
    D. Fibula
    E. Metatarsals

73. The muscle in the upper extremity that is used as an injection site is the
    A. Deltoid
    B. Biceps brachii
    C. Triceps brachii
    D. Trapezius
    E. Gluteus medius

74. The pacemaker of the heart is the
    A. Septum
    B. SA node
    C. AV node
    D. Left atrium
    E. Mitral valve

75. Gas exchange in the lungs takes place in the
    A. Pharynx
    B. Bronchi
    C. Trachea
    D. Bronchiole
    E. Alveoli

76. The liver
    A. Makes bile
    B. Detoxifies harmful substances
    C. Produces heparin
    D. Stores glycogen
    E. All of the above

77. The fertilized ova implants into the
    A. Cervix
    B. Endometrium
    C. Myometrium
    D. Epimetrium
    E. Oviducts

78. Testosterone is produced in the
    A. Ovaries
    B. Testes
    C. Epididymis
    D. Seminal vesicles
    E. Prostate gland

79. The largest portion of the brain is the
    A. Cerebrum
    B. Cerebellum
    C. Medulla oblongata
    D. Brain stem
    E. Hypothalamus

80. There are _____ pairs of spinal nerves
    A. 100
    B. 10
    C. 12
    D. 25
    E. 31

81. Gustatory receptors are located in the
    A. Mouth
    B. Nose
    C. Eye
    D. Ear
    E. Skin

82. Insulin
    A. Is produced by the liver
    B. Controls metabolism
    C. Increases blood sugar levels
    D. Decreases blood sugar levels
    E. Controls blood calcium levels

83. A decrease in the total number of white blood cells
    A. Leukocyte
    B. Leukoderma
    C. Leukocytosis
    D. Anemia
    E. Leukopenia

84. The abbreviation meaning "immediately" is
    A. prn
    B. stat
    C. qod
    D. ad lib
    E. dc

85. The physician is legally obligated to report
    A. Deaths
    B. Births
    C. Communicable diseases
    D. Abuse
    E. All of the above

86. The prefix "brady-" denotes
    A. Slow
    B. Fast
    C. Hard
    D. Soft
    E. Difficult

87. The opposite of superficial is
    A. Ventral
    B. Proximal
    C. Deep
    D. Distal
    E. Dorsal

88. An authorization in advance to withdraw artificial life support is
    A. Assault
    B. Battery
    C. An advance directive
    D. Uniform Anatomical Gift Act
    E. Good Samaritan Act

89. Unconsciously avoiding the reality of an unpleasant event is
    A. Regression
    B. Denial
    C. Repression
    D. Suppression
    E. Rationalization

90. "Tell me more about it" is an example of
    A. An open-ended statement
    B. A closed statement
    C. Clarification
    D. Feedback
    E. Reflection

91. The study of the cause of disease is
    A. Epidemiology
    B. Pathology
    C. Etiology
    D. Symptomology
    E. Risk management

92. Nonverbal communication may be conveyed by
    A. Touch
    B. Eye contact
    C. Body position
    D. Silence
    E. All of the above

93. Bulimia is
    A. A mass of food
    B. An eating disorder
    C. Loss of appetite
    D. A blood condition
    E. An arrhythmia

94. A cerebral vascular accident can also be called a(n)
    A. Arrhythmia
    B. Heart attack
    C. Aneurysm
    D. Stroke
    E. Thrombus

95. Rubeola is
    A. Herpes simplex I
    B. Scarlet fever
    C. Whooping cough
    D. Measles
    E. Chicken pox

96. A sexually transmitted disease caused by a protozoal infestation is
    A. Herpes
    B. Gonorrhea
    C. Trichomoniasis
    D. Crabs
    E. Syphillis

97. An electrolyte that has an important influence of the activity of the heart muscles is
    A. Chloride
    B. Magnesium
    C. Peptase
    D. Phosphorus
    E. Potassium

98. Which of the following respiratory disorders is characterized by a loss of lung capacity?
    A. Asthma
    B. Emphysema
    C. Bronchitis
    D. Tuberculosis
    E. Psoriasis

99. The type of membrane that lines cavities of the body that open to the outside is
    A. Cutaneous
    B. Synovial
    C. Mucous
    D. Pleural
    E. Peritoneum

100. Another name for an open fracture is a
    A. Communated fracture
    B. Closed fracture
    C. Simple fracture
    D. Greenstick fracture
    E. Compound fracture

101. Which of the following types of scheduling is *not* a good type of time management?
    A. Same-day appointments
    B. Double-booking
    C. Wave
    D. Modified wave
    E. Grouping

102. What piece of mail should be placed on top when sorting the physician's mail?
    A. First-class mail
    B. Journals
    C. Special delivery letter

D. Envelope marked "personal"
E. Bills and statements

103. Open punctuation is characterized by
A. Enclosure notation
B. Absence of punctuation after the salutation and a comma after the complimentary close
C. Modified block style
D. Use of a colon after the salutation
E. Block style

104. The federal insurance program that provides for the medically indigent is
A. CHAMPUS
B. Medicare
C. Blue Shield
D. Medicaid
E. HMO

105. The process of transferring an amount from the day sheet to the ledger is
A. Journalizing
B. Charting
C. Posting
D. Crediting
E. Debiting

106. A numeric filing system requires the use of
A. Lateral files
B. An alphabetical cross-reference
C. Color-coding
D. A tickler file
E. Subject headings

107. The file folder label for Jennie Holmes-Mathis should be
A. Jennie, Holmes-Mathis
B. Mathis, Jennie Holmes
C. Holmes, Jennie-Mathis
D. Holmes-Mathis, Jennie
E. Mathis, Jennie (nee Holmes)

108. Third-party participation in an office indicates the relationship between the physician,
A. Patient and medical assistant
B. Medical assistant and insurance company
C. Patient and insurance company
D. Hospital and insurance
E. Patient and hospital

109. A claim may be rejected by an insurance company because of the omission of
A. Complete diagnosis
B. Policy number
C. Patient birth date
D. Itemization of charges
E. All of the above

110. How much postage is required for a first-class letter that weighs 3 oz if the first ounce costs $0.34 and each additional ounce is $0.25?
A. $1.00
B. $0.50
C. $0.34
D. $0.84
E. $0.75

111. When the word "Confidential" is to be typed on the envelope, it should be placed
A. In the lower right corner
B. Below the zip code
C. In the lower left corner
D. Below the return address
E. Both C and D

112. The most formal of complimentary closings is
A. Very truly yours
B. Warm wishes
C. Sincerely
D. Sincerely yours
E. As always

113. When making an appointment, which of the following is *not* needed?
A. Patient's name
B. Phone number
C. Reason for visit
D. Insurance information
E. Availability

114. This type of call allows more than one person in more than one place to talk simultaneously:
A. Person-to-person
B. Conference call
C. Three-party billing
D. Appointment call
E. Collect call

115. This procedure protects against the loss of data:
A. Buffering
B. Debugging
C. Backing-up
D. Initializing
E. Formatting

116. A tickler file is
A. A guide for processing insurance claims
B. A list of procedures for equipment maintenance
C. A type of color-coding
D. A physician referral service
E. Future events arranged in chronological order

117. All of the following would require a CPT code *except*
A. Diarrhea
B. Mastectomy

C. Otoplasty
D. Hysterectomy
E. Sigmoidoscopy

118. Which of the following characteristics of a receptionist could make an impression on a patient?
   A. Appearance
   B. Professionalism
   C. Manners
   D. Attitude
   E. All of the above

119. A direction to consider additional codes is
   A. NEC
   B. NOS
   C. See also
   D. See condition
   E. See category

120. A "V" code
   A. Refers to specific health conditions
   B. Refers to specific body systems
   C. Refers to factors that influence health status
   D. Refers to neoplasms
   E. Refers to injuries

121. Mail that is opened accidentally should be
   A. Hand-delivered immediately
   B. Put at the bottom of the stack
   C. Left as-is
   D. Resealed with tape, and noted as "opened in error"
   E. Placed in another envelope

122. Which of the following are E/M descriptors?
   A. Physical exam
   B. School physical
   C. Well-baby check-up
   D. Pre-op physical
   E. All of the above

123. Which is an example of a third-party payer?
   A. HMO
   B. Medicare
   C. PPO
   D. Patient's spouse
   E. Patient's parent

124. In the POMR system, the initial database includes
   A. A list of past medical problems
   B. A complete physical exam
   C. A numbered list of present problems
   D. The patient's progress
   E. A list of social problems

125. A trial balance is a comparison of
   A. Cash on hand and cash received
   B. Daily charges and payments

C. Balance sheet and income sheet
D. Ledger card totals and account-receivable balance
E. Owners' equity and liabilities

126. When adding information to the medical record, new notes are added
   A. In alphabetical order
   B. In subject order
   C. Newest to the front
   D. Newest to the back
   E. To a newly created file

127. Which of the following calls require immediate transfer to the physician?
   A. A young child with a high fever
   B. A patient with a possible medical allergy
   C. Another physician
   D. An adult with a low-grade fever
   E. A patient with questions about a mammogram

128. Appointments should be scheduled
   A. For 15 minutes each with 15-minute open slots in between
   B. Every 15 minutes
   C. Either all in the morning or all in the afternoon
   D. In consecutive order without large gaps
   E. So that patients with similar problems are seen on the same day

129. Which is *not* part of basic information obtained at the patient's first visit?
   A. Insurance information
   B. Name, address, phone number
   C. Name of person who referred the patient
   D. Business address and business phone number
   E. Diagnosis

130. Standard size paper and envelope for business correspondence is
   A. 8-½ × 11; no. 10 envelope
   B. 7-¼ × 10-½; no. 7-¾ envelope
   C. 5-½ × 8-½; 3-½ × 6 envelope
   D. 6-¼ × 9-¼; no. 6-¾ envelope
   E. 11 × 14; no. 10 envelope

131. Patient's ledger cards should be kept
   A. With the patient's chart
   B. In a general ledger
   C. In a separate ledger file
   D. In a job ledger
   E. With insurance forms

132. The bank statement is reconciled with
   A. The checkbook
   B. The day sheet

C. Accounts receivable
D. The payment record
E. Both A and D

133. The record of the proceedings of a meeting is the
A. Agenda
B. Roberts Rules
C. Itinerary
D. Minutes
E. Format

134. Which of the following protects data from loss?
A. Booting-up the system
B. Initializing disks
C. Backing-up
D. Virus check
E. Debugging

135. The scheduling system based on scheduling similar appointments or procedures together is called
A. Wave
B. Modified wave
C. Grouping
D. Double-booking
E. Open scheduling

136. Appropriate information to include in a patient information brochure would be
A. Information about the scope of the practice
B. Physician's fees
C. Billing information
D. Employee's names and telephone numbers
E. Coding information

137. A new employee must complete which of the following?
A. 501 form
B. W-4 form
C. W-3 form
D. W-2 form
E. FICA form

138. Which of the following abbreviations is *not* correct?
A. pH
B. mEq
C. PKU
D. HGB
E. Kg

139. Patient information that is released without patient's authorization could result in legal charge of
A. Fraud
B. Battery
C. Invasion of privacy
D. Abandonment
E. Libel

140. A correctly addressed envelope includes
A. Omission of all punctuation
B. Periods after abbreviation
C. Periods after initials
D. Comma between city and state
E. Comma between street name and numbers

141. Which of the following circumstances would waive the need for a written release of medical records?
A. Requested from other practices
B. A subpoena
C. Attorney request
D. Hospital request
E. Insurance company request

142. In double-entry bookkeeping, the original entry is put onto the
A. Patient ledger card
B. Daily log
C. General ledger
D. Account ledger
E. Appointment book

143. The correct way to indicate an enclosure notation is
A. encl:
B. Enclosure
C. enclosure
D. enc
E. encl

144. A superbill provides which of the following?
A. Insurance claim
B. Fee schedule
C. Deposit slip
D. Dictation
E. Abnormal test results

145. Which of the following is the purpose of records management?
A. Storage
B. Arranging
C. Accessibility
D. Classifying
E. All of the above

146. Which coding system is *not* associated with medical procedures?
A. CPT
B. ICD-9-CM
C. HCPCS
D. RVS
E. RBRVS

147. Which is *not* an indexing rule?
  A. Unit 1 is the surname
  B. A hyphen is disregarded
  C. Initials come after complete names
  D. Apostrophes are disregarded
  E. Names are divided into units

148. ICD-9-CM codes that refer to factors that may influence the patient's health status are
  A. HIV codes
  B. Volume I codes
  C. Volume II codes
  D. E-codes
  E. V-codes

149. The smallest piece of information that the computer can process is a(n)
  A. Output
  B. Bit
  C. Byte
  D. Font
  E. Icon

150. The index of files on a disk is the
  A. Window
  B. Menu
  C. Byte
  D. Directory
  E. Icon

151. The appointment system of the office should take into account the needs of the
  A. Staff
  B. Physician
  C. Patients
  D. A and B only
  E. B and C only

152. "Dear Mrs. May:" is an example of
  A. Open punctuation
  B. Mixed punctuation
  C. Block punctuation
  D. Semiblock punctuation
  E. Modified block

153. A master list of equipment inventory includes all of the following *except* the
  A. Date of purchase
  B. Cost
  C. Operating manuals
  D. Estimated life of the piece
  E. Description

154. Which of the following hospital records may be released by the authorization of the attending surgeon only?
  A. Nurses' notes
  B. Operative notes
  C. Lab reports
  D. Radiology reports
  E. Billing information

155. An illness that existed before an insurance policy is written is known as a(n)
  A. Special risk
  B. Exclusion
  C. Preexisting condition
  D. Waiting period
  E. Prior authorization required

156. A patient has not been seen in the office for two years. His record would be found in the
  A. Basement
  B. Active files
  C. Open files
  D. Inactive files
  E. Closed files

157. An important consideration when deciding how to position the computer monitor at the reception desk is
  A. Patient confidentiality
  B. Staff access
  C. Lighting
  D. Position of the printer
  E. Availability of patient records

158. Which group of patients should be escorted to the exam room and given instructions on what they are to do?
  A. Children
  B. New patients
  C. Established patients
  D. Elderly
  E. All of the above

159. Which information is *not* essential for the surgery scheduler when requesting a surgery date?
  A. Type of procedure
  B. Name of the assisting physician
  C. Name of patient
  D. Age of patient
  E. Telephone number of the patient

160. The notation "c: Julia Jones, MD" means
  A. A copy is made for Dr. Jones
  B. A copy of the letter is sent to Dr. Jones
  C. The receiver had been advised that a copy has been sent to Dr. Jones
  D. Dr. Jones will answer the letter
  E. The copy was sent to Dr. Jones by Certified Mail

161. A "History and Physical" usually contains all of the following *except*
  A. Results of lab tests
  B. Reason for the visit

C. Vital signs
D. Review of body systems
E. General appearance of patient

162. Under a managed care plan, the physician agrees to
    A. Set fees within certain ranges provided by the plan
    B. Accept predetermined fees
    C. Charge fees based on community average
    D. Base fees based on national average
    E. Limit the number of patients seen

163. Which type of insurance organization uses the fee-for-services concept?
    A. HMO
    B. Managed Care
    C. Independent Practice Association
    D. PPO
    E. Medicaid

164. Which factor is *not* included when determining the level of service for E and M codes?
    A. Cost of services
    B. Level of decision making required of the physician
    C. Health history of patient
    D. Type of examination
    E. Type of lab tests

165. When money is placed in an account, which of the following documents is prepared?
    A. Check
    B. Statement
    C. Debit slip
    D. Credit slip
    E. Deposit slip

166. The most common color-coding system color codes the
    A. Patient's Social Security number
    B. Patient's date of birth
    C. Patient's given name
    D. Patient's surname
    E. Patient's account number

167. Who is the legal owner of the information in a patient's medical record?
    A. The physician
    B. The patient
    C. The insurance company
    D. The patient and physician
    E. The physician and the insurance company

168. Standard Precautions are designed to be used for
    A. Patients known to be infected
    B. Patients suspected of being infected

C. All patients
D. Patients recovering from an infectious disease
E. Infected healthcare workers

169. Disposable single-use gloves should be worn
    A. When taking a blood pressure
    B. When handling specimens
    C. When performing venipuncture
    D. All of the above
    E. B and C

170. Normal oral temperature, in degrees, is
    A. 96.8 F
    B. 97.6 F
    C. 98.6 F
    D. 36 C
    E. 38 C

171. Normal respiratory rate for an adult is
    A. 10-16 breaths per minute
    B. 14-20 breaths per minute
    C. 20-26 breaths per minute
    D. 30-38 breaths per minute
    E. 30-60 breaths per minute

172. Vital signs include
    A. Temperature
    B. Blood pressure
    C. TPR
    D. A and B
    E. B and C

173. The pulse rate is
    A. Usually higher in adults than children
    B. Usually higher in children than adults
    C. The same for both
    D. Lower at birth than at one year
    E. Higher in adults over 60 than in a child under 7

174. Pulse rate is decreased by
    A. Sleep
    B. Brain injury, causing increased pressure
    C. Hypothyroidism
    D. A and B
    E. All of the above

175. A high fever occurs when the body temperature, in degrees, is
    A. 98-99 F
    B. 99-101 F
    C. 101-103 F
    D. 103-105 F
    E. 38.3-39.5 C

176. The pulse pressure is
    A. The difference between the systolic and diastolic blood pressure
    B. An occasional missed beat

C. Absence of a carotid pulse
D. Alternating weak and strong beats
E. The difference between apical and radial pulses

177. A patient who weighs 45 kg also weighs how many pounds
A. 45
B. 99
C. 105
D. 145
E. 150

178. A patient who is 72 inches tall is
A. 6 feet
B. 6 feet, 2 inches
C. 6 feet, 4 inches
D. 5 feet, 2 inches
E. 5 feet, 6 inches

179. During a physical exam, percussion is most commonly used to examine the
A. Chest and back
B. Mouth and throat
C. Eyes and ears
D. Breasts
E. Nose and neck

180. A patient's reaction to stress, use of defense mechanisms, and resources for support would be recorded under
A. Chief complaint
B. Past history
C. History of present illness
D. Social history
E. Family history

181. Subjective findings include
A. How the patient feels
B. Information about the patient's family
C. Previous pregnancies
D. All of the above
E. A and B

182. Visual acuity is
A. Pressure in the eyeball
B. Nearsightedness
C. Farsightedness
D. Color vision
E. Clearness of vision

183. The purpose of a proctoscopy is to examine the
A. Prostate gland
B. Uterus
C. Rectum
D. Sigmoid colon
E. Esophagus

184. A patient in the Sims' position is lying on the
A. Right side, with left leg flexed
B. Left side and chest, with right leg flexed
C. Back, with both legs bent
D. Right side, with right leg flexed
E. Left side, with left leg flexed

185. A patient lying flat on the abdomen is in the
A. Dorsal position
B. Lithotomy position
C. Supine position
D. Prone position
E. Fowler's position

186. The physician uses which of the following to examine the patient's eyes?
A. Ophthalmoscope
B. Percussion hammer
C. Tonometer
D. Otoscope
E. Speculum

187. The patient should be placed in which of the following positions for examination of the head and neck?
A. Standing
B. Sitting
C. Prone
D. Supine
E. Sims'

188. For an obstetrics exam, urine is routinely checked for the presence of
A. Glucose and protein
B. Glucose and ketones
C. HCG
D. Protein and ketones
E. Blood and glucose

189. A patient should be taught that the best time to perform a self-breast exam is about
A. One week after her period
B. The sixth day of every month
C. One week before her period
D. Two weeks after her period
E. Two weeks before her period

190. An infection that has a rapid onset, severe symptoms, and subsides in a short period of time is called
A. Acute
B. Chronic
C. Local
D. Systemic
E. Contagious

191. Sterile wrapped items can be safely stored, and considered sterile, for up to
    A. 7-14 days
    B. 14-21 days
    C. 21-28 days
    D. 28-35 days
    E. Indefinitely

192. When removing a pack from the autoclave, you notice that the sterilization indicator has not changed color. You should
    A. Do nothing
    B. Place the pack back in the autoclave and resterilize
    C. Place a new indicator on the pack and resterilize
    D. Place the pack back in the autoclave but in a different location
    E. Unwrap the pack; rewrap the pack; replace the indicator; resterilize

193. Scrubbing an item with soap and water before sterilization is
    A. Cleaning
    B. Sanitization
    C. Disinfection
    D. Sterilization
    E. Antisepsis

194. The type of immunity that develops from having the disease is
    A. Natural active
    B. Natural passive
    C. Acquired active
    D. Acquired passive
    E. Congenital

195. When opening a sterile pack, the top flap should be opened
    A. Toward the body
    B. Away from the body
    C. Toward the right-side
    D. Toward the left-side
    E. In any direction

196. The finest suture material of the following list is
    A. 0
    B. 00
    C. 000
    D. 4-0
    E. 8-0

197. A type of instrument that is used to grasp or hold tissues or objects is a
    A. Probe
    B. Scalpel
    C. Scissors
    D. Forceps
    E. Retractor

198. Betadine (providone-iodine) should not be used on the skin of a patient who is allergic to
    A. Alcohol
    B. Metal
    C. Iodine
    D. Soap
    E. Latex

199. Wound drainage that contains pus is charted as
    A. Serous
    B. Normal
    C. Serosanguinous
    D. Sanguinous
    E. Purulent

200. The angle for the insertion of the needle for an ID injection is
    A. 10-15 degrees
    B. 20-30 degrees
    C. 45 degrees
    D. 90 degrees
    E. Not important

201. A medication that is placed under the tongue is being administered by which technique?
    A. By mouth
    B. Buccal
    C. Sublingual
    D. Instillation
    E. Topical

202. To administer an intramuscular injection, which needle would you use?
    A. 1 inch, 25 gauge
    B. 1 ½ inch, 21 gauge
    C. 1 inch, 18 gauge
    D. ½ inch, 22 gauge
    E. 2 inch, 20 gauge

203. A type of drug that increases urinary output is
    A. Emetic
    B. Diuretic
    C. Miotic
    D. Cathartic
    E. Antibiotic

204. The physician orders 250 mg amoxicillin IM. The vial reads "500 mg per 1 ml." How much would be given to the patient?
    A. 0.5 ml
    B. 1 ml
    C. 2 ml
    D. 3 ml
    E. 5 ml

205. When a specimen is placed in a centrifuge, a tube of similar size containing a liquid of similar weight should be placed
  A. On the counter
  B. Directly opposite the specimen
  C. Directly beside the specimen
  D. In all empty spaces in the centrifuge
  E. To the right side of the specimen

206. Microscopic examination of a urine sample should be performed
  A. Within ½ hour of collection
  B. Within 1 hour of collection
  C. Within 1 ½ hours of collection
  D. Within 2 hours of collection
  E. Within 3 hours of collection

207. The absence of urine formation is termed
  A. Anuria
  B. Polyuria
  C. Dysuria
  D. Oliguria
  E. Ketonuria

208. Normal specific gravity is generally between
  A. 1.000 and 1.005
  B. 1.010 and 1.050
  C. 1.025 and 1.500
  D. 1.005 and 1.050
  E. 1.010 and 1.025

209. A CBC includes
  A. Platelet count
  B. Hemoglobin and hematocrit
  C. WBC count
  D. All of the above
  E. A and C

210. Capillary blood is usually obtained
  A. From a skin puncture
  B. From a venipuncture
  C. From an arterial puncture
  D. All of the above
  E. B and C

211. A cholecystogram is used to view the
  A. Urinary bladder
  B. Liver
  C. Gallbladder
  D. Kidneys
  E. Ureters

212. Heat application
  A. Dilates blood vessels
  B. Constricts blood vessels
  C. Elevates blood pressure
  D. Decreases respiration
  E. Produces weight loss

213. The wave on an EKG that represents contraction of the atria is
  A. P
  B. QRS
  C. T
  D. V
  E. R

214. The pacemaker of the heart is the
  A. Myocardium
  B. Sinoatrial node
  C. Atrioventricular node
  D. Purkinje fibers
  E. Bundle of His

215. A standard EKG has how many leads?
  A. 4
  B. 8
  C. 10
  D. 12
  E. 14

216. The standard speed for recording an EKG is
  A. 5 mm/sec
  B. 10 mm/sec
  C. 20 mm/sec
  D. 25 mm/sec
  E. 50 mm/sec

217. To cauterize a small lesion on the oral mucosa, the physician may use an applicator with
  A. Silver nitrate
  B. Alcohol
  C. Formalin
  D. Betadine
  E. Zephirin chloride

218. A common lab test that may be ordered for a patient on Coumadin therapy is
  A. Pro time
  B. Sed rate
  C. WBC count
  D. Hematocrit
  E. CBC

219. Which one of the following types of suture material is absorbable?
  A. Steel
  B. Cotton
  C. Catgut
  D. Nylon
  E. Silk

220. The minimum number of cells to be counted in a differential blood smear is
    A. 50
    B. 100
    C. 150
    D. 200
    E. Unlimited, count them all

221. A hemoglobin of 10 g/dL is approximately equivalent to a hematocrit of
    A. 10%
    B. 20%
    C. 30%
    D. 36%
    E. 40%

222. Which of the following lab results should be called to the attention of the physician?
    A. WBC count: 7,200/mm(3)
    B. RBC count: 4.4 million/mm(3)
    C. Hemoglobin: 12 g/dL
    D. Sed rate: 30 mm/hr
    E. Total cholesterol: 180 mg

223. The stain used to identify bacteria is the
    A. Gram stain
    B. Wright's stain
    C. Grimsa stain
    D. India ink
    E. All of the above

224. On standing for a long time, a urine sample becomes
    A. Clear
    B. Alkaline
    C. Acid
    D. Neutral
    E. Darker

225. A blood sample for serum is collected in which of the following tubes?
    A. Blue-stoppered
    B. Lavender-stoppered
    C. Green-stoppered
    D. Red-stoppered
    E. Black-stoppered

226. Which of the following are categories to classify instruments used in surgery?
    A. Probing and dilating
    B. Cutting and dissecting
    C. Grasping and clamping
    D. Retracting
    E. All of the above

227. The first thing that should be done in an emergent situation involving an unconscious person is to
    A. Assess victim's airway
    B. Control any bleeding
    C. Apply a tourniquet
    D. Call for help
    E. Give breaths

228. A physical examination of a urine sample includes
    A. Odor
    B. Color
    C. Transparency
    D. Specific gravity
    E. All of the above

229. Most drugs are metabolized in the
    A. Lungs
    B. Blood
    C. Stomach
    D. Liver
    E. Intestines

230. The Ishihara test
    A. Tests for visual acuity
    B. Tests for glaucoma
    C. Tests for color-blindness
    D. Tests for presbyopia
    E. Tests for nerve deafness

231. Which is *not* a common symptom of a myocardial infarction?
    A. Nausea
    B. Angina
    C. Dyspnea
    D. Diaphoresis
    E. Polyuria

232. Hemostats are a type of
    A. Forceps
    B. Probe
    C. Applicator
    D. Scissors
    E. Retractors

233. The normal ratio for respiration to pulse is
    A. 1 to 6
    B. 1 to 2
    C. 1 to 4
    D. 2 to 4
    E. 4 to 1

234. Symptoms of insulin shock include
    A. Restless and confusion
    B. Cold, clammy skin
    C. Profuse sweating
    D. Rapid, weak pulse
    E. All of the above

235. Which is the most important route for the elimination of drugs from the body?
    A. Kidneys
    B. Skin

C. Mammary glands
D. Lungs
E. Digestive system

236. Prozac is an example of an
A. Antihistamine
B. Antidiuretic
C. Antidepressant
D. Antifungal
E. Antibiotic

237. The two most important factors in performing an effective handwash are
A. Temperature of water and soap
B. Friction and running water
C. Position of hands and hot water
D. Length of time and soap
E. Friction and soap

238. At which age is the first MMR vaccination recommended?
A. Birth
B. Two months
C. Four months
D. Twelve months
E. Five years

239. If a patient describes an aura before the onset of a severe headache, this is often a sign of
A. CVA
B. Migraine
C. Hay fever
D. Brain tumor
E. Seizure

240. A function of hemoglobin is
A. To repair cells
B. To destroy cells
C. To prevent blood loss
D. To carry oxygen and carbon dioxide
E. To fight off infection

241. A quality assurance program in the lab
A. Ensures the accuracy of results
B. Requires less paperwork
C. Eliminates outside labs
D. Increases convenience
E. Provides quick results

242. The reaction of the PPD test is read
A. 12–24 hours after it is administered
B. 48–72 hours after it is administered
C. Immediately after it is administered
D. 24–36 hours after it is administered
E. 4–8 hours after it is administered

243. The abbreviation for "both ears" is
A. AS
B. AD

C. AU
D. BE
E. AS/AD

244. The blood type known as the "universal donor" is
A. A
B. B
C. AB
D. O
E. All of the above

245. A lower GI series is performed to outline the
A. Esophagus
B. Stomach
C. Ileum
D. Duodenum
E. Colon

246. A technique that provides soft tissue images in three dimensions is
A. Ultrasound
B. CT scan
C. Myelography
D. Tomography
E. IVP

247. Massive and prolonged exposure to radiation can result in
A. Cancer
B. Increased number of WBCs
C. Increased number of RBCs
D. Arthritis
E. Death

248. The first group of leads to be recorded on an EKG are
A. Augmented leads
B. Leads I, II, and III
C. aVR, aVL, and aVF
D. Leads V(1) through V(3)
E. Leads V(1) through V(6)

249. Streptococci are arranged in
A. Clusters
B. Chains
C. Circles
D. Pairs
E. Fours

250. Pulse rate may be increased in all of the following except
A. Fear
B. Anger
C. Anxiety
D. Increasing age
E. Exercise

251. The electrode that is used for grounding in an EKG is
   A. LA
   B. RA
   C. LL
   D. RL
   E. C

252. Which federal agency oversees the safety of health facilities?
   A. OSHA
   B. CLIA '88
   C. CDC
   D. DEA
   E. COLA

253. A drug reference contains all of the following information *except*
   A. Description
   B. Indications
   C. Contraindications
   D. Dosage
   E. Cost

254. Ibuprofen has analgesic and antipyretic properties and is used to treat
   A. Pain
   B. Arthritis
   C. Headache
   D. Dysmenorrhea
   E. All of the above

255. Which of the following patient instructions is critical for a successful Holter Monitor recording interpretation?
   A. Avoid stress
   B. Refrain from exercise
   C. Keep a written recording of all daily activities
   D. Wear the monitor for five days
   E. Do not take any medications

256. The involuntary muscular action that moves food along the GI tract is called
   A. Digestion
   B. Indigestion
   C. Mastication
   D. Peristalsis
   E. Deglutition

257. The first dose of DTP (DTaP) vaccine should be administered at
   A. Two months
   B. Four months
   C. Twelve months
   D. Five years
   E. Twelve years

258. A ligament
   A. Connects muscle to bone
   B. Connects muscle to muscle
   C. Connects joint to bone
   D. Connects bone to bone
   E. Connects muscle to organ

259. Tissue samples removed during a biopsy would be sent to which department of the lab?
   A. Serology
   B. Cytology
   C. Histology
   D. Chemistry
   E. Microbiology

260. Which of the following would be *least* likely to contaminate the sterile field?
   A. Talking over the field
   B. Hair not pulled back
   C. Nonsterile person entering the room
   D. A sterile instrument touching the edge of the field
   E. Moisture on the sterile field

261. An antihistamine that may be used to treat an allergic reaction is
   A. Bactrim
   B. Motrin
   C. Benadryl
   D. Inderal
   E. Indorin

262. Each of the following abbreviations is correctly defined *except*
   A. bid—twice a day
   B. tid—three times a day
   C. OD—right eye
   D. qod—every day
   E. ac—before meals

263. Surgical asepsis should be maintained when performing which of the following?
   A. Dipstick urinalysis
   B. Pelvic exam
   C. Snellen test
   D. Needle biopsy
   E. Blood pressure

264. How often should quality control tests be performed in the lab?
   A. Daily
   B. Weekly
   C. Monthly
   D. When necessary
   E. Before each test

265. This type of nerve conducts impulses toward the brain
    A. Afferent
    B. Efferent
    C. Superior
    D. Inferior
    E. Spinal

266. Sweat glands are termed
    A. Oil glands
    B. Sudoriferous glands
    C. Pores
    D. Sebaceous glands
    E. Pustules

267. An infectious inflammatory skin disease caused by staphylococci and characterized by vesicles that later crust is called
    A. Vitiligo
    B. Impetigo
    C. Tinea
    D. Cellulitis
    E. Acne

268. A decrease in bone density may indicate
    A. Osteolysis
    B. Osteoclasis
    C. Osteoporosis
    D. Crepitus
    E. Osteomyelitis

269. The largest portion of the brain is the
    A. Cerebrum
    B. Cerebellum
    C. Brain stem
    D. Cerebral cortex
    E. Hypothalamus

270. An impairment of vision due to old age is
    A. Macular degeneration
    B. Hyperopia
    C. Myopia
    D. Presbyopia
    E. Astigmatism

271. An infection of the middle ear may be charted as
    A. Otitis media
    B. Tennitis
    C. Conjunctivitis
    D. Mastoiditis
    E. Tympanitis

272. The valve located between the right atrium and left ventricle is the
    A. Tricuspid
    B. Bicuspid
    C. Mitral
    D. Cardiac
    E. Semilunar

273. The medical term for whooping cough is
    A. Croup
    B. Percussion
    C. Pertussis
    D. Tuberculosis
    E. Epistaxis

274. The region between the lungs that contains the heart, aorta, esophagus, and bronchial tubes is the
    A. Pleural cavity
    B. Cardiac cavity
    C. Septum
    D. Mediastinum
    E. Peritoneum

275. Inflammation of the nasal mucosa results in
    A. Rhinitis
    B. Sinusitis
    C. Laryngitis
    D. Bronchitis
    E. Pneumonitis

276. A disease that is characterized by muscle rigidity, a shuffling gait, and progressive tremors is
    A. Alzheimer's disease
    B. meningitis
    C. Bell's palsy
    D. Parkinson's disease
    E. Cerebral palsy

277. Which of the following accessory organs of digestion stores and concentrates bile?
    A. Spleen
    B. Liver
    C. Pancreas
    D. Gallbladder
    E. Appendix

278. Micturition is a synonym for
    A. Urination
    B. Defecation
    C. Dialysis
    D. Oliguria
    E. Anuria

279. Which of the following indicates an aggravation of symptoms?
    A. Remission
    B. Etiology
    C. Exacerbation
    D. Recession
    E. Dominance

280. A woman who has given birth to two or more children may be called
   A. Nullipara
   B. Multipara
   C. Unipara
   D. Bipara
   E. Multigravida

281. The release of an ovum from the ovary is
   A. Ovulation
   B. Parturition
   C. Fertilization
   D. Amenorrhea
   E. Placenta previa

282. Male sterilization is
   A. Circumcision
   B. Vasoligation
   C. Prostatectomy
   D. Vasectomy
   E. Vasotomy

283. Which of the following are ways in which pathogens can be spread?
   A. Transmission by a vector
   B. Person-to-person contact
   C. Environmental contact
   D. Object-to-person contact
   E. All of the above

284. The "colored" portion of the eye is known as the
   A. Retina
   B. Pupil
   C. Cornea
   D. Sclera
   E. Iris

285. All of the following are bones of the middle ear *except* the
   A. Incus
   B. Pinna
   C. Malleus
   D. Stapes
   E. B and C

286. The combining form for "bone" is
   A. Arthro-
   B. Osteo-
   C. Uro-
   D. Onco-
   E. Adeno-

287. Slow heartbeat is also called
   A. Murmur
   B. Tachycardia
   C. Sinus rhythm
   D. Arrythmia
   E. Bradycardia

288. A temporary absence of respiration is
   A. Infiltration
   B. Apnea
   C. Dyspnea
   D. Hyperpnea
   E. Atelectasis

289. A collection of blood in the pleural cavity is called a(n)
   A. Hemothorax
   B. Pneumothorax
   C. Pyothorax
   D. Pyoneumothorax
   E. Hemoneumothorax

290. An endoscopic examination of the rectum is charted as a(n)
   A. Sigmoidoscopy
   B. Proctoscopy
   C. Endoscopy
   D. Bronchoscopy
   E. Barium enema

291. The downward projection from the lower edge of the soft palate is the
   A. Uvula
   B. Frenulum
   C. Tonsil
   D. Adenoid
   E. Larynx

292. The combining form "labio-" means
   A. Gum
   B. Tongue
   C. Lip
   D. Mouth
   E. Tooth

293. The hollow, muscular organ that temporarily stores urine is the
   A. Kidney
   B. Urethra
   C. Ureter
   D. Urinary bladder
   E. Urinary meatus

294. The secretion from an endocrine gland is called a(n)
   A. Catalyst
   B. Hormone
   C. Enzyme
   D. Protein
   E. Chromosome

295. Progesterone is produced by the
  A. Corpus luteum
  B. Testes
  C. Prostate
  D. Uterus
  E. Anterior pituitary

296. The region between the vagina and anus is termed the
  A. Perimetrium
  B. Perineum
  C. Placenta
  D. Peritoneum
  E. Puerpera

297. Which of the following is *not* a part of the axial skeleton?
  A. Scapula
  B. Cranial bones
  C. Vertebrae
  D. Ribs
  E. Sternum

298. A wound that barely penetrates the skin is charted as being
  A. Superior
  B. Superficial
  C. Proximal
  D. Distal
  E. Deep

299. A surgical opening into the eardrum to avoid rupture is a(n)
  A. Tympanoplasty
  B. Myringoplasty
  C. Myringotomy
  D. Otoplasty
  E. Otoclesis

300. An antipyretic agent works against
  A. Fever
  B. Rash
  C. Toothaches
  D. Poison
  E. Acne

1. **B** Hypertrophy
RATIONALE: The suffix *-trophy* means development, growth. The prefix *hyper-* means above, excessive. The prefix *a-* means lack of; the prefix *dys-* means abnormal or painful; the prefix *hypo-* means deficient. Visceral pertains to internal organs.

2. **B** An osteoblast
RATIONALE: The prefix *osteo-* means bone. The suffix *-blast* means immature form, stage of development. *-Erythr/o* pertains to the color red (red blood cells); *-neur/o* means nerve; *-my/o* means muscle. The suffix *-clast* means something that breaks.

3. **A** OD
RATIONALE: *OD* is the abbreviation for right eye; *OS* is the abbreviation for left eye; *OU* is the abbreviation for both eyes; *AD* is the abbreviation for right ear; *AS* is the abbreviation for left ear.

4. **B** Listen to breath sounds
RATIONALE: A stethoscope is an instrument used to listen to the sounds produced by the body. A sphygmomanometer measures blood pressure; an otoscope examines the external ear.

5. **E** Spirometry
RATIONALE: The volume of air moving in and out of the lungs is measured by an instrument called a spirometer. The process is known as spirometry. A tracheostomy is an opening through the neck into the trachea; thorocentesis is the insertion of a needle into the chest; intubation is the insertion of a tube into a body opening or hole; bronchoscopy is the examination of the bronchi using a bronchoscope.

6. **D** Fasting blood glucose
RATIONALE: Diabetes is a metabolic disease caused by the body's inability to utilize carbohydrates (glucose). Blood glucose levels would be high. Abnormal results of the other lab tests listed aren't commonly indicative of diabetes mellitus.

7. **A** Oncologist
RATIONALE: An oncologist specializes in the treatment of patients with cancer. A cardiologist specializes in the heart; a gynecologist specializes in the female reproductive system; an ENT physi-

cian deals with the ear, nose, and throat; a pediatrician treats children.

8. **D** Leukopenia
RATIONALE: The root word *leuko-* refers to white blood cells. The suffix *-penia* means decrease. The suffix *-osis* with the combined form *leuko/cy-* means an abnormal increase in white blood cells; the suffix *-emia* means blood condition; the prefix *-an* means a lack of.

9. **C** Hyperpyrexia
RATIONALE: Pyrexia refers to fever. The prefix *hyper-* means excessive. The other word forms using the prefix *-hyper* refer to other abnormalities.

10. **D** -phagia
RATIONALE: The suffix *-phagia* means to eat. *-cardia* means heart; *-phasia* means to speak; *-algia* means pain; *-dipsia* means thirst.

11. **A** -lysis
RATIONALE: The suffix *-lysis* means to break apart or destroy. *-desis* means binding, fusing together; *-pexy* means fixation; *-plasty* means surgical repair; *-rrhaphy* means suturing.

12. **B** Kidneys, ureters, bladder
RATIONALE: A KUB is a radiological study of the kidneys, ureters, and bladder.

13. **C** Hirsutism
RATIONALE: Hirsutism is a condition in which there is excessive hairiness. Alopecia is partial or complete hair loss; myopia is nearsightedness; vitiligo is a skin disorder; urticaria is the medical term for hives.

14. **C** Deglutition
RATIONALE: Deglutition is the act of swallowing or passing food down the throat. Obstipation is extreme and persistent constipation; peristalsis is the contraction of intestinal muscles that propel digestion; herniation is the protrusion of a body organ through an abnormal opening in a membrane, muscle, or other tissue; regurgitation describes a backward flow from the normal direction, as in the return of swallowed food into the mouth.

15. **D** Scar on the back of the knee
RATIONALE: A cicatrix is the result of a healed

wound or scar. The popliteal area is the area of the body in back of the knee.

16. **A** Arthrocentesis

RATIONALE: Arthrocentesis is the puncturing of a joint cavity. Arthritis is an inflammatory condition of the joints; arthroplasty is the reconstruction or replacement of a joint; tympanocentesis involves the tympanic membrane; thoracocentesis involves the chest.

17. **D** Fat

RATIONALE: Adipose tissue is the section of subcutaneous tissue that stores fat.

18. **E** Idiopathic

RATIONALE: Idiopathic refers to a disease process without a recognizable cause. Diastolic refers to the dilatation of the heart and ventricles; epidemic refers to the sudden occurrence of disease in excess of normal expectancy; biologic pertains to life and living organisms in general; etiologic pertains to the causes of disease.

19. **B** Seeing

RATIONALE: The optic nerve, Cranial Nerve II, is responsible for the sense of vision.

20. **B** Nose

RATIONALE: *Rhino-* is the root word meaning nose. *-plasty* is a suffix meaning surgical repair.

21. **E** Urology

RATIONALE: Urology is the study of urine, urinary systems of both males and females, and the diseases of the male reproductive system. Nephrology is the study of the kidney; oncology is the study of tumors; proctology is the study of the rectum and anus; hematology is the study of the blood.

22. **B** Bronchoscopy

RATIONALE: A bronchoscopy is the procedure which utilizes a scope to view the internal surface characteristics of the bronchus. A bronchogram is a roentgenogram obtained by bronchography; cholecystography involves the gallbladder; endoscopy is the visual inspection of any cavity of the body by means of an endoscope.

23. **E** Hives

RATIONALE: Urticaria is a skin reaction in which there is intense itching near pale, irregular, raised patches of skin (wheals). This is commonly known as hives.

24. **E** Peritoneum

RATIONALE: The peritoneum is the membrane that lines the abdominal cavity and encloses the abdominal organs. The perineum; the pericardium is the sac that surrounds the heart; the endocardium is the lining of the heart; the endometrium is the lining of the uterus.

25. **B** Mucous

RATIONALE: Mucous membranes line the digestive, respiratory, urinary, and reproductive tracts. The other membrane types line internally contained cavities.

26. **A** Posterior

RATIONALE: Dorsal refers to the back (posterior) of the body. Anterior refers to the front; medial refers to the middle; lateral refers to the side; superior is a term pertaining to above, or directed upward.

27. **E** Thoracic

RATIONALE: The thoracic cavity (chest) is the part of the body between the neck and the diaphragm. The pleural spaces contain the lungs only.

28. **B** Abduction

RATIONALE: To abduct means to move away from the midline or middle. To adduct means to move toward the midline of the body; rotation is the process of turning around an axis.

29. **D** Sagittal

RATIONALE: The sagittal plane vertically divides the body into right and left portions. The frontal and coronal planes divide the body into front and back portions; the transverse and horizontal planes divide the body into top and bottom halves.

30. **B** Reye's Syndrome

RATIONALE: Reye's Syndrome is an acute and sometimes fatal illness characterized by fatty invasion of internal organs and swelling of the brain. The cause is unknown, but has been linked to the use of aspirin and viral diseases in young children.

31. **A** Cervical

RATIONALE: The vertebral column is divided into five sections: cervical (neck), thoracic (chest), lumbar (lower back), sacral (below the lumbar), and coccygeal (tailbone).

32. **E** Melanoma

RATIONALE: Malignant melanoma is the most serious type of skin cancer. The tumor arises from the melanocytes. Often, this tumor comes from a mole, causing changes in the mole's size, color, and shape ("ABCs" or asymmetry, border, color). The tumor can quickly spread to the lymphatic system and may metastasize to all organs of the body.

33. **B** Psoriasis

RATIONALE: Psoriasis is a chronic inflammatory disease of the integumentary system characterized by silvery scaly patches. The cause is unknown. The patches generally occur on the elbows, knees, and scalp.

34. **A** Frontal
RATIONALE: The frontal bone is located at the front of the skull. The ethmoid bone is found at the base of the cranium; the temporal bone forms part of the lower cranium; the occipital bone is found at the back of the skull; the mandible is the lower jaw.

35. **C** 12
RATIONALE: The 12 pairs of cranial nerves arise from the brainstem and are named for the function they carry out.

36. **C** Cerebrum
RATIONALE: The cerebrum is the largest portion of the brain, divided into right and left hemispheres. It is responsible for controlling voluntary movements and coordination of mental activity. The other portions of the brain are smaller than the cerebrum.

37. **C** Pernicious
RATIONALE: Pernicious anemia is a severe anemia characterized by the lack of intrinsic factor in the lining of the stomach leading to the malabsorption of Vitamin B_{12}. Vitamin B_{12} is necessary for the production of red blood cells. This decrease in the production of red blood cells results in an anemia.

38. **A** Asthma
RATIONALE: Asthma is an obstructive lung disease characterized by the constriction of the bronchi. This constriction results in wheezing, shortness of breath, and difficulty breathing. The remaining diseases listed present other signs and symptoms.

39. **B** Tympanic membrane
RATIONALE: The tympanic membrane is the membrane between the external and middle ear. It vibrates in response to sound waves. The remaining choices listed represent other structures of the middle and internal ear.

40. **C** Inferior vena cava
RATIONALE: The inferior vena cava is one of the great veins of the body. It drains blood from the lower part of the body and empties it into the right side of the heart. The remaining choices listed represent veins that return blood to the heart from areas above the diaphragm.

41. **A** Sino-atrial node
RATIONALE: Specialized masses of tissue in the heart wall form the conduction or electrical system of the heart. These structures include masses called nodes, and their branches. The SA node (sino-atrial node) is one of these nodes and is located in the upper wall of the right atrium. Its function is to act as pacemaker because it initiates the heartbeat and sets the rate of heart contractions.

42. **D** Potassium
RATIONALE: Electrolytes are electrically charged particles (ions) and are an important constituent of all body fluids. Potassium is a major positive ion. It is important in the regulation of neuromuscular excitability and muscle contraction. Heart muscle requires this electrolyte for its electrical system which regulates the heartbeat and heart rate.

43. **D** Flexion
RATIONALE: Voluntary muscle action is action which we can consciously control. We can consciously control flexion of joints. Breathing, heartbeat, peristalsis, and pupil dilation are all involuntary muscle actions, beyond our control.

44. **E** Away from
RATIONALE: Each of these prefixes can mean away from, opposite, or derivation from. Prefixes for against are *anti-* or *contra-*; prefixes for before are *ante-*, *pre-*, or *pro-*; prefixes for within are *eso-*, *intra-*, or *endo-*; prefixes for outside are *e-* or *ecto-*.

45. **B** Esophagus
RATIONALE: The esophagus (food tube) extends from the pharynx (throat) to the stomach. It is a direct passage into the stomach. The salivary glands and tongue aid in mastication; the trachea is the airway that leads to the lungs; the tonsils are found in the throat, but do not aid in mastication or swallowing.

46. **D** Scoliosis
RATIONALE: Scoliosis is the sideways bending of the spine beyond the limits of the natural curve. Kyphosis is also known as ''hunchback''; spondylosis is stiffness of the vertebral joints; lordosis characterizes a bent forward position of the spine; ankylosis is the fixation of any joint in an abnormal position.

47. **C** Insulin
RATIONALE: Insulin is the hormone secreted by the beta cells of the islands of Langerhans in the pancreas. Insulin is important for the transport of glucose across the cell wall, thus lowering blood glucose levels.

48. **E** Colostomy
RATIONALE: A colostomy is a surgical procedure that brings a portion of the colon through the abdominal wall to create an artificial anus. A colectomy is the removal of part or all of the colon; a gastrostomy is a surgical procedure that creates an artificial opening into the stomach through the abdomen; a cholecystectomy is the removal

of the gallbladder; gastropexy is the surgical fixation of the stomach.

49. **D** Olfactory
RATIONALE: The olfactory nerve, Cranial Nerve I, is associated with the sense of smell.

50. **B** Tibia and fibula
RATIONALE: The tibia and fibula make up the bones of the lower leg. The radius and ulna are bones of the forearm; the femur, trochanter, and patella are bones of the upper leg and kneecap; the humerus and scapula are bones of the upper arm and shoulder.

51. **D** Following long-term illnesses
RATIONALE: All states require documentation of death. A coroner/medical examiner must be consulted in deaths that may be suspicious or violent. Imminent deaths are not required to be reported.

52. **E** Sincerely yours
RATIONALE: The complimentary close is the writer's way of saying good-bye. The words used are determined by the formality of the salutation (introductory greeting).

53. **D** Invasion of privacy
RATIONALE: Invasion of privacy is the divulging of patient information without the patient's consent.

54. **B** Asking relevant questions
RATIONALE: Anxiety is the state or feeling of apprehension, uneasiness, agitation, uncertainty, and/or fear. Anxiety can result as a response to a certain situation that produces tension. Signs of anxiety can include decreased attention span, urinary urgency, and increased perspiration.

55. **E** Informed consent
RATIONALE: Negligence is the commission of an act that a prudent person would not do. Duty owed, dereliction of duty, direct cause, and damages make up the "4 Ds" of negligence.

56. **C** Immediately after the initial visit
RATIONALE: The first report of the injury should be completed in quadruplicate at the first visit and distributed to the patient's chart, employer, compensation carrier, and the State Workers' Compensation Board. Filing deadlines vary by state, but generally range from twenty-four hours to ten days after the initial visit.

57. **C** Use care, diligence, and skill in treatment
RATIONALE: A duty is an obligation or commitment to act in a certain way. The physician has a duty to do no harm, act to create good, meet the patient's reasonable expectation, and tell the truth.

58. **A** A six-year-old child
RATIONALE: Consent is voluntary permission that is granted by someone who is legally able to do so to receive medical treatment. A minor (under the age of 18) requires the consent of a parent or guardian.

59. **D** A medical assistant who administers an incorrect medicine
RATIONALE: "Respondeat Superior" is the doctrine that makes employers such as physicians liable for the conduct of their employees while serving within the scope of their employment. While a medical assistant may be directly employed by a physician, pharmacists, hospital lab techs, hospital interns, and insurance companies generally are not.

60. **A** The most important information is given first
RATIONALE: A patient may be showing signs of anxiety such as a decrease in attention span or a decrease in the ability to follow directions. The patient will most likely receive the message before he/she is affected by these signs of anxiety.

61. **B** Speak naturally
RATIONALE: The medical assistant should position herself/himself directly in front of the patient and speak naturally but slowly. Speaking quickly or using medical terminology can confuse the hearing impaired patient; not maintaining eye contact may be considered rude, speaking loudly is unnecessary.

62. **B** To accept the fee approved by Medicaid as payment in full
RATIONALE: Medicaid is a federal insurance program administered by each state and available to patient's with income below the poverty level. A physician who elects to treat Medicaid patients must accept the reimbursement as payment in full without further billing the patient.

63. **D** Past surgical history
RATIONALE: Subjective information is data related to the patient's signs, symptoms, and feelings as described by the patient or the personal data supplied by the patient on the first visit. The patient would reveal past medical information, such as previous surgeries, during the patient interview or health history.

64. **D** Give the patient a copy of the original records
RATIONALE: The patient owns the information in the medical record, but the physician owns the record.

65. **E** Noise
RATIONALE: Noise is anything that interferes with the communication process. The source is the sender of the message. The message is the content of the communication. The channel is the means by which the message is sent. The receiver is the destination of the message.

66. **A** The five stages of dying
RATIONALE: Dr. Kubler-Ross described five stages that dying clients experience. These include denial, anger, bargaining, depression, and acceptance. The hierarchy of needs was established by Maslow.

67. **C** Breach of contract
RATIONALE: A tort is a civil wrong committed against another person or property. A tort can be unintentional (negligence) or intentional (assault and battery, abandonment, invasion of privacy)

68. **B** Licensure
RATIONALE: A license is the strongest form of professional regulation. It is a mandatory process by which a state verifies that the individual has met minimum standards required by law. Certification and registration are voluntary processes that identify an individual as having achieved standards set forth by an accrediting agency.

69. **C** Medial
RATIONALE: Lateral indicates away from the midline of the body. Medial indicates toward the midline of the body. Anterior means toward the front; proximal means nearer the trunk or point of attachment; distal means farther away from the trunk or point of attachment; posterior means toward the back.

70. **A** The process of sharing meaning
RATIONALE: Communication is defined as the process that involves the sharing of meaning. This sharing can be accomplished in many ways and through different means, such as talking, explaining nonverbal action, and analysis.

71. **E** All of the above
RATIONALE: The patient's medical record is a legal document that provides a chronological record of his/her medical care. It can also provide legal protection and documentation of evidence for litigation. It must be complete, accurate, and up-to-date. Falsification of medical records is a criminal offense.

72. **A** Cell
RATIONALE: The cell is the fundamental unit of all living tissues. Tissues, organs, and organ systems are made up of many cells; a nucleus is the control center of a cell.

73. **D** Tissue
RATIONALE: Tissues are composed of a group of cells that are similar in structure and functions. Tissues make up organs, organ systems, and glands; organelles are found within cells.

74. **D** Periosteum
RATIONALE: The periosteum is composed of fibrous connective tissue. It covers the outer surface of the bone excluding the epiphysis. Diaphy-

sis is the shaft of a long bone; epiphysis is the end of a long bone; endosteum is the inner lining of the marrow cavity of a long bone; marrow is the connective tissue that occupies the spaces in bone.

75. **E** A, B, and C
RATIONALE: Smooth muscle tissue makes up involuntary muscles. Cardiac muscle tissue is found only in the heart. Skeletal muscle tissue makes up voluntary muscles.

76. **B** Myocardium
RATIONALE: The myocardium is the thick, muscular layer of the heart wall. The endocardium is the inner lining of the heart wall; the pericardium is membrane that partially encloses the heart; the epicardium is one of the three layers of tissue forming the heart wall; a ventricle is a heart cavity.

77. **B** Larynx
RATIONALE: The larynx is commonly known as the voicebox. It is located between the root of the tongue and the upper trachea. It is made up of cartilage and contains the vocal cords. The pharynx is the throat.

78. **C** Small intestine
RATIONALE: The small intestine occupies most of the abdominal cavity. It functions to complete chemical digestion and is the primary site of absorption of nutrients into the bloodstream. The large intestine deals with unabsorbable food material.

79. **D** Production of insulin
RATIONALE: The urinary system functions to eliminate liquid and nitrogenous waste products, balances water gains and losses, regulates gains and losses of hydrogen and bicarbonate ions and levels of sodium, potassium, and chloride. Insulin is made in the pancreas.

80. **B** Perineum
RATIONALE: The area between the vaginal orifice and the rectum is the perineum. This area may be torn during childbirth. The peritoneum is the membrane located in the abdominal cavity; the hymen is the membrane that partially covers the entrance to the vagina; fimbriae are fingerlike projections at the opening of the fallopian tube near the ovary; the labia majora are the outer skin folds of the female genitalia.

81. **C** Vas deferens
RATIONALE: Vasectomy is a surgical procedure for sterilization of the male patient. It is performed by surgically removing a section of each vas deferens. Fallopian tubes are a part of the female reproductive system, and are surgically altered when a female undergoes sterilization.

82. **C** Brain and spinal cord
RATIONALE: The central nervous system (CNS) is made up of the brain and spinal cord. It integrates sensory information to achieve a responsive action.

83. **E** All of the above
RATIONALE: The midbrain is the upper portion of the brainstem and connects it to the cerebrum. The pons is inferior to the midbrain and links the cerebellum to the rest of the nervous system. The Medulla oblongata is the lowest portion and is attached to the spinal cord just superior to the foramen magnum.

84. **B** Nose
RATIONALE: Olfaction is the special sense of smell. It is stimulated by olfactory receptors located in the nasal cavity.

85. **C** Pituitary gland
RATIONALE: The pituitary gland (hypophysis) is located on the inferior surface of the brain. It is divided into anterior and posterior sections. It secretes hormones which regulate or stimulate other endocrine glands, like the thyroid. The hypothalamus controls the secretion of the pituitary gland.

86. **B** Cytologist
RATIONALE: Cytology is the study of cells. A cytologist is one who specializes in the study of cells, using special techniques to aid in diagnoses. Histology and histologists specialize in the structure of organ tissues; pathologists specialize in the study of disease.

87. **C** qid
RATIONALE: Bid means two times a day; tid means three times a day; qod means every other day; q4h means every four hours.

88. **D** Euphoria
RATIONALE: Euphoria is the feeling or state of well-being or elation.

89. **B** Below
RATIONALE: *Hypo-* means below, under, or decreased. Other prefixes for below are *hypo-, infra-,* or *sub-*. Prefixes for above are *supra-, hyper-,* or *epi-*; prefix for excessive is *hyper-*; prefixes for skin are *cutane-* or *derm-*; prefixes for before are *ante-, pre-,* or *pro-*.

90. **D** Diagnoses and treats cancers
RATIONALE: An oncologist diagnoses and treats tumors and cancerous growths. Their specialty is oncology. Gynecologists diagnose and treat female reproductive disorders; obstetricians deliver babies; pediatricians care for infants and children; anesthesiologists administer anesthesia.

91. **B** Battery
RATIONALE: Battery is defined as intentional physical contact with another without that person's consent. A physician who fails to secure some formal expression of consent before treating a patient could be charged with trespass or battery.

92. **A** Duty
RATIONALE: A duty is the obligation or commitment of a person to act in certain ways. It is a basic principle of ethics—judgments of right and wrong. Duties include beneficence, nonmaleficence, veracity, fidelity, and justice.

93. **D** Verified the patient's signature
RATIONALE: A physician must have consent to treat a patient. This consent can be implied, which is sufficient for procedures that involve little risk, or this consent can be informed when more complex procedures are involved. Informed consent implies an understanding of what is to be done, why it is to be done, risks involved, expected benefits, alternative treatments, and risks involved. This should be done by discussion between the patient and physician, and a form may be signed. The Medical Assistant witnesses the signature of the patient on this form by signing and dating it.

94. **D** Nonverbal communication
RATIONALE: Nonverbal communications are messages conveyed without the use of words. They can be transmitted by body language and can include grooming, eye contact, facial expressions, hand gestures, and posture. Therapeutic and nontherapeutic communication involves the influence of a patient or helping a patient to a better understanding through verbal or nonverbal communication.

95. **A** Negligence
RATIONALE: Negligence is an unintentional tort that is characterized by an omission or commission of an act that a reasonably prudent person would or would not do in a given situation. Negligence can be in the form of failure to act, improper performance of an act that results in harm, or the performance of an illegal act.

96. **C** Tinea pedis
RATIONALE: Tinea is a group of fungal skin infection caused by dermatophytes. Tinea pedis is a chronic, superficial fungal infection of the skin between the toes and on the soles. Tinea cruris involves the groin; pediculosis is the infestation of lice; moniliasis is an infection caused by a species of *Candida*; an abrasion is a scrape or rub.

97. **B** Petichiae
RATIONALE: Petechiae (sing: petechia) are tiny purple or red spots that appear on the surface of the skin as a result of tiny hemorrhages under

the skin. Petechiae can range in size from pinpoint to pinhead size, and are flush with the surface of the skin.

98. **D** Pus formation
RATIONALE: Suppuration is the production of purulent material or pus. Pus is a thick, yellowish or greenish-yellow exudate that is the result of a bacterial infection. It consists mainly of dead and living leukocytes, skin cells, and bacteria. Its color, quantity, consistency, and odor may be of diagnostic importance.

99. **C** Eclampsia
RATIONALE: Eclampsia is a form of toxemia of pregnancy. Dermatitis is an inflammation of the skin. Urticaria is hives. Impetigo is an infectious bacterial inflammation of the skin. Psoriasis is a chronic skin condition.

100. **A** The common cold
RATIONALE: The common cold is a viral infection characterized by inflammation of the mucous membranes of the nose and a nasal discharge (coryza).

101. **C** Times not available
RATIONALE: To develop the matrix in the appointment book, block out the times the physician(s) will be unavailable. All else revolves around the physicians' availability.

102. **D** Grouping/scheduling
RATIONALE: Grouping is scheduling similar appointments together during a day. For example, all complete physical exams are scheduled for Friday morning. This type of scheduling is a method of time management.

103. **A** Extensive editing capability
RATIONALE: The computer, as a document production tool, permits efficient preparation and editing of written documents. Spell-check and column layout are simply added benefits. Storage capacity relates to the computer as a whole, and is not specific to word processing.

104. **A** Insurance coverage is available
RATIONALE: Certified mail requires the receiver's signature as proof of delivery and receipt. Any mail in which First Class postage is paid can be accepted as Certified Mail.

105. **D** Personal letters and postcards
RATIONALE: First class mail includes sealed or unsealed handwritten or typed material, such as letters, postcards, and business reply mail. There are a variety of mailing options available for other mailable materials.

106. **E** The estate is billed
RATIONALE: Estate claims are made against the estate of a deceased patient. Once the office receives notification of the patient's death, the office must submit a claim for the unpaid balance to the administrator of the estate. Each state has different rules and regulations concerning the filing of estate claims.

107. **A** Immediately
RATIONALE: Endorsement is a signature or writing on the back of a check by which the endorser transfers all rights of the check to another party. All checks received as payments should be restrictively endorsed (for deposit only) immediately to safeguard against loss or theft.

108. **E** Andrew Stephen
RATIONALE: In alphabetical filing, a person's name is indexed with the surname as unit 1, the given name as unit 2, and the middle name as unit 3. Names are alphabetized according to the first unit letter by letter.

109. **B** Is a form designed to help in filing insurance claims
RATIONALE: A superbill is a combination charge slip, statement, and insurance reporting form. It is given to the patient at each visit. It lists the charges for procedures performed including CPT-4 codes, and ICD-9-CM codes.

110. **E** David Roberts, M.D.
RATIONALE: The inside address includes the name, title, and address of the receiver. When addressing a letter to a physician, omit the courtesy title and type the physician's name followed by his/her academic degree.

111. **E** A license must be obtained from the Post Office
RATIONALE: A postage meter is an efficient way of stamping large amounts of mail. Postage is prepaid and applied directly to the envelope or on adhesive strips. The other choices are all true about postage meters.

112. **B** NE
RATIONALE: The use of standard two-letter abbreviations aids in the reading, coding, sorting, and canceling of the mail. The U.S. Postal Service has issued a list of two-letter state abbreviations to be used with zip codes. None of the other choices represent a US state abbreviation.

113. **C** Full block style
RATIONALE: The full block style places all lines flush at the left margin. The other choices vary indentation of the margin(s).

114. **C** Complimentary close
RATIONALE: A memorandum is a written communication among persons within an office or organization. It uses guide words that indicate the date, sender, receiver(s), and subject.

115. **C** Name, page number, and date
RATIONALE: The second and continuous pages

of a letter or report are placed on plain paper that matches the letterhead in weight, color, and fiber content. The heading of the subsequent pages must contain the name of the addressee, page number, and date.

116. **A** Two
RATIONALE: The complimentary close is placed on the second line below the last line of the body of the letter.

117. **B** Software
RATIONALE: Software is the programming necessary to direct the hardware of a computer system. It consists of sets of instructions placed on disks and is necessary for the computer to function.

118. **D** Physician charges
RATIONALE: A fee profile is established by compiling and averaging the usual charges for services of the physician over a given period of time. This profile is then used to determine the amount of third-party liability.

119. **B** Date of birth
RATIONALE: Demographics relate to the statistical characteristics of a population. It includes the name, date of birth, marital status, children, occupation, education, and social information of the patient.

120. **D** Irritable bowel syndrome
RATIONALE: ICD-9-CM (International Classification of Diseases, 9th Revision, Clinical Modification) assigns numeric codes to diseases, illnesses, injuries, and health-related conditions. The coding system is used to establish medical necessity to facilitate payment for health care services and to translate written terminology or descriptions into numbers to provide a universal common language.

121. **B** 1:00 P.M.
RATIONALE: The United States is divided into four time zones: Pacific time (WA, OR, NV, and CA), Mountain time (MT, UT, ID, WY, CO, NM, AZ, and parts of ND, SD, NE, and KS), Central time (MN, WI, IA, MO, AR, OK, TX, LA, MS, IL, AL, and parts of TN, KY, ND, SD, NE, and KS), and Eastern time (all others). Central, Mountain, and Pacific time zones are one or more hours behind Eastern time. Pacific time is 3 hours behind Eastern time; when it is 1:00 Pacific time, it is 4:00 Eastern time.

122. **E** CHAMPUS
RATIONALE: CHAMPUS (Civilian Health and Medical Program of the Uniformed Services) is a federal medical aid program to benefit military dependants and veterans only. PPOs, Workers' Compensation, and Medicaid programs can in-

clude nonmilitary families. CHAMPVA is a program for dependents of military veterans.

123. **A** Second ring
RATIONALE: If possible, the telephone should be answered on the first ring, and always by the third ring.

124. **A** Refers to external causes
RATIONALE: An E-code is a classification of ICD-9-CM coding. It is used to describe environmental events, circumstances, and conditions as the external cause of injury, poisoning, and other adverse effects.

125. **D** HCFA-1500
RATIONALE: The HCFA-1500 is a universal claim form developed by the HCFA that standardizes the data required by most insurance carriers to process insurance claims.

126. **D** At the end of the day
RATIONALE: Patients who are habitually late for appointments should be scheduled at the end of the day so as not to disrupt the workflow.

127. **A** A PPO
RATIONALE: A Preferred Provider Organization (PPO) preserves the fee-for-service concept. An insurer contracts with a group of physicians who agree on a predetermined list of charges for all services. Care is not prepaid. The physician treats the patient and bills the PPO.

128. **C** Draw a single line through the error, write the word "error," make the correction, date and initial the entry
RATIONALE: Corrections are made in the medical record by drawing a single line through the error, writing the word "error" next to it, making the correction, and dating and initialing the correction (SLIDE rule)

129. **D** Problem-oriented progress notes
RATIONALE: SOAP is an organized way of charting progress notes. SOAP stands for Subjective, Objective, Assessment, and Plan.

130. **A** A referral to another physician
RATIONALE: The physician must notify the patient of his/her intention to terminate the relationship to protect the physician against abandonment. The physician is not required to refer to another physician.

131. **E** Should be squeezed in for a brief visit so the physician can decide what the next treatment step should be
RATIONALE: If the patient requires immediate attention, he/she should be accommodated. If the patient does not need immediate care, a brief visit with the physician and a scheduled appointment at a later date may be the best policy. The

patient should be told that the office runs on an appointment basis.

132. **B** Immediately offer a new appointment time
RATIONALE: Attempt to reschedule the appointment while the patient is on the phone. Canceled appointments may be filled by patients with advance appointments.

133. **B** Low-pitched and expressive voice
RATIONALE: The telephone voice should be warm, friendly, and natural. Pronunciation and enunciation should be clear and distinct. A normal tone of voice carries best. Variance in tone brings out the meaning of words and adds vitality to what is said. The other choices present opportunities for disconcertion, confusion, or miscommunication.

134. **D** A write-it-once system
RATIONALE: The pegboard system generates all the necessary financial records for each patient transaction with one writing. The perforated forms, aligned one on top of the other, are held in place by a row of pegs along the side or top of a board. One writing enters a transaction on the daysheet, gives the patient a receipt for payment, brings the patient's account up to date, provides a current statement of account for the patient, and gives the patient a reminder of the next appointment.

135. **B** Posting
RATIONALE: Posting is the term used to describe the process of transferring an amount from one record to another. All charges and payments for professional services are posted to the ledger daily. The ledger then becomes a source for reliable patient account information.

136. **B** To deal with the collection agency
RATIONALE: After an account has been released to a collection agency, the medical office makes no further attempts at collection. No more statements are sent. The patient's ledger is marked so that the office knows it is in the hands of an agency. Refer the patient to the agency if he/she contacts the office in regard to the account. Any payments should be reported to the agency.

137. **B** Formatting
RATIONALE: Formatting magnetically creates tracks on a disk where information can be stored. RAM is an acronym for Random Access Memory; merging is related to data records and field formats (databases or word processing programs).

138. **D** Word processing
RATIONALE: Word processing is the system used to process written communications. It is a document production tool. Telecommunications in-

volve verbal communication; documentation, interfacing, and formatting are not types of computer systems.

139. **B** Enclosed packing slip
RATIONALE: All orders received should be compared with the original purchase order and the invoice included with the shipment. The order should be checked for correct items, sizes, styles, and amounts.

140. **C** The patient pays in advance
RATIONALE: A credit balance is the amount of advance payment or overpayment on an account. The amount of receipts exceeds the amount charged.

141. **B** Restrictive
RATIONALE: An endorsement is a signature on the back of the check by which the endorser transfers all rights in the check to another party. A restrictive endorsement specifies the purpose of the endorsement. A restrictive endorsement is used in preparing checks for deposit into the physician's account. An example of a restrictive endorsement is "For Deposit Only."

142. **E** bl pr
RATIONALE: BP is the accepted charting abbreviation for blood pressure.

143. **A** Medicaid
RATIONALE: Some patients may be covered by both Medicare and Medicaid (Medi-Medi). Assignment must always be accepted since Medicaid will not pay a claim unless the office accepts assignment on the Medicare portion of the claim. In this case, Medicare is the primary carrier and is billed first, and Medicaid is the payer of last resort.

144. **D** Have a single line drawn through it and marked "not done"
RATIONALE: The patient's medical chart is a chronological record of that patient's medical care. It is used to establish a database on each patient. All patient contact related to medical care should be documented correctly in the chart. Improper or false inclusions in the medical record can be as legally damaging as an omission.

145. **A** "Return to school" forms
RATIONALE: Routine correspondence may be stamped with the physician's signature. Nonroutine correspondence such as insurance forms, operative notes, reports, and discharge summaries must have an original physician's signature.

146. **D** Simplified
RATIONALE: The simplified style is the same as the full block style except there is no salutation or complimentary close.

147. **A** Payments made to the patient
RATIONALE: Most commercial carriers will reimburse the patient unless instructed to do otherwise. The patient indicates assignment of benefits by completing a form or signing the appropriate place on the insurance claim form.

148. **B** Five
RATIONALE: Each disease entry has been assigned a three-digit code. Further specificity is identified by adding a fourth-digit and fifth-digit modifier.

149. **E** All of the above
RATIONALE: The medical record is a legal document owned by the physician. The information contained in the record is confidential and is owned by the patient. Any information concerning the contents of the record requires consent from both the patient and physician before it can be released unless the information is subpoenaed by the courts. Omission of information can be legally damaging.

150. **C** Copayment
RATIONALE: A copayment is a fixed dollar amount that the insured person must pay each time service is received. It must be paid to cover some portion of the bill. The copayment amount is set by the insurance company.

151. **E** Express
RATIONALE: Express mail is available seven days per week, 365 days per year. It features next-day/overnight delivery to most metropolitan areas. Other delivery options can take two or more days to reach their destination.

152. **C** Conditioning
RATIONALE: A filing of materials involves five basic steps: conditioning (documents are checked for damage and repaired), releasing (some mark is placed on the document so it can be filed), indexing and coding (where to file the document and the caption to be used), sorting (arranging the documents), and storing and filing (placing the documents).

153. **A** Carrier
RATIONALE: Medical insurance is a protection against the chance of catastrophic loss of finances due to illness or injury. The carrier (insurer) is the insurance company that sells and administers an insurance contract (policy). The subscriber (insured) pays a premium to the carrier to keep the policy in force.

154. **D** All of the above
RATIONALE: An overdraft is the issuing of a check without sufficient funds to cover it. A postdated check is a check dated after the date it was written. It is not considered payable until the date written on the check. Not sufficient funds (NSF) checks are refused due to insufficient funds deposited in the account.

155. **A** Salutation
RATIONALE: The salutation is the opening greeting of a letter.

156. **E** Caller's Social Security number
RATIONALE: The information recorded on a telephone message includes the date and time of call, name of person called, caller's name and phone number, reason for the call/message, and the taker's initials.

157. **C** Patient's surname
RATIONALE: Color-coding uses colored tabs to represent information about a chart or a patient at a glance. Most systems use letters of the patient's surname to identify charts. A misfiled chart is easy to find.

158. **B** Independent commercial carriers
RATIONALE: Except for independent carriers, Medicaid, Title 19, CHAMPUS, and Workers' Compensation patients are covered by federally funded programs. If a physician elects to treat these patients, he/she must accept the reimbursement as payment in full.

159. **D** Salutation
RATIONALE: The salutation is the opening greeting to the person being addressed. The words will vary depending on the letter's degree of formality.

160. **B** Writing "canceled" in the appointment book
RATIONALE: All canceled appointments should be noted in the appointment book. Choices A and C are extraneous and unnecessary.

161. **C** Difficulty in retrieving
RATIONALE: As files expand, more time is required for filing or retrieving each folder because of the greater number of folders involved in the search.

162. **B** Received on account
RATIONALE: Proving the correctness of the general ledger is called taking the trial balance. It includes listing all account balances to determine if the credit balances equal the debit balance.

163. **A** It is unpredictable
RATIONALE: An allergy may alter medication and/or treatment procedures, and should always be documented in the patient's chart.

164. **A** A request for a change in appointment time
RATIONALE: A change in appointment time is not, in most cases, directly related to the type or quality of patient care, while the other choices are.

165. **C** The attitude and appearance of the receptionist

RATIONALE: The receptionist is the first person a patient comes in contact with in the office, either by phone or in person. The disposition of the receptionist can set the tone for the office visit. Receptionists should show pride in themselves and their work.

166. **D** The person who will pay the bill
RATIONALE: The responsible person is one who is responsible for payment. This is usually the patient if an adult, or the parent of a minor child.

167. **A** Hours of hospital rounds
RATIONALE: The matrix is the base upon which to build. To establish the matrix in the appointment book, block off those time slots when the physician is routinely not available to see patients. All else revolves around the physicians' availability.

168. **C** December 30, 2000
RATIONALE: The date line consists of the name of the month written in full, followed by the day and year. The other date formats are considered less formal and not appropriate for a business letter.

169. **A** Correctly spelled words may be used incorrectly
RATIONALE: Spell-check is an added word processing application that checks for misspelled words, but not necessarily the use of those words. Proofreading is the process by which copy is determined to be exactly what it was intended to be.

170. **D** The place to replace a file
RATIONALE: An OUT guide is used to temporarily replace a chart that has been removed from the shelf. It identifies the location of the record.

171. **B** The patient
RATIONALE: A copay is a fixed dollar amount that the insured person must pay each time service is received.

172. **C** The patient
RATIONALE: Preauthorization is the permission by the insurance carrier obtained prior to giving certain treatment to a patient. If the carrier does not give permission, the carrier will not pay, and the patient is then responsible for payment of services.

173. **D** Printer
RATIONALE: An input device allows for the input of data into the computer. These devices include the keyboard, light pen, mouse, and joystick. Output devices allow data to be displayed or recorded. These include monitors and printers.

174. **B** High blood pressure
RATIONALE: Objective findings are perceptible to a person other than the patient. They are signs that the physician or medical assistant detects when examining the patient. Health habits, medical insurance, family history, and previous illnesses are typically obtained directly from the patient, and can be highly subjective.

175. **C** Summary of amount owed physician by patients
RATIONALE: Accounts receivable are the amounts owed to the physician. This includes the fees owed by the patient to the provider for services rendered.

176. **A** Handling all blood and body fluids as if they are infected
RATIONALE: Standard Precautions is the application of the concept that all blood, body fluids, secretions, excretions, and most body substances be treated as if contaminated. Measures taken to practice this concept include wearing personal protective equipment such as gloves, washing hands, and handling "infected" items with care.

177. **A** Remove infectious microorganisms
RATIONALE: Medical asepsis is the destruction of organisms after they leave the body. Practicing medical asepsis means directing efforts at prevention of reinfection. Handwashing is the most important defense against this reinfection. Proper handwashing requires both friction and running water.

178. **B** A sharps container
RATIONALE: Contaminated sharps (anything that can cut or puncture) should be placed in a clearly labeled, puncture-resistant, leak-proof container immediately after use. Bending, breaking, or recapping is not allowed in order to prevent needle-stick injuries.

179. **A** 60–80 beats per minute
RATIONALE: Average pulse rate for an adult can range from 60 to 80 beats per minute. Normal limits are between 60 to 100 beats per minute.

180. **B** Usually higher in children than adults
RATIONALE: The pulse rate may vary as a result of a person's age, body size, sex, and health status. Children and infants normally have a faster pulse than do adults due to the faster rate of the hearbeat.

181. **E** Both arms
RATIONALE: For a new patient, the blood pressure should be taken on both arms. If a discrepancy exists between the two readings, the arm with the higher pressure is used in future recordings. The discrepancy is noted in the chart. The arm that is used is also noted.

182. **E,** B, C, and D
RATIONALE: Fear, fever, and physical activity can cause an increase in the pulse rate. This is due to

an increase in heart rate. Hyperthyroidism typically does not cause the pulse or heart rate to increase.

183. **E** 1°F
RATIONALE: The rectal temperature registers 1°F higher than an oral temperature because the mucous membrane lining of the rectum is not exposed to the air.

184. **C** At the right and left sides of the neck
RATIONALE: The carotid arteries are located between the larynx and the sternocleidomastoid muscle in the front and to the side of the neck. It can be felt by pushing the muscle to the side and pressing against the larynx. It is a common site to take a pulse, and is most frequently used in emergency situations.

185. **C** 67.5 kg
RATIONALE: To convert pounds to kilograms, multiply the number of pounds by 0.45.
(1 pound = 0.45 kilograms)

186. **B** 5 feet, 5 inches
RATIONALE: 12 inches equals one foot. Five feet equals 60 inches. Therefore 65 ÷ 12 = 5.41 feet, or 5 feet 5 inches.

187. **D** Prognosis
RATIONALE: A prognosis is a statement made by the physician indicating the probable or anticipated outcome of a disease process in a patient. A prodrome is an early sign or the earliest phase of a developing condition or disease; a diagnosis is the identification of a disease or condition; a syndrome is a complex of signs and symptoms resulting from a common cause; a cure is the restoration to health of a person afflicted with a disease or disorder.

188. **A** Auscultation
RATIONALE: Auscultation is the process of listening to sounds produced in the body as the organs perform their functions. This is done with the use of a stethoscope. Palpation involves feeling certain body parts with the hands; meansuration is the process of measuring; percussion involves tapping the body with the fingertips or fist to evaluate internal organs; inspection involves visual analysis of body parts.

189. **D** CBC
RATIONALE: A CBC (complete blood count) is a routine blood test that can be used to monitor the health status of the patient. An EEG (electroencephalogram), BUN (blood urea nitrogen), O& P (ova and parasites), and an IVP (intravenous pyelogram) are specific and specialized tests.

190. **A** Unusual cell growth on the cervix
RATIONALE: The Papanicolaou smear or test (Pap smear) is commonly done on a cervical

scraping to detect abnormal cells in the mucus. The smear is examined microscopically.

191. **E** 24–48 hours
RATIONALE: The patient should be instructed not to put any creams or foams in the vagina, not to douche, and not to have sexual intercourse for 24 to 48 hours before having a Pap smear taken. These circumstances can interfere with the specimen and can make the test invalid.

192. **B** 20
RATIONALE: The standard testing distance for visual acuity is 20 feet.

193. **A** Lithotomy position
RATIONALE: In the lithotomy position, the patient is supine with the knees flexed, and feet placed in stirrups. The buttocks are moved to the edge of the table and legs are spread apart. This position is most commonly used for gynecological and obstetrical examinations.

194. **C** Hearing
RATIONALE: Audiometry is a test used to measure hearing acuity. The test uses an electronic instrument called an audiometer. The audiometer produces different tones at selected frequencies and intensities. It is commonly used in schools to evaluate hearing levels in young children.

195. **A** Sims'
RATIONALE: The Sims' position is used for rectal examinations. The patient lies on the left side and chest with the left leg slightly flexed and the left leg sharply flexed on the abdomen. The buttocks are brought up to the edge of the table.

196. **D** The left eye at 20 feet what a normal eye can read at 40 feet
RATIONALE: *OS* is the abbreviation for left eye. 20/40 means that the patient can read at only 20 feet what a normal eye can read at 40 feet.

197. **D** CBC, blood type and Rh, VDRL, HIV, and rubella titer
RATIONALE: A CBC assesses the general health status of the mother. A VDRL tests for syphilis. Type and Rh are needed to detect blood type of the mother for possible Rh complications. A rubella titer determines the mother's immunity. HIV can detect if the mother has been exposed to the virus.

198. **C** Antiseptic
RATIONALE: An antiseptic is a substance capable of inhibiting the growth or actions of microorganisms without necessarily killing them. It is safe for use on body tissues. Germicides kill microorganisms; disinfectants are typically used on inanimate surfaces, like countertops.

199. **B** Temp: 250°F; pressure: 15 lbs
RATIONALE: The autoclave operates on the prin-

ciple of steam under pressure. The recommended temperature of 250°F and steam pressure of 15 pounds is recommended to kill pathogens and spores.

200. **D** Sterilization
RATIONALE: Sterilization is defined as the complete destruction of all forms of microbial life. This process includes the use of physical or chemical means. Sterilization plays a vital role in protecting the health of patients and health care professionals.

201. **A** Immediately
RATIONALE: Because the instruments are unwrapped, there is a greater chance of contamination. Instruments should not sit too long after sterilization because of this risk.

202. **B** Active
RATIONALE: Artificial active immunity is acquired through vaccination with an inactivated (dead) or attenuated (weakened) organism. Natural active immunity results from being a carrier, recovering from, or having a disease.

203. **D** Artificial active
RATIONALE: Artificial active immunity is acquired through vaccination with an inactivated or attenuated organism in the form of vaccination. Natural active immunity results from being a carrier, recovering from, or having a disease; artificial passive immunity is acquired through the transfer of antibody or lymphocytes from an immune donor.

204. **E** 0
RATIONALE: The size, or gauge, of most suture material is labeled in terms of 0s. 0 is the thickest, then 00, 000, and so on up to 10–0.

205. **D** Together, and facing downwards
RATIONALE: Sterile forceps are used to handle sterile instruments and supplies when sterile gloves are not worn. They are kept in a container that contains a chemical disinfectant/germicide. The forceps handle is not sterile; the prongs are sterile. If the tips are turned upward, any solution will run onto the nonsterile area and then back down over the sterile end, contaminating the sterile end. Keeping the prongs together keeps them from touching the sides of the container.

206. **C** Disinfecting the skin at the surgical site
RATIONALE: Betadine is the preferred skin antiseptic. Since skin cannot be sterilized, the presurgical scrub should remove as many microorganisms as possible to reduce the chance of infection.

207. **B** Incisional biopsy
RATIONALE: A biopsy is the removal of tissue from the body for examination. An incisional biopsy removes a portion of the lesion. An excisional biopsy removes the entire lesion.

208. **D** 90 degrees
RATIONALE: The main objective when administering an intramuscular medication is to inject it deep into the muscle. A 90-degree angle helps ensure the needle is in muscle tissue.

209. **C** 45 degrees
RATIONALE: The objective of a subcutaneous injection is to deposit a relatively small amount of the medication under the skin. A 45-degree angle helps deliver the medication to this area.

210. **B** Is applied to the skin
RATIONALE: A topical medication is externally applied to the skin or mucous membranes.

211. **E** ⅝ inch, 25 gauge
RATIONALE: A ⅝-inch needle is long enough to reach subcutaneous tissue. 25 gauge is large enough to handle aqueous solutions used in this area.

212. **D** Analgesic
RATIONALE: An analgesic is an agent that relieves the sensation of pain. Antidotes counteract poisons; antidepressants prevent or relieve depression; anesthetics produce a complete or partial loss of feeling; antiemetics prevent or alleviate nausea and vomiting.

213. **B** 2 capsules
RATIONALE:

$$\frac{\text{dosage ordered}}{\text{available strength}} \times \text{dosage form} = \text{dosage given}$$

Therefore: $\dfrac{500 \text{ mg}}{250 \text{ mg}} \times 1 \text{ capsule} = 2 \text{ capsules}$

214. **D** Given to the physician to review
RATIONALE: The physician should review lab results before they are filed in the patient's chart.

215. **D** Upper gastrointestinal bleeding
RATIONALE: In conditions in which the patient is having bleeding from the upper GI system, such as an ulcer, the stool can appear black and tarry. In lower GI bleeding, such as a hemorrhoid, the stool will appear bright red and bloody.

216. **C** Aspirin
RATIONALE: Aspirin, vitamin C in excess, and anti-inflammatory drugs may interfere with accurate readings because they can cause GI irritation and bleeding in some patients.

217. **C** Pus in urine
RATIONALE: *Py-* is a prefix/root word meaning pus. *-uria* is the suffix meaning urine.

218. **B** Glycosuria
RATIONALE: Diabetes mellitus is a complex disorder of carbohydrate, fat, and protein metabolism. It is due to the lack of insulin secretion in the pancreas. Signs and symptoms include polyuria (excessive urination), polydipsia (excessive thirst), polyphagia (excessive hunger), glycosuria (sugar in the urine), and weight loss.

219. **C** Cephalic and basilic veins
RATIONALE: The basilic and cephalic veins are located in the antecubital space. The vessels are usually large and close to the surface in this area. The other veins are much harder to access.

220. **B** Hematology studies
RATIONALE: Tubes containing EDTA are recommeded for use when doing hematology studies. White blood cells and platelets are best preserved in this type of tube, and red blood cell morphlogy is best obtained.

221. **E** Mammography
RATIONALE: A mammogram is an x-ray examination of the breast. It can identify breast lesions or tumors. It is the most effective method for determining early and curable breast cancer along with SBE. Thermography is a technique for sensing and recording on film hot and cold areas of the body by means of an infrared detector that reacts to blood flow; CAT scans, tomography, and xeroradiography are diagnostic x-ray techniques, but are not specific to breast examination.

222. **B** Cryotherapy
RATIONALE: Cryotherapy is the local application of cold. It is applied with dry or moist applications. Diathermy and thermotherapy involve the use of heat; electrotherapy involves the use of electrical current; hydrotherapy involves the use of water.

223. **A** Tachycardia
RATIONALE: Tachycardia is an abnormally rapid heart action. It is characterized by a pulse rate greater than 170 beats per minute. Bradycardia characterizes an abnormally slow heartbeat; fibrillation and defibrillation are terms that characterize disruptions in the normal heartbeat; a myocardial infarction is the medical term for a heart attack, of which tachycardia is typically a sign.

224. **B** QRS
RATIONALE: The normal EKG cycle consists of waves that have been labeled P, QRS, and T waves. Each wave corresponds to a particular part of the cardiac cycle. The P wave reflects contraction of the atria. The QRS wave (QRS complex) reflects the contraction of the ventricles. The T wave reflects ventricular recovery.

225. **B** 0.8 second
RATIONALE: Each cardiac cycle takes approximately 0.8 second. With this time limit, there are 75 heartbeats per minute.

226. **B** 10 mm
RATIONALE: The diagnostic value of an EKG depends on an accurate reading. Standard techniques have been adapted worldwide so that a recording can be interpreted anywhere. The universal standard is 1 millivolt of cardiac electrical activity will deflect the stylus 10 mm (1 cm) high. This is equal to 10 small blocks on the EKG paper.

227. **D** Distilled water
RATIONALE: Distilled water contains no additives or chemicals that may leave deposits in the chamber and interfere with the process. Tap water contains additives and purifiers that can leave deposits; saline contains salt.

228. **C** The desired temperature is reached
RATIONALE: When the temperature gauge reaches 250°F and the pressure gauge indicates 15 pounds of steam pressure, the load of articles to be sterilized can be timed for the recommended length of time.

229. **E** Potassium determination
RATIONALE: Lasix is a diuretic. Diuretics promote the formation and excretion of urine. They are prescribed to reduce the volume of extracellular fluid in the body. Potassium is a major electrolyte found in extracellular fluid, and can be lost with diuretic therapy.

230. **E** Sterile saline
RATIONALE: Sterile saline can be used to moisten a dressing that has adhered to a wound or is difficult to remove. Sterile saline will not contaminate the wound or cause discomfort to the patient.

231. **E** Brachial
RATIONALE: The brachial artery is the principal artery of the upper arm. It can be easily palpated at the antecubital space opposite the elbow. This area is easily accessible for ausculation.

232. **C** Volume of packed cells
RATIONALE: Hematocrit represents the volume percentage of red blood cells present in whole blood.

233. **A** Bevel-up, about ½ inch penetration
RATIONALE: The bevel of the needle should be facing upwards. This ensures the sharpest point of the needle is inserted first. A ½ in penetration depth should be sufficient to enter the vein.

234. **B** Casts
RATIONALE: A urine dipstick is used for the chemical examination of urine. Tests include glu-

cose, bilirubin, ketones, blood, protein, urobilino-gen, nitrite, and leukocytes. Casts are identified on microscopic examination.

235. **C** Radial
RATIONALE: Palpating a peripheral pulse gives the rate and rhythm of the heartbeat. A pulse can be taken at any artery that is near the surface of the body and can be pressed against a bone. The radial artery is located on the inner aspect of the wrist area on the thumb side. This site is the one most frequently used and accessible.

236. **E** First morning specimen
RATIONALE: The first morning specimen is the most concentrated specimen, and the hormone level would be at its highest, making pregnancy more accurately detectable.

237. **C** 1,000
RATIONALE: Total magnification equals the magnification of the ocular multiplied by the magnification of the objective. $100 \times 10 = 1,000$.

238. **E** Inflammation
RATIONALE: The erythrocyte sedimentation rate (ESR, sed rate) measures the rate at which antico-agulated RBCs will fall when allowed to settle in a special tube. Inflammation causes an alteration of the blood proteins, which makes the red blood cells aggregate, becoming heavier than normal. The speed with which they fall to the bottom of the tube corresponds to the degree of inflammation.

239. **A** Three times the hemoglobin value
RATIONALE: The hemoglobin and hematocrit values are related. Each 1% of hematocrit contains 0.34 gm of hemoglobin; the hematocrit should equal three times the hemoglobin.

240. **D** Artifacts
RATIONALE: Artifacts are considered to be contaminants. They can include hair, cloth fibers, mucous threads, and other contaminants. Casts, RBCs, and WBCs can be found in limited numbers in normal urine.

241. **C** Grains
RATIONALE: Grains, which include bread, cereal, rice, and pasta, are at the base of the food pyramid guide. 6–11 servings of this group are recommended per day.

242. **A** Depth
RATIONALE: Pulse characteristics include the rate (number of beats per minute), rhythm (interval of time between beats), volume (force or strength of the pulse), and texture of the artery wall (smooth and soft).

243. **B** Hypovolemic shock
RATIONALE: Shock is a physiological response to sudden illness/trauma. It is characterized by inad-equate peripheral circulation that can deprive vital organs to a blood supply. Hypovolemic shock occurs when there is a sudden blood or body fluid loss. Cardiogenic shock is characterized by low cardiac output associated with acute myocardial infarction and congestive heart failure. Anaphylactic shock is a hypersensitivity reaction to a substance, such as a drug, specific food, allergen, etc., and is usually marked by respiratory distress and vascular collapse. Cardiogenic shock results from peripheral vascular dilation.

244. **D** Yeast infection
RATIONALE: *Candida albicans* is found in the normal flora of the bowel and skin. It can cause opportunistic infections especially in the mouth (thrush) and vagina.

245. **B** Fourth intercostal space right of the sternum
RATIONALE: Lead V1 is the first precordial (chest) lead. The precordial leads provide a point of reference on the chest wall. They can differentiate between left-sided and right-sided events.

246. **B** Generic name
RATIONALE: A drug can have up to three names: chemical, generic, and trade. The generic name of a drug is the official name assigned to it. It is much simpler than the chemical name, and it is not protected by a copyright like the trade name. There are many brand names for each generic drug.

247. **A** 19 gauge
RATIONALE: The width of the needle is its gauge. The smaller the number of the gauge, the larger the width of the needle.

248. **B** Antibiotic
RATIONALE: An antibiotic kills or inhibits the growth of microorganisms. They are used in the treatment of bacterial invasions/infections. Antifungals destroy fungi; antitussives are used to suppress nonproductive coughs; anti-inflammatories are used to reduce inflammation; antipyretics are used to reduce fever.

249. **A** Lead V1
RATIONALE: The rhythm strip is the recording of Lead V1. It is used to determine the rhythm of the heartbeat (fast, slow, regular, irregular). This data can be a useful screening tool for frequent arrhythmias.

250. **E** A and B
RATIONALE: The label should be affixed to the requisition form and to the specimen container. The lid to the container could be lost, along with the label, if it were affixed to the lid.

251. **D** Ulcers
RATIONALE: *Helicobacter pylori* is a gram-

negative spiral bacterium that can cause gastritis and pyloric ulcers.

252. **B** Aspirin
RATIONALE: Reye's syndrome has been linked to the use of aspirin for febrile illnesses in pediatric patients. The other medications listed are not linked to Reye's syndrome.

253. **C** Dysuria
RATIONALE: The prefix *dys-* refers to pain. The root word *-uria* means urination. The prefix *-hema* means blood (the presence of blood in the urine); *-an* means none or lack of (lack of urination); *-poly* means many (frequent urination); pyuria is the presence of white blood cells in the urine.

254. **A** Platelets
RATIONALE: Platelets (thrombocytes) are the smallest of the formed elements in the blood. They are responsible for the clotting (coagulation) of the blood.

255. **B** By injection
RATIONALE: A parenteral drug is given by injection through a needle. The routes for parenteral administration include intradermal, subcutaneous, intramuscular, and intravenous. Dermal medications are administered via application to the skin; enteral medications can be given via the mouth.

256. **D** Cerumen
RATIONALE: Cerumen is the waxy secretion produced by the ceruminous glands in the external ear canal. Sebum is the oily secretion of the sebaceous glands of the skin.

257. **C** 37%–47%
RATIONALE: The hematocrit measures the percentage of packed cells in the total blood volume. Normal values for adult females are between 37% and 47%. Normal values for men are between 42% and 52%.

258. **D** Anemia
RATIONALE: Anemia is a disorder characterized by a decrease in hemoglobin in the blood. It can be caused by blood loss, decrease in hemoglobin or RBC production, or an increase in RBC destruction. Polycythemia is an increase in the number of erythrocytes; infection is usually accompanied by an increase in white blood cells; leukemia involves abnormal numbers and forms of immature white blood cells; diabetes is a metabolic disorder.

259. **A** Upper GI series
RATIONALE: Barium sulfate, a contrast medium, is administered by mouth before an upper GI series is taken to visualize the esophagus and stomach.

260. **D** Anteroposterior
RATIONALE: In the anteroposterior (AP) position, the rays from the machine enter the anterior of the body and exit the posterior before hitting the film.

261. **C** Treat muscle sprains and strains
RATIONALE: Ultrasound uses high frequency sound waves as a deep-heating agent for soft tissues of the body. Deep-heating can be used to treat muscle injuries, like sprains or strains.

262. **A** Monocytes
RATIONALE: WBCs are classified as granulocytes (containing granules in the cytoplasm) or agranulocytes (containing no granules in the cytoplasm). The granulocytes include neutrophils, eosinophils, and basophils. The agranulocytes include monocytes and lymphocytes.

263. **B** A type of respiration
RATIONALE: Cheyne-Stokes is an abnormal pattern of respiration characterized by alternating periods of apnea and deep, rapid breathing. These are often a sign of impending death, but may also be observed during deep sleep.

264. **E** Vitamin K
RATIONALE: Vitamin K, a fat-soluble vitamin, is essential for the synthesis of prothrombin in the liver. Prothrombin is the precursor of thrombin, a protein necessary for blood clotting. In the diet, it is found in green leafy vegetables, fruit, dairy, and grain products. It is also formed by bacteria in the colon.

265. **C** CLIA '88
RATIONALE: The Clinical Laboratory Improvement Amendments (CLIA) was passed in 1988 to improve the quality of laboratory testing. It consists of federal regulations that govern all facilities that perform lab testing for diagnosis, prevention, or treatment of disease. These regulations include quality control and assurance, record-keeping, and personnel requirements.

266. **B** Antibiotic
RATIONALE: An antibiotic drug kills or inhibits the growth of microorganisms. Amoxicillin (Amoxil) is a synthetic penicillin used to treat bacterial infections.

267. **B** Antidepressants
RATIONALE: An antidepressant drug treats the symptoms of depression. Zoloft and Paxil are examples of a seratonin selective reuptake inhibitor, a type of antidepressant.

268. **E** All of the above
RATIONALE: The "Seven Rights" of drug administration include: right patient, right drug, right dose, right time, right route, right technique, and right documentation.

269. **B** Cones
RATIONALE: The rods and cones are photoreceptors located on the retina of the eye. Cones allow a person to visualize colors. Rods tend to detect visual motion and serve night vision. Rods and cones are found in the retina.

270. **D** Diarrhea
RATIONALE: Diarrhea is the frequent passage of loose, watery stools. Children lose large amounts of water and electrolytes with the passage of these stools, and can be in danger of dehydration if these fluids are not quickly replaced.

271. **D** Lumbar puncture
RATIONALE: A lumbar puncture is the introduction of a hollow needle into the subarachnoid space of the lumbar portion of the spinal canal. It is used to obtain cerebrospinal fluid (CSF) for analysis. CT scans, MRIs, EEGs, and EKGs are all noninvasive procedures.

272. **C** Ensure the accuracy of the test results
RATIONALE: Quality control in the laboratory is used to ensure the accuracy of test results while detecting and eliminating error. Control samples are tested daily along with patient samples. The results of these control samples must be within a preestablished range before patient tests can be run.

273. **E** Squeezing the finger to encourage blood flow
RATIONALE: Squeezing the finger after puncture can lead to contamination of the sample from tissue fluid. Blood should be allowed to flow naturally to the puncture site.

274. **E** All of the above
RATIONALE: Any unwanted movement of the stylus on the paper produced by outside interference is called an artifact; artifacts on the tracing that can result from loose electrodes, poor grounding, muscle tremors, or electrical interference can make interpretation of the recording difficult.

275. **D** Coumadin
RATIONALE: An anticoagulant drug delays or blocks the clotting of blood. Coumadin (warfarin sodium) is an oral anticoagulant. It is used for treatment of thrombosis (blood clots).

276. **C** IV
RATIONALE: The intravenous (IV) route delivers medication directly into the bloodstream producing the quickest effect. Other routes take more time to be absorbed into the body and to take effect.

277. **C** 46
RATIONALE: All body cells contain 46 chromosomes. This includes 22 pairs of autosomes and one pair of sex chromosomes. One member of each pair comes from each parent.

278. **C** Thoracic/abdominal
RATIONALE: The diaphragm is a dome-shaped muscle that separates the thoracic and abdominal cavities. It aids in respiration by moving up and down.

279. **C** Second degree
RATIONALE: A second-degree burn is characterized by involvement of the epidermis and superficial dermis. It produces blisters and redness. First-degree burns involve the epidermis only; third-degree burns involve deep tissue damage. Excoriation is an injury to a surface of the body caused by trauma, such as scratching, abrasion, or a chemical or thermal burn.

280. **C** Ligament
RATIONALE: A ligament is a band of fibrous connective tissue that binds joints together and connects various bones and cartilages. A fascia is a connective tissue membrane that covers individual skeletal muscles or certain organs; articulation is the joining of structures at a joint; an epiphysis is the end of a long bone; a tendon is a strong band of connective tissue that anchors muscle to bone.

281. **E** Hemiplegia
RATIONALE: Paralysis of one side of the body is hemiplegia. (*hemi-* means half; *-plegia* means paralysis.) This type of paralysis is most often associated with a cerebrovascular accident or brain tumor.

282. **B** Hyperopia
RATIONALE: Farsightedness (hyperopia) is a condition resulting from an error of refraction. The light rays enter the eye and are brought into focus behind the retina. Emmetropia is the state of normal vision; myopia is nearsightedness; nystagmus is involuntary, rhythmic movements of the eyes; astigmatism is when light rays cannot be focused clearly in a point on the retina because the spheric curve of the cornea is not equal, thereby causing blurred vision.

283. **D** Eustachian tube
RATIONALE: The Eustachian tube joins the nasopharynx and tympanic cavity. It is lined with a mucous membrane, and allows equalization of the air pressure in the inner ear with the atmospheric pressure.

284. **A** Embolus
RATIONALE: An embolus is a foreign object, air, tissue, or thrombus (blood clot) that circulates in the bloodstream. A thrombus is a blood clot formed within a blood vessel or a heart chamber; an occlusion is a blockage in a canal, vessel, or

passage of the body; thrombocyte is another name for a platelet; an aneurysm is the dilation of the wall of a blood vessel.

285. **B** Hemostasis
RATIONALE: The root word *hemo-* means blood. The suffix *-stasis* means to control or stop.

286. **A** Epistaxis
RATIONALE: Epistaxis is bleeding from the nose caused by local irritation of mucous membranes, trauma, hypertension, fragility of the venous walls, or by picking of the nose. Rhinorrhea is otherwise known as a runny nose.

287. **C** Rales
RATIONALE: Rales is a common abnormal respiratory sound heard on auscultation during inspiration. It is characterized by bubbling or rattling noises.

288. **B** Anorexia
RATIONALE: Anorexia is the lack or loss of appetite. This condition may result from illness or psychological causes. Polyphagia is excessive, uncontrolled eating; bulimia is often characterized by food binging and purging; ascites is an abnormal intraperitoneal accumulation of fluid.

289. **E** Ileum
RATIONALE: The ileum is the distal portion of the small intestine, extending from the jejunum to the cecum.

290. **D** Cholelithiasis
RATIONALE: The root word *chole-* means pertaining to bile. The root word *lith-* means a stone or calculus. The suffix *-iasis* means abnormal condition of. Cholecystitis is the inflammation of the gallbladder; cholangitis is inflammation of the bile ducts; cholecystectomy is the surgical removal of the gallbladder; choledochiasis relates to the common bile duct.

291. **B** Nephron
RATIONALE: A nephron is the structural and functional unit of the kidney, which forms urine. Each kidney contains about one million nephrons.

292. **B** A gene
RATIONALE: A gene is unit of genetic material and inheritance. It occupies a specific place on a chromosome. A gene is a segment of DNA.

293. **A** Mitosis
RATIONALE: Mitosis is the type of cell division that occurs in somatic cells. It results in the formation of two identical daughter cells.

294. **E** Salpingo-oophorectomy
RATIONALE: The suffix *-ectomy* means surgical removal. *Salping/o-* means Fallopian tubes. *Oophor-* means ovary. A panhysterectomy is the removal of the uterus and cervix; a hysterectomy is the removal of the uterus; a salpingectomy is the removal of one or both fallopian tubes; a hysterosalpingectomy is the removal of one or both fallopian tubes and the uterus.

295. **A** Embryo
RATIONALE: An embryo is the stage of prenatal development between the time of implantation of the fertilized ovum until the end of the seventh or eighth week. An embryo is characterized as a fetus typically after the eight week of development. A neonate is an infant from birth to 28 days of age.

296. **C** Amenorrhea
RATIONALE: The prefix *a-* means absence of, without, lack of. *-Menorrhea* refers to the menstrual flow or menses.

297. **C** Viruses
RATIONALE: Viruses are microscopic intracellular parasites, and are the smallest pathogens. They require a host to carry out their activities.

298. **B** Skin
RATIONALE: The skin is the largest barrier against infection. As long as it remains intact, the skin is the first and main physical barrier to microorganisms. The skin also contains chemical barriers such as an acid pH and sweat, which can inhibit bacterial infection. If microorganisms breach the skin barrier, other body defense mechanisms may combat them, such as WBCs, mucous membranes, and immunity.

299. **C** Right atrium
RATIONALE: The superior vena cava is the second largest vein of the body. It returns deoxygenated blood from the upper half of the body to the right atrium.

300. **E** Cardio-
RATIONALE: *Cardio-* means heart. *Hemo-* means blood. *Cranio-* means cranium. *Electro-* refers to electricity or electrical activity. *Neuro-* means nerve.

1. **B** Atrophy
   RATIONALE: The prefix *a-* means without, lack of. The suffix *-trophy* means development.

2. **C** Myoblast
   RATIONALE: The root word *myo-* means muscle. The suffix *-blast* means immature cell, form.

3. **A** AD
   RATIONALE: AD is the abbreviation for right ear (auris dextra). *AS* is the abbreviation for left ear, *AU* for both ears, *OD* for right eye, and *OS* for left eye.

4. **B** Inspect the exterior ear canal
   RATIONALE: An otoscope is a lighted instrument used to visually examine the outer ear and tympanic membrane.

5. **D** Thoracentesis
   RATIONALE: A thoracentesis is the surgical puncture of the chest wall and pleural space. Fluid or air can then be withdrawn.

6. **B** Hematocrit/hemoglobin
   RATIONALE: Anemia is a disorder characterized by a decrease in hemoglobin or a decrease in the total number of red blood cells.

7. **C** Endocrinologist
   RATIONALE: Hyperparathyroidism is an abnormal endocrine condition in which an excess of parathyroid hormone is secreted. An endocrinologist diagnoses and treats diseases and disorders of the endocrine system.

8. **D** Leukocytosis
   RATIONALE: A leukocytosis is an increase in the total numbers of circulating white blood cells. *Leuko-* refers to white. *-cyt* refers to cells. *-osis* is an abnormal condition.

9. **A** Hyperpnea
   RATIONALE: Hyperpnea is deep or rapid breathing. The prefix *hyper-* means above. The root word *-pnea* refers to breathing.

10. **D** -algia
    RATIONALE: The suffix *-algia* means pain, painful condition.

11. **C** -plasty
    RATIONALE: The suffix *-plasty* means surgical repair.

12. **C** Breast
    RATIONALE: A mammogram is an x-ray film of the soft tissue of the breast. *Mammo-* refers to breast. The suffix *-gram* refers to a record (x-ray).

13. **D** Baldness
    RATIONALE: Alopecia is the partial or complete lack of hair. This can be due to normal aging, an endocrine disorder, chemotherapy, or a skin disease.

14. **A** Mastication
    RATIONALE: Mastication is the chewing, tearing, or grinding of food with the teeth while it becomes mixed with saliva.

15. **E** Mole on the inside of the elbow
    RATIONALE: A nevus is a mole. The antecubital area is located on the inner aspect of the elbow.

16. **D** Arthritis
    RATIONALE: The root word *arth-* means joint. The suffix *-itis* means inflammation.

17. **B** Adipose tissue
    RATIONALE: Adipose tissue is made up of fat cells arranged in globules. It is found under the skin, and serves as a reserve energy source and for insulation.

18. **C** Pathology
    RATIONALE: Pathology is the study of the characteristics, causes, and effects of disease on the structure and function of the body.

19. **C** Smelling
    RATIONALE: The olfactory nerve, Cranial Nerve I, is one of two pairs of nerves associated with the sense of smell.

20. **B** Ovaries
    RATIONALE: An oophorectomy is the surgical removal of one or both ovaries. The root word *oophor-* means ovary. The suffix *-ectomy* means surgical removal.

21. **C** Urology
    RATIONALE: Urology is the branch of medicine concerned with the urinary tract in men and women, and the male genital tract. The physician who specializes in urology is a urologist.

22. **D** Cystoscopy
    RATIONALE: Cystoscopy is the direct visualization of the urinary tract and/or bladder by means of a cystoscope inserted in the urethra.

23. **A** Urticaria
    RATIONALE: Urticaria is a pruritic skin eruption characterized by wheals (hives) of various shapes and sizes. This can be caused by allergic reactions to drugs, insect bites, and foods.

24. **C** Pericardium
    RATIONALE: The pericardium is the serous membrane that surrounds the heart.

25. **D** Lines body cavities that open to the outside
    RATIONALE: A mucous membrane lines body cavities or spaces of the body which open to the outside including the mouth, digestive tract, respiratory tract, and genitourinary tract.

26. **D** Anterior
    RATIONALE: The ventral area of the body is towards the front of the body (anterior).

27. **C** Abdominal
    RATIONALE: The abdominal cavity is part of the ventral cavity of the body. It contains the stomach, small and large intestines, spleen, liver, gallbladder, and pancreas.

28. **C** Adduction
    RATIONALE: Adduction is the movement of a limb or body part towards the body.

29. **A** Frontal
    RATIONALE: The frontal plane is the vertical plane that divides the body or a structure into anterior and posterior portions.

30. **A** Can follow a viral illness in children
    RATIONALE: Reye's syndrome is an acute and sometimes fatal illness characterized by fatty invasion of internal organs and swelling of the brain. The cause is unknown, but has been linked to the use of aspirin and viral illnesses in children.

31. **C** Lumbar
    RATIONALE: The vertebral column is divided into five sections: cervical (neck), thoracic (chest), lumbar (lower back), sacral (below the lumbar), and coccygeal (tailbone).

32. **A** Impetigo
    RATIONALE: Impetigo is an infection of the skin caused by staph, strep, or a combination of the two. The lesions usually begin around the mouth and nose and spread locally. The lesions blister and crust.

33. **D** Occipital
    RATIONALE: The occipital bone of the skull is located at the back of the skull. It articulates with the two parietal bones and contains the foramen magnum (opening for the spinal cord).

34. **C** Greenstick fracture
    RATIONALE: A greenstick fracture is an incomplete fracture. The bone is bent but fractured only on the outer arc of the bend.

35. **E** 31
    RATIONALE: The peripheral nervous system is made up of the motor and sensory nerves and ganglia located outside the brain and spinal cord. It consists of 12 pairs of cranial nerves and 31 pairs of spinal nerves.

36. **A** Brainstem
    RATIONALE: The brainstem is the portion of the brain made up of the midbrain, pons, and medulla. It performs sensory, motor, and reflex functions. Vital centers that regulate internal body functions are located here.

37. **A** Aplastic
    RATIONALE: Aplastic anemia results from a failure of blood cell production due to the failure of bone marrow to produce cells. The cause is unknown.

38. **C** Hiatal hernia
    RATIONALE: A hernia is the abnormal protrusion of an organ or tissue through the structures that normally contain it. A hiatal hernia is the protrusion of the upper portion of the stomach upward through the esophageal opening in the diaphragm.

39. **D** Eardrum
    RATIONALE: The tympanic membrane is the membrane between the external and middle ear. It is commonly called the eardrum.

40. **D** Aorta
    RATIONALE: The aorta is the main trunk of the systemic arterial circulation. Blood is pumped out of the left ventricle through the aortic valve into the aorta. The aorta then branches and carries blood all over the body.

41. **C** Is the pacemaker of the heart
    RATIONALE: The sinoatrial (SA) node of the heart is located in the right atrium. The electrical impulse that initiates the heartbeat originates here.

42. **B** Radius and ulna
    RATIONALE: The radius is the lateral lower arm bone on line with the thumb. The ulna is the medial lower arm bone.

43. **E** All of the above
    RATIONALE: Involuntary (smooth) muscle is muscle that is not under a person's conscious or voluntary control. These muscle actions include muscles of the heart and muscles of the intestines, stomach, and other visceral organs.

44. **A** Liver
    RATIONALE: The right upper quadrant (RUQ) of the abdominopelvic area contains the liver, gallbladder, part of the pancreas, and parts of the small and large intestines.

45. **D** Phrenic
RATIONALE: The diaphragm is stimulated by the phrenic nerve from the cervical plexus. The diaphragm aids in respiration by moving up and down.

46. **C** Scoliosis
RATIONALE: Scoliosis is a lateral curvature of the spine commonly seen in childhood. Unequal heights of hips and shoulders may be a sign of this condition.

47. **B** Glucagon
RATIONALE: Glucagon is a hormone produced by the alpha cells in the Islets of Langerhans in the pancreas. It stimulates the conversion of glycogen to glucose in the liver.

48. **C** Cholecystectomy
RATIONALE: The root word *cholecyst-* means gallbladder. The suffix *-ectomy* means surgical removal.

49. **E** Optic
RATIONALE: The optic nerve (Cranial Nerve II) is a sensory nerve that is involved with the sense of vision.

50. **D** 32
RATIONALE: There are 32 adult (permanent) teeth that replace the deciduous (baby) teeth. These include four central incisors, lateral incisors, cuspids, first and second premolars, first molars, second molars, and third molars (wisdom teeth).

51. **E** May refuse to accept a patient if he or she chooses
RATIONALE: Physicians have the right to determine whom they will accept as patients. Patient load may be as large as one person can adequately care for, and the decision may be made to limit new patients.

52. **D** Is a detailed outline of a trip
RATIONALE: An itinerary is detailed information about a trip. It includes the date and time of departure, flight numbers, mode of transportation to hotel, name, address and telephone number of hotel, date, and time of return.

53. **B** Staying calm when dealing with angry patients
RATIONALE: Professional qualities that a medical assistant must have include a friendly and pleasant attitude, ability to maintain confidentiality, courtesy, ability to control temper, consideration, respect and kindness, dependability, and accuracy.

54. **B** Empathy
RATIONALE: Empathy is the ability to recognize the emotions and state of mind of another person.

55. **B** The physician
RATIONALE: The physician owns the medical record but the patient owns the information.

56. **A** Denial
RATIONALE: Denial is the unconscious avoidance of the reality of an unpleasant or disturbing situation.

57. **E** All of the above
RATIONALE: Personality is the pattern of behavior each person develops as a means of adapting to a particular environment and its standards. Age, life experiences, heredity, and environment all play a part in this development.

58. **B** Impatient
RATIONALE: The professional services of a medical assistant are extremely personal, and the manner in which these services are performed can affect the health and well-being of the patient. An impatient person could negatively affect the patient.

59. **E** Young children react differently to stressful situations
RATIONALE: Stereotyping is a preconceived generalized belief. Young children do react differently to stressful situations than adults react.

60. **C** The patient must sign a release form
RATIONALE: The patient must sign a release of information form before information from the medical record can be released to anyone. This preserves the patient's confidentiality.

61. **E** HIV
RATIONALE: The physician has a legal duty to report communicable diseases to the county health department. This helps the state to provide for the public's health, safety, and welfare.

62. **B** Vital signs
RATIONALE: Objective data is data determined by someone other than the patient such as the physician or medical assistant. Vital signs are considered to be objective.

63. **A** Another physician
RATIONALE: A call from another physician or professional colleague should be transferred to the physician immediately.

64. **C** Social need
RATIONALE: Maslow believed that lower level needs must be satisfied before higher level needs could be satisfied. These levels, from lowest to highest, include physiological needs, safety needs, social needs, self-esteem needs, and self-actualization needs.

65. **D** Delay treatment and inform/consult the physician
RATIONALE: A physician must have consent to

treat a patient even though this consent is usually implied. A physician who fails to secure some formal type of consent could be charged with assault and battery or trespass.

66. **E** All of the above
RATIONALE: A contract is an agreement that creates an obligation. To be valid or enforceable, the contract must have four basic elements: an offer/acceptance, consideration, capacity, and legality.

67. **D** Posterior
RATIONALE: The anterior of a structure is the front of the structure. The posterior of a structure is the back of the structure.

68. **E** All of the above
RATIONALE: Informed consent must be obtained from the patient when a complex procedure is to be performed. Informed consent implies an understanding of what is to be done, why it should be done, the risks involved, the expected outcomes, alternative treatments including failure to treat, and the risks involved.

69. **E** Providing atypical care
RATIONALE: The license to practice medicine may be revoked or suspended under certain circumstances. Grounds for revoking or suspending a license generally falls within one of three categories: conviction of a crime, unprofessional conduct, or personal/professional incapacity.

70. **C** Nucleus
RATIONALE: The nucleus is the control center of every cell. It contains DNA which is the genetic material.

71. **E** All of the above
RATIONALE: The subcutaneous tissue is a layer of connective tissue that is found between the skin and the deep fascia. It contains a fatty layer. Hypodermic injections into this tissue is usually on the upper arm, thigh, or abdomen.

72. **B** Humerus
RATIONALE: The humerus is the largest bone of the upper arm. The femur is the bone of the thigh; the tibia and fibula make up the lower leg; the metatarsals form the arch of the foot.

73. **A** Deltoid
RATIONALE: The deltoid is a large, thick, triangular muscle that covers the shoulder.

74. **B** SA node
RATIONALE: The SA (sino-atrial) node is a cluster specialized cells located in the right atrial wall of the heart. It generates impulses which travel throughout the muscle fibers of the atria and cause them to contract.

75. **E** Alveoli
RATIONALE: The alveoli are small saclike structures at the terminal ends of the bronchioles. They are the functional units of respiration. They are composed of a single layer of epithelium which allows oxygen and carbon dioxide to be easily exchanged with the surrounding capillaries.

76. **E** All of the above
RATIONALE: The liver is the largest gland of the body. Its main functions include production of bile, detoxification of toxins and wastes, metabolism of proteins and carbohydrates, storage of vitamins and glycogen, production of heparin, and recycling of worn-out red blood cells.

77. **B** Endometrium
RATIONALE: The endometrium is the innermost layer of the uterus. The fertilized ovum implants into this layer where it develops until delivery.

78. **B** Testes
RATIONALE: Testosterone, the male hormone, is manufactured in the interstitial cells of the testes.

79. **A** Cerebrum
RATIONALE: The cerebrum is the largest portion of the brain. It is divided into two hemispheres which are further divided into lobes. Its outer surface (cortex) is made up of gray matter.

80. **E** 31
RATIONALE: There are 31 pairs of spinal nerves which are connected to the spinal cord. They are numbered according to which vertebra they emerge from.

81. **A** Mouth
RATIONALE: The gustatory sense is the sense of taste. The receptors are located on the tongue within papillae (taste buds).

82. **D** Decreases blood sugar levels
RATIONALE: Insulin is a hormone manufactured by the beta cells in the pancreas. Its main function is to metabolize glucose and thus reduce blood sugar levels.

83. **E** Leukopenia
RATIONALE: A leukopenia is an abnormal decrease in the number of white blood cells to fewer than 5,000 cells per cu mm of blood. *Leuko-* means white, or white blood cell. *-penia* means a decrease.

84. **B** Stat
RATIONALE: STAT is the abbreviation for "statim" meaning immediately.

85. **E** All of the above
RATIONALE: The physician has a legal duty to report information that may have an effect on the health, safety, or welfare of the public. This information includes births, deaths, communicable diseases, abuse, criminal acts, and professional misconduct.

86. **A** Slow
RATIONALE: The prefix *brady-* means slow.

87. **C** Deep
RATIONALE: Superficial pertains to the skin or another surface. Deep refers to away from the surface.

88. **C** An advance directive
RATIONALE: An advance directive is a legal document that gives persons the right to determine what medical procedures they want provided if they become unable to make those decisions.

89. **B** Denial
RATIONALE: Unconscious defense mechanisms serve to protect the mind from guilt or anxiety. Denial is the unconscious avoidance of the reality of an unpleasant or disturbing feeling, thought, or event.

90. **A** Open-ended statement
RATIONALE: An open-ended statement or question helps the patient to decide what is relevant. It also encourages the patient to continue discussion.

91. **C** Etiology
RATIONALE: Etiology is the study of all factors that may be involved in the development of a disease. This can include the susceptibility of the patient, the nature of the disease-causing agent, and the way the patient's body is invaded by the agent.

92. **E** All of the above
RATIONALE: Nonverbal communications are messages conveyed without the use of words. They are transmitted by body language. Body language involves grooming, dress, eye contact, facial expression, hand gestures, space, tone of voice, posture, and touch.

93. **B** An eating disorder
RATIONALE: Bulimia is an insatiable craving for food characterized by binge eating and self-induced vomiting.

94. **D** Stroke
RATIONALE: A cerebrovascular accident (CVA) or brain attack is an abnormal condition of the blood vessels of the brain characterized by an occlusion that results in an ischemia of the brain tissue. Paralysis, weakness, speech defect, aphasia, or death may occur.

95. **D** Measles
RATIONALE: Measles (rubeola) is an acute, highly contagious viral infection. It involves the respiratory tract and is characterized by a spreading cutaneous rash. It is caused by the paramyxovirus and is transmitted by droplets.

96. **C** Trichomoniasis
RATIONALE: Trichomoniasis is a vaginal infection caused by the protozoan *Trichomonas vaginalis*. It is transmitted by sexual intercourse.

97. **E** Potassium
RATIONALE: Potassium is necessary to the life of all animals. It is the major intracellular cation, and helps to regulate neuromuscular excitability and muscle contraction.

98. **B** Emphysema
RATIONALE: Emphysema is an abnormal condition of the pulmonary system. It is characterized by overinflation and destructive changes of the alveoli. This results in a loss of lung elasticity and a decreased gas exchange.

99. **C** Mucous
RATIONALE: A mucous membrane is a major kind of body membrane that covers or lines cavities or canals that open to the outside.

100. **E** Compound fracture
RATIONALE: An open or compound fracture is a fracture in which the broken end of the bone tears open the skin.

101. **B** Double-booking
RATIONALE: Double-booking is the practice of scheduling two patients to come in at the same time to see the physician.

102. **D** Envelope marked "personal"
RATIONALE: Incoming mail should be sorted according to importance and urgency. The order of importance is the physician's personal mail, ordinary First Class mail, periodicals and newspapers, and lastly, all other pieces.

103. **B** Absence of punctuation after the salutation and a comma after the complimentary close
RATIONALE: Open punctuation style uses no punctuation at the end of any line outside of the body of the letter unless the line ends with an abbreviation. This type of punctuation is used with the simplified block letter style.

104. **D** Medicaid
RATIONALE: Medicaid is a federally funded insurance program. It was set up by the federal government in 1965 to provide for the medically indigent. It is regulated by each state.

105. **C** Posting
RATIONALE: Posting is the transfer of information from one record to another. Transactions are posted from the day sheet to the ledger.

106. **B** An alphabetical cross reference
RATIONALE: Numeric filing involves filing records, correspondence, or cards by number. It is an indirect filing system, and requires the use of alphabetical cross-reference in order to find a given file.

107. **D** Holmes-Mathis, Jennie
RATIONALE: Hyphenated elements of a name,

whether first name, middle name, or surname, are considered as one unit.

108. **C** Patient and insurance company
RATIONALE: A third-party payer is someone other than the patient, spouse, or parent who is responsible for paying all or part of the patient's medical costs.

109. **E** All of the above
RATIONALE: If a claim form is not sufficiently detailed, complete and accurate, it may be rejected by the insurance company. Reasons for claim rejection could include: missing/incomplete diagnosis, incorrectly coded diagnosis, charges not itemized, patient's group, member, or policy number missing, patient signature missing, patient date of birth missing, dates missing/incorrect, or physician signature missing.

110. **D** $0.84
RATIONALE: The first ounce would cost $0.34, and the two additional ounces would total $0.50. $0.34 + $0.50 = $0.84.

111. **D** Below the return address
RATIONALE: Any notation on the envelope directed toward the addressee (such as *Personal* or *Confidential*) should be typed and underlined on the third line below the return address. It should be aligned with the return address on the left edge of the envelope.

112. **A** Very truly yours
RATIONALE: The complimentary close is the writer's way of saying goodbye. The words used are determined by the formality used in the salutation.

113. **D** Insurance information
RATIONALE: The patient's insurance information is obtained at the time of the first visit to the office. Necessary information includes the patient's name, phone number, reason for coming to the office, and times available for the appointment.

114. **B** Conference call
RATIONALE: A conference call allows more than two persons to participate in a conversation at one time. Each person can hear or talk to all others participating.

115. **C** Backing-up
RATIONALE: A back-up is a tape or disk for storage of files to prevent their loss in the event of hard disk failure.

116. **E** Future events arranged in chronological order
RATIONALE: A tickler file is a chronological file used as a reminder that something must be taken care of on a certain date. This type of file is frequently used as a follow-up method.

117. **A** Diarrhea
RATIONALE: CPT (current procedural terminol-

ogy) is a listing of descriptive terms and identifying codes used for reporting medical services and procedures performed by the physician. All of the above are procedures except diarrhea.

118. **E** All of the above
RATIONALE: The receptionist is usually the first person in the medical office that the patient has contact with. The appearance, professionalism, attitude, and manners of the receptionist, and the appearance of the reception area as a whole, can influence the patient's perception of the entire practice.

119. **C** See also
RATIONALE: "See also" is the coding convention that gives the direction to the coder to consider another code.

120. **C** Refers to factors that influence health status
RATIONALE: V codes (V01-V82) are codes referring to factors that influence health status. A definite diagnosis is not stated, but there is a valid reason for seeking medical care. These reasons can include annual physical exams, well-baby checks, and preoperative physicals. These codes are part of the ICD-9-CM coding system.

121. **D** Resealed with tape, and noted as "opened in error"
RATIONALE: All offices should have a procedure to follow regarding incoming mail. Personal mail should be left unopened. Should it be opened in error, fold and replace it inside the envelope, reseal the envelope, and write across the outside "opened in error" followed by the opener's initials.

122. **E** All of the above
RATIONALE: E/M descriptors (evaluation and management) include basic diagnostic and treatment services such as office visits and physical exams. These descriptors are part of the CPT coding system.

123. **B** Medicare
RATIONALE: A third-party payer is any person, insurance company, or government agent other than the patient or the patient's family who pays the patient's account.

124. **C** A numbered list of present problems
RATIONALE: The problem-oriented medical record (POMR) is a system to organize the patient's medical record and the information it contains. The system utilizes four parts: the database, the problem list, the treatment plan, and the progress notes. The database includes the chief complaint, present illness or illnesses, and the patient profile.

125. **D** Ledger card totals and account receivable balance

RATIONALE: A trial balance is a method of checking the accuracy of accounts. It should be done once a month after all posting has been completed and before preparing monthly statements. The purpose of a trial balance is to disclose any discrepancies between the ledger cards and accounts receivable. It does not prove the accuracy of the accounts.

126. **C** Newest to the front
RATIONALE: The medical record is a chronological system for recording a patient's medical care. Its continuity ensures the best medical care. By filing the most current information to the front, it provides a quick current reference of the patient's care and management.

127. **C** Another physician
RATIONALE: The person answering the telephone is expected to screen all incoming calls. Good judgment in deciding whether to put through a call comes with experience. Calls from other physicians should be put through at once if the physician is available to take the call.

128. **D** In consecutive order without large gaps
RATIONALE: Appointment scheduling is the process that determines which patients will be seen by the provider, dates and times of the appointments, and how much time will be allotted to each patient based on the complaint and the availability of the provider. Most providers find that efficient scheduling and time management is one of the most important factors in the success of the practice.

129. **E** Diagnosis
RATIONALE: At an initial visit, the patient's diagnosis may not be made. At the first visit, the patient may complete a patient information form which will include name, address, and phone number, insurance information, business information, and referral information.

130. **A** 8½ × 11; no. 10 envelope
RATIONALE: Standard letterhead (8½ in × 11 in) is used for general business and professional correspondence. Standard ways of folding and inserting letters are used so the letter fits properly and is easy to remove. A size #10 envelope is used for a standard-size letter.

131. **C** In a separate ledger file
RATIONALE: A ledger card is prepared for each patient (or family) at the time of the first visit. It is the record of all charges and payments for each patient. It is kept in a separate file for ease of access and billing purposes.

132. **A** The checkbook
RATIONALE: A bank statement is periodically sent by the bank to the customer. It shows the status of the account on a given date. The bank statement balance and the checkbook balance should be the same or they will need to be reconciled (disclosure of any errors in the checkbook or bank statement).

133. **D** Minutes
RATIONALE: The record of the proceedings of a meeting is called the minutes. The minutes contain a record of what was done at a meeting, not what was said by the members. Minutes should be signed by the secretary and kept on file according to the procedure of the organization.

134. **C** Backing up
RATIONALE: Backing up is the process of using a tape or floppy disk for storage of files to prevent their loss in the event of hard drive failure.

135. **C** Grouping
RATIONALE: Grouping or clustering allows the provider to use good use of time by seeing patients with the same needs at the same time. An example of grouping may be that the provider only performs complete physical exams on Wednesday mornings.

136. **A** Information on the type of practice
RATIONALE: Each office should have an attractive brochure which can be used to welcome new patients and to furnish general information about the practice. This can include name and type of practice, name(s) of physicians, address and location map, appointment procedures, office hours, comments on billing, charges, and insurance, and a statement concerning the confidentiality of medical records. Any more specific information should be discussed with the appropriate person.

137. **B** W-4 form
RATIONALE: The W-4 form is the Employee's Withholding Allowance Certificate. It is filled out by the employee and allows him/her to determine the number of withholding allowances.

138. **D** HGB
RATIONALE: The correct abbreviation for hemoglobin is Hgb.

139. **C** Invasion of privacy
RATIONALE: Invasion of privacy is the act of divulging patient information that has been acquired through privileged interaction (provider/patient communication) without the consent of the patient. This is an intentional tort. Information shared between the provider and patient is confidential. A release of information form must be signed before this information can be shared.

140. **A** Omission of all punctuation
RATIONALE: The U.S. Postal Service attempts to read, code, sort, and cancel all mail electroni-

cally. The success of this system depends on the correct format that can be read by the automatic equipment. This format includes: all addresses typed in block format in the correct area of the envelope, everything in the address capitalized, all punctuation eliminated, states abbreviated using the standard two-letter code, and ZIP code must be included in the last line.

141. **B** A subpoena

RATIONALE: A subpoena duces tecum is an order to provide records or documents to the court. Authority to release information from the medical record lies solely with the patient unless required by law.

142. **B** Daily log

RATIONALE: The double-entry system provides a comprehensive picture of the medical practice and its effect on the physician's net worth. It requires skill and time, and is not frequently used in a small practice. The medical assistant generally maintains only the daily log.

143. **B** Enclosure

RATIONALE: The enclosure notation identifies any material that may be accompanying the correspondence. The notation is placed two lines below the signature line. If there is more than one enclosure, specify the number (e.g., Enclosures 2).

144. **A** Insurance claim

RATIONALE: A superbill is a combination charge slip, statement, and insurance reporting form. It is completed and given to the patient at each visit.

145. **E** All of the above

RATIONALE: Complete and accurate records are essential to a well-managed medical practice. Health information management includes not only the assembling of the record, but also having an efficient system for saving, retrieving, protecting, transferring, storing, retaining, and destroying these records.

146. **B** ICD-9-CM

RATIONALE: ICD-9-CM (International Classification of Diseases, 9th Revision, Clinical Modification) is the coding system used to code diagnosis or disease conditions. CPT (Current Procedural Terminology), HCPCS (HCFA Common Procedural Coding System), RVS (Relative Value Scale), and RBRVS (Resource-based Relative Value System) are systems used to code medical procedures.

147. **C** Initials come after complete names

RATIONALE: Indexing rules are standardized and are based on current business practices. The rule that applies to initials states "that initials precede a name beginning with the same letter." For example, the chart for M. Johnson would be filed BEFORE the chart for Mary Johnson.

148. **E** V-codes

RATIONALE: V codes (V01 to V82) are the codes that refer to factors that influence the health status of the patient. A definite diagnosis cannot be stated, but there is a valid reason for seeing the provider (e.g., well-baby check, annual physical exam).

149. **B** Bit

RATIONALE: A bit is a binary digit. It is the smallest piece of information that can be processed by a computer.

150. **D** Directory

RATIONALE: The directory is the index of files on a disk. It shows the names of the documents that are saved on that disk. The operator can then choose a file and open it.

151. **E** B and C only

RATIONALE: The scheduling system chosen by the facility must be individualized for each specific practice. Important factors that determine the best system include patient need, physician preferences and habits, and the facilities available.

152. **B** Mixed punctuation

RATIONALE: Mixed (standard) punctuation is appropriate for use with block or modified block letter styles. It places a colon after the salutation, and a comma after the complimentary closing. It is the most commonly used punctuation pattern.

153. **C** Operating manuals

RATIONALE: An inventory of all capital items (equipment) should be prepared every year. For each item, the name, serial number, date of purchase, price, and any warranty information. Operating manuals should be kept separate and readily accessible.

154. **B** Operative notes

RATIONALE: Operative notes are considered to be part of the physician's records and can only be released by the physician. Nurse's notes, lab reports, radiology reports, and billing are hospital generated documents and belong to the institution.

155. **C** Pre-existing condition

RATIONALE: A pre-existing condition is a physical condition of a person that existed before the insurance policy was issued.

156. **D** Inactive files

RATIONALE: Inactive files generally are those of patients whom the provider has not seen for six months or longer. When the patient returns for care, their chart is replaced in the active file.

157. **A** Patient confidentiality
RATIONALE: The patient is entitled to complete confidentiality with regards to his/her medical records and release of information. Computer technology allows for the gathering and storage of vast amounts of information. This information can then be accessible to a variety of individuals. The monitor displays information, and should be positioned away from others that may be at the desk.

158. **E** All of the above
RATIONALE: All patients should be escorted to the exam or treatment room. All patients are generally more cooperative and less anxious if they understand what is expected of them.

159. **B** Name of the assisting physician
RATIONALE: Surgery is scheduled by type of procedure and availability of facilities. Important information includes the name of the procedure, expected length of the procedure in hours, type of anesthesia, patient's name, age, and telephone number.

160. **B** A copy of the letter is sent to Dr. Jones
RATIONALE: The copy notation ("c:") indicates that a copy of the document was sent to a third party or parties. The notation is placed one to two lines below the enclosure notation.

161. **A** Results of lab tests
RATIONALE: The history and physical are valuable tools in diagnosis. They are a way for the physician to gather information about the physical and psychological condition of the patient. The history is the record of the information provided by the patient. The physical involves a thorough examination of the patient from head to toe. Labs may be ordered after the physical if needed for diagnosis.

162. **B** Accept pre-determined fees
RATIONALE: Managed Care is a type of pre-paid health plan. It was developed to provide health care services at a low cost. Managed Care includes HMOs (Health Maintenance Organizations) and IPAs (Independent Practice Associations). The traditional HMO builds a group of physicians who agree to be paid on a per-patient basis instead of a fee-for-service basis.

163. **D** PPO
RATIONALE: The PPO (Preferred Provider Organization) uses a fee-for-service concept. Providers agree on a predetermined list of charges for all services. Care is not prepaid. There are deductibles that the patient must pay.

164. **A** Cost of services
RATIONALE: E & M (evaluation and management) codes include basic diagnostic and treatment services such as office visits and examinations. The type of history, the type of examination and the complexity of medical decision making must be determined in order to properly select the correct code.

165. **E** Deposit slip
RATIONALE: Deposit slips are itemized documents of cash, checks, and other funds that a depositor presents to the bank with the money to be credited to an account. All deposits must be accompanied by a deposit slip. A copy of the slip is kept on file.

166. **D** Patient's surname
RATIONALE: One system of color coding files is the alphabetic color coding system. This system uses different colored tabs to represent a different segment of the alphabet. The chart is coded by the patient's last name (surname).

167. **B** The patient
RATIONALE: The physician owns the medical record, but the patient owns the information contained in the chart. Any information concerning the contents of the chart requires consent from both the patient and the physician before it can be released.

168. **C** All patients
RATIONALE: Standard precautions apply to the handling of all potentially infectious body fluids and tissues. Health care workers should take nondiscriminatory precautions to protect themselves.

169. **E** B and C
RATIONALE: Gloves are considered to be a barrier precaution and should be used when contact with blood or other body fluids is anticipated.

170. **C** 98.6°F
RATIONALE: Normal adult oral temperature is between 97 to 99 degrees F.

171. **B** 14–20 breaths per minute
RATIONALE: Normal adult rate can be from 14 to 20 breaths per minute.

172. **E** B and C
RATIONALE: Temperature, pulse, respiration, and blood pressure are considered to be the vital signs. They are the measurements that indicate the state of general health of the patient.

173. **B** Usually higher in children than adults
RATIONALE: The normal pulse rate for a child is between 80 and 120 beats per minute. Normal values for an adult is 60 to 100 beats per minute.

174. **E** All of the above
RATIONALE: The pulse rate is decreased by conditions such as depression, chronic pain, CNS disorders, and hypothyroidism.

175. **D** 103–105°F
RATIONALE: Fever is a temperature over 100 de-

grees F. A high fever is over 103 degrees F. Untreated high fever can result in brain damage or death.

176. **A** The difference between the systolic and diastolic blood pressure
RATIONALE: The pulse pressure is the difference between the systolic and diastolic blood pressures. It reflects the volume of circulating blood. Less than 30 points or more than 50 points is considered normal.

177. **B** 99
RATIONALE: To convert kilograms to pounds, multiply the number of kilograms by 2.2. (45 kilograms times 2.2 = 99 pounds)

178. **A** 6 feet
RATIONALE: Height is measured in inches. Using the conversion factor of 12 inches = 1 foot, divide 72 inches by 12 inches. 72 divided by 12 is 6.

179. **A** Chest and back
RATIONALE: Percussion is the use of tapping or striking the body to elicit sounds. This is usually done with the fingers or small hammer. Percussion aids in the determination of the size, position, and density of the underlying organ or cavity.

180. **D** Social history
RATIONALE: The social history gives information regarding the patient's lifestyle, hobbies, education, occupation, sleeping habits, methods of exercise, sex life, and coping skills.

181. **D** All of the above
RATIONALE: Subjective findings (symptoms) are perceptible only to the patient, or known only to the patient.

182. **E** Clearness of vision
RATIONALE: Visual acuity using the Snellen chart is a common distance acuity screening test.

183. **C** Rectum
RATIONALE: Proctoscopy is the use of a scope to examine the rectum and the distal portion of the colon.

184. **B** left side and chest, with right leg flexed
RATIONALE: The Sims position is the position in which the patient lies on the left side with the right knee and thigh drawn up toward the chest. It is sometimes called the lateral position and can be used for rectal exams and some pelvic exams.

185. **D** Prone position
RATIONALE: The prone position is the position in which the patient is lying face down on the table.

186. **A** Ophthalmoscope
RATIONALE: The ophthalmoscope is an instrument used to inspect the inner structures of the eye. It has a handle containing batteries, and an attached head equipped with a light and magnifying lenses.

187. **B** Sitting
RATIONALE: In the sitting position, the patient is sitting upright on the examination table. This position is useful in the examination and treatments of the head, neck, and chest.

188. **A** Glucose and protein
RATIONALE: On all subsequent visits, a urine sample is obtained and tested for the presence of sugar (glucose) and albumin (protein). The presence of glucose could be a warning sign of a prediabetic state or diabetes. The presence of protein could be an early warning sign of toxemia. Both of these conditions would require careful medical supervision and treatment.

189. **A** One week after her period
RATIONALE: A monthly self-breast exam can detect early signs of breast cancer. The exam should be performed once a month about one week before the menstrual period since the breasts are usually not tender or swollen at that time.

190. **A** Acute
RATIONALE: Disease is a pathologic process that in some way alters the normal function, structure, or metabolism of an organism. An acute disease process or acute infection begins abruptly with sharp intensity and then subsides after a short period of time.

191. **C** 21–28 days
RATIONALE: Double-wrapped sterile packs are considered sterile up to 28 days from the date of sterilization. They should be stored in a clean, dry, dust-free place. When a pack expires, the contents must be reprocessed.

192. **E** Unwrap the pack, rewrap the pack, replace the indicator, resterilize
RATIONALE: A sterilization indicator shows that the proper combination of steam, time, and temperature has been achieved. It does not prove that the contents are sterile. Failure of an indicator to change color could indicate that there is an error in the sterilization technique. The pack should be redone in order to correct any problem that may have caused the improper sterilization.

193. **B** Sanitization
RATIONALE: Instruments and other items used in the office must be carefully cleaned before proceeding with disinfection or sterilization. This cleaning process is sanitization. It is used to re-

move microorganisms, blood, and debris that could interfere with the sterilization process.

194. **C** Acquired active
RATIONALE: Immunity is the body's resistance to pathogenic microorganisms. It is classified as either natural or acquired. Natural immunity is a genetic feature specific to a person's race, sex, and ability to respond. Acquired immunity means that the body has developed an ability to defend itself. Acquired immunity can be active or passive. Active immunity results when a person has been exposed to or has had the disease. Passive is gained from receiving immune substances, thus bypassing the body's immune system.

195. **B** Away from the body
RATIONALE: Unfolding the top flap away from the body avoids the necessity of reaching over the sterile field and causing contamination. It also helps to avoid touching a person or uniform.

196. **E** 8-0
RATIONALE: The size or gauge of most sutures is labeled in terms of 0s. 0 is the thickest, and the numbers of 0s decrease up to 10-0, which is the thinnest. (The more 0s, the thinner the material.)

197. **D** Forceps
RATIONALE: Forceps are instruments of varied sizes and shapes used for grasping, compressing, or holding tissues and/or objects. They are two-pronged instruments with either a spring handle or a ring handle with a ratchet closure.

198. **C** Iodine
RATIONALE: Betadine is an antiseptic solution often used to disinfect the skin before a minor surgical procedure. It contains iodine, and a patient allergic to iodine will have a reaction to the solution.

199. **E** Purulent
RATIONALE: When a dressing is changed, it and the wound must be inspected for the amount and character of drainage. Drainage that is described as purulent consists of or contains pus.

200. **A** 10-15 degrees
RATIONALE: The objective of an ID (intradermal) injection is to inject a minute amount of solution between the layers of the skin. The needle is inserted at a 10-15 degree angle in order to deliver the solution to the correct area. When given correctly, the injection produces a wheal on the skin surface.

201. **C** Sublingual
RATIONALE: A sublingual route of administration places the drug under the patient's tongue. It is then left to dissolve and be absorbed.

202. **B** 1½ inch, 21 gauge
RATIONALE: The main objective when administering an IM injection is to inject the medication into deep muscle tissue for gradual and optimal absorption. The longer length of the needle allows this to occur. The gauge allows for thicker medications to be injected easily.

203. **B** Diuretic
RATIONALE: A diuretic medication promotes the formation and excretion of urine. They can be prescribed to reduce the volume of extracellular fluid in the treatment of many disorders including hypertension, edema, and congestive heart failure.

204. **A** 0.5 ml
RATIONALE: Use the following formula:

$$\frac{\text{dosage ordered}}{\text{available strength}} \times \text{dosage form} = \text{dosage given}$$

$$\frac{250 \text{ mg}}{500 \text{ mg}} \times 1 \text{ ml} = 0.5 \text{ ml}$$

205. **B** Directly opposite the specimen
RATIONALE: A centrifuge is a piece of laboratory equipment used to separate specimens by using centrifugal force. When a specimen tube is placed in the centrifuge, it must be counterbalanced with a tube of similar design and weight for balance. An unbalanced load can cause the centrifuge to vibrate and ruin the specimen.

206. **A** Within ½ hour of collection
RATIONALE: The microscopic examination of urine consists of categorizing and counting cells, casts, crystals, and miscellaneous constituents of the sediment. Chemical and cellular components change rapidly in a urine sample if they are allowed to sit at room temperature. These changes can be avoided by refrigerating the specimen if the analysis cannot be performed within 30 minutes after collection.

207. **A** Anuria
RATIONALE: Normal volume of urine produced every 24 hours is about 750-2,000 ml with an average of 1,500 ml. Anuria is the complete suppression of urine formation by the kidney. It can be caused by renal obstruction or renal failure.

208. **E** 1.010 and 1.025
RATIONALE: Specific gravity is the weight of a substance compared with the weight of an equal volume of distilled water. In urinalysis, it is the rough measurement of the concentration of substances dissolved in urine. Most urine samples fall between 1.010 and 1.025. This reading indicates the ability of the kidney to concentrate the specimen, and is one of the first indications of kidney disease.

209. **D** All of the above
RATIONALE: A CBC is a complete blood count. It

is one of the most common laboratory tests ordered on blood. It gives a complete look at the blood components thus giving a wealth of information about a patient's condition. Tests performed in a CBC include RBC count, WBC count, hemoglobin and hematocrit, differential, platelet number estimation, and RBC morphology.

210. **A** From a skin puncture
RATIONALE: Capillary or peripheral blood is obtained by performing a skin puncture on the fingertip, earlobe, or great toe or heel of an infant. This method allows for a minimal amount of blood to be collected, but is sufficient for many lab tests.

211. **C** Gallbladder
RATIONALE: A cholecystogram is an x-ray of the gallbladder. It is made after the ingestion or injection of a radiopaque substance. The test is useful in the diagnosis of cholecystitis (inflammation of the gallbladder), cholelithiasis (gallstones), and tumors.

212. **A** Dilates blood vessels
RATIONALE: Thermotherapy (application of heat) produces local vasodilation and increases circulation. These results of heat application speed up the inflammatory process, promote local drainage, relaxes muscles, and relieves pain.

213. **A** P
RATIONALE: Electrocardiography is the procedure that records the electrical activity of the heart. The EKG (ECG) records a series of waves or deflections above or below a baseline. Each wave or deflection corresponds to a particular part of the cardiac cycle. The P wave reflects contraction of the atria.

214. **B** Sinoatrial node
RATIONALE: The sinoatrial node (SA node) is a specialized tissue found in the right atrial wall near the superior vena cava. It initiates each heartbeat and sets its pace (pacemaker).

215. **D** 12
RATIONALE: The standard EKG (ECG) consists of 12 separate leads or recordings of the electrical activity of the heart from different angles. Each lead must be marked or coded for the physician to know which angle has been recorded. The 12 leads include Lead I, II, and III (standard or bipolar leads), leads aVR, aVL, aVF (augmented leads), and leads V1, V2, V3, V4, V5, and V6 (chest or precordial leads).

216. **D** 25 mm/sec
RATIONALE: The paper used in an EKG machine is a specialized graph paper with internationally accepted increments for measuring the cardiac cycle. As the paper advances, the heat-sensitive stylus moves along the vertical line and intersects with a vertical line. The paper advances at a speed of 25 mm/sec.

217. **A** Silver nitrate
RATIONALE: Silver nitrate ($AgNO_3$) is a caustic solution that is used to promote the healing process after surgery. It is available in solution form or coated on an applicator stick.

218. **A** Prothrombin time (PT, protime)
RATIONALE: The drug Coumadin (warfarin sodium) is an anticoagulant and keeps the blood from clotting. The protime is a test for detecting coagulation deficits. A prolonged protime can indicate a deficiency in the normal blood clotting mechanism and can help monitor anticoagulation therapy.

219. **C** Catgut
RATIONALE: The purpose of sutures is to hold the edges of a wound together until healing can occur. Absorbable sutures, usually used on deeper tissues, do not have to be removed because they are absorbed or digested by body fluids and tissues during the healing process. An example of this type of suture material is surgical gut (catgut). Nonabsorbable sutures used on outer skin surfaces are removed after the wound is healed.

220. **B** 100
RATIONALE: The differential white blood cell count is a test that determines the percentage of each of the five different types of white blood cells in the blood. The procedure involves examining a specific area of a stained blood smear under the microscope. 100 cells are counted and classified, and a tally is kept.

221. **C** 30%
RATIONALE: Hemoglobin and hematocrit values are related. Each 1% hematocrit contains 0.34 gm of hemoglobin. The hematocrit should equal three times the hemoglobin within 3%.

222. **D** Sed rate: 30 mm/hr
RATIONALE: The normal value for a sedimentation rate is 0–20 mm/hr. An increased sed rate could indicate inflammation.

223. **A** Gram stain
RATIONALE: Because bacteria are small and possess little color, staining is necessary to observe them under the microscope. The Gram stain is used most often. The dyes in the stain are taken up differently in each type of bacterial cell, and they stain different colors. Bacteria are identified as Gram-negative (stain red) or Gram-positive (stain purple).

224. **B** Alkaline
RATIONALE: pH expresses the degree of acidity

or alkalinity of a solution. Usually, freshly voided urine is acidic. Upon sitting, bacteria contaminate the sample and cause it to become alkaline.

225. **D** Red-stoppered
RATIONALE: Blood collection tubes are color-coded depending on the additive it contains or does not contain. Red-stoppered tubes contain no additives so the blood collected in these tubes clot and serum can be removed.

226. **E** All of the above
RATIONALE: Surgical instruments have clearly identifiable parts and can easily be differentiated from one another. Instruments are classified according to their uses, and most belong to one of four main groups: cutting and dissecting, grasping and clamping, retractors, and probes and dilators.

227. **A** Assess victim's airway
RATIONALE: Check the victim for responsiveness. If unconscious, assess "ABCs": airway, breathing, and circulation.

228. **E** All of the above
RATIONALE: A complete urinalysis is composed of three parts: the physical exam that includes assessment of color, clarity, odor, amount, and specific gravity; the chemical exam that can include using a reagent strip to test for the presence of glucose, ketones, leukocytes, blood, nitrates, pH, urobilinogen, protein, and bilirubin; and the microscopic exam for cells, bacteria, casts, and artifacts.

229. **D** Liver
RATIONALE: After a drug is absorbed into the body and transported to the cells or tissues it is intended, it is again picked up by the blood stream and transported to the liver, the site of metabolism and/or biotransformation. There, the drug is broken down and prepared for elimination from the body.

230. **C** Tests for color-blindness
RATIONALE: Color-blindness is tested with use of Ishihara plates. The Ishihara color test uses a series of plates on which are printed round dots in a variety of colors and patterns. Patients with normal color vision are able to discern specific patterns on the plates. Patients with a deficiency in color perception cannot.

231. **E** Polyuria
RATIONALE: Signs and symptoms of a myocardial infarction (MI, heart attack) is an occlusion of a coronary artery that results in loss of blood flow and necrosis to the myocardium. The onset is characterized by crushing chest pain. The patient becomes ashen, clammy, short of breath, and nauseated.

232. **A** Forceps
RATIONALE: Hemostatic forceps are a type of clamping instrument. They are used to stop bleeding, clamp severed vessels, and hold tissue.

233. **E** 4 to 1
RATIONALE: A fairly constant ratio of four pulse beats to one respiration exists. As a general rule, both pulse and respiration rates normally respond to exercise or emotional upsets. Normal pulse rate for an adult is between 60 and 80 beats per minute. Normal respiratory rate for an adult is between 14 and 20 breaths per minute.

234. **E** All of the above
RATIONALE: Insulin shock is caused by too much insulin intake, decrease in food intake, or excessive exercise. It is characterized by sweating, trembling, chills, nervousness, irritability, hunger, hallucinations, and pallor. If uncorrected, it can progress to convulsions, coma, and death. Treatment requires an immediate dose of glucose.

235. **A** Kidneys
RATIONALE: The kidneys are the most important route for the excretion (elimination) of drugs from the body. Most drugs are filtered out of the circulation, broken down into harmless substances, and then excreted in the urine.

236. **C** Antidepressant
RATIONALE: Drugs can be classified according to their actions in the body. An antidepressant medication is used as a mood elevator, and is used to treat depression. Prozac (fluoxetine) is an example of an antidepressant.

237. **B** Friction and running water
RATIONALE: Hands must be washed, using the correct technique, before and after each patient is examined or treated. Proper handwashing depends on two factors: running water and friction. Friction is the firm rubbing of skin surfaces to loosen debris. Running water washes away the debris.

238. **D** Twelve months
RATIONALE: MMR is the vaccination for mumps, measles, and rubella. It is recommended that the first dose be given between 12 and 15 months of age. The second dose is recommended between ages 6 and 12 years.

239. **B** Migraine
RATIONALE: Migraine headaches are paroxysmal attacks of headaches that may be completely incapacitating. They are frequently characterized by nausea, vomiting, visual disturbances, throbbing pain in one side of the head, and an aura. An aura is some type of visual disturbance such as lines or spots across the visual field.

240. **D** To carry oxygen and carbon dioxide
RATIONALE: Hemoglobin, which is made up of iron and protein, is a main constituent of red blood cells. It carries oxygen to the cells from the lungs, and carbon dioxide away from the cells to the lungs for excretion. Normal hemoglobin values vary throughout life, and are affected by age, sex, diet, altitude, and disease.

241. **A** Ensures the accuracy of results
RATIONALE: Quality assurance is a major component of the CLIA '88 regulations relating to laboratory standards. It is a comprehensive set of policies and procedures developed to ensure the quality of laboratory testing. It includes quality control, personnel orientation, laboratory documentation, knowledge of instrumentation, and enrollment in a proficiency-testing program.

242. **B** 48–72 hours after it is administered
RATIONALE: The Mantoux test is used for routine screening and diagnosis of tuberculosis. The test uses a purified protein derivative (PPD) from a live tuberculin culture to test for antibodies. The results should be read 48–72 hours after the test is given by intradermal injection. Extent of induration is measured and recorded.

243. **C** AU
RATIONALE: The abbreviation for both ears is AU. It comes from the latin "auris unitas."

244. **D** O
RATIONALE: Patients with type O blood are considered to be universal donors. Type O blood contains no antigens on the red blood cells, so it will not agglutinate in the presence of anti-A and anti-B antibodies in the plasma.

245. **E** Colon
RATIONALE: A lower GI series (barium enema) is an x-ray examination of the colon. Contrast medium (barium) is instilled into the colon through an enema. The colon can then be visualized by x-ray.

246. **B** CT scan
RATIONALE: A CT scan (computed tomography) is a radiographic technique that produces a film that represents a detailed cross-section of a tissue structure. The technique uses a narrow beam of x-ray that rotates in a continuous 360-degree motion around the patient. The pictures obtained from this method are very detailed and simulate a three-dimensional appearance.

247. **A** Cancer
RATIONALE: Massive or excessive exposure to radiation can cause tissue damage and various side effects. This can include damage to blood cells, skin cells, eyes, and reproductive cells. Overexposure can result in decreased red and white blood cell counts, burns, and a higher incidence of cancers.

248. **B** Leads I, II, and III
RATIONALE: The first three leads recorded are the standard or bipolar leads (leads I, II, and III). They each use two limb electrodes to record electrical activity.

249. **B** Chains
RATIONALE: Bacteria may be classified by morphology (size and shape). Streptococci are bacteria that are spherical in shape and arranged in chains.

250. **D** Increasing age
RATIONALE: Normal pulse rates normally vary as a result of a person's sex, age, body size, posture, activity level, health status, nervous system function, emotional state, and the volume and composition of the blood. Pulse normally decreases with age.

251. **D** RL
RATIONALE: The leads of an EKG measure the electrical activity from the frontal and horizontal planes of the body. The right leg acts as the grounding as electrical activity is recorded from the right arm, left arm, and left leg.

252. **A** OSHA
RATIONALE: The Occupational Safety and Health Act was established by the federal government in 1970 to set standards and protocols for occupational health and safety. The regulations must be known and followed. They include hazard exposure plans, medical waste management, personal protective measures, general safety precautions, fire safety, staff development, and blood-bourne pathogen regulations.

253. **E** Cost
RATIONALE: A drug reference provides information about medications. Most references include the following information about the medication: action, indication, side effects, adverse effects, precautions, contraindications, dosage, and administration. These references include the PDR, package inserts, US Pharmacopeia/National Formulary, and other published references.

254. **E** All of the above
RATIONALE: An analgesic medication lessens the sensory function of the brain. They are used for pain relief. Analgesics can be classified as narcotic (morphine, codeine, Demerol) or nonnarcotic (aspirin, Tylenol, ibuprofen).

255. **C** Keep a written recording of all daily activities
RATIONALE: A Holter monitor is a portable monitoring system used to record the cardiac activity of the patient for a 24-hour period. It is important for the patient to keep a written diary of all

activities during the day that causes stress. Examples include driving in traffic, stair climbing, and bowel movements. Symptoms associated with possible heart problems should also be included.

256. **D** Peristalsis
RATIONALE: Peristalsis is the involuntary wave-like movement that moves food downward through the gastrointestinal tract. Peristalsis is activated when the food mass is swallowed and enters the esophagus.

257. **A** Two months
RATIONALE: The schedule for childhood immunizations begins with the first doses of DTP (DtaP), IPV, HIB, and HepB being administered at age 2 months.

258. **D** Connects bone to bone
RATIONALE: Ligaments are strong fibrous connective tissues that connect bone to bone at the joint and enclose the joint capsule.

259. **C** Histology
RATIONALE: Histology involves the preparation and study of specimens of tissue from any source in the body. Changes in the tissue form and/or structure are observed microscopically.

260. **C** A nonsterile person entering the room
RATIONALE: Surgical asepsis, or sterile technique, is the practice used when an area and supplies in that area are to be made and kept sterile. The goal of surgical asepsis is to prevent the introduction of microorganisms into the body. Talking over the sterile field can introduce microorganisms onto it. Hair that is not pulled back or inside a cap could also introduce microorganisms. Moisture contaminates the sterile field. A one-inch edge around the entire sterile field is considered not sterile.

261. **C** Benadryl
RATIONALE: An antihistamine drug counteracts the effects of histamine by blocking the action in the tissues. Antihistamines are used for relief of allergies. An example of an antihistamine is diphenhydramine (Benadryl).

262. **D** qod—every day
RATIONALE: The abbreviation "qod" means "every other day." The abbreviation "qd" means "every day."

263. **D** Needle biopsy
RATIONALE: Surgical asepsis is defined as the destruction of organisms before they enter the body. The technique is used for any procedure that punctures, pierces, or incises the skin or mucous membranes. Everything that comes in contact with the patient should be sterile, including instruments, drapes, and gloved hands. A needle

biopsy is a procedure that breaks the skin and thus requires surgical asepsis.

264. **A** Daily
RATIONALE: Quality control is the operational procedure used to implement the quality assurance program. The objective of quality control is to assure accuracy of test results while detecting errors. It is mandated by law. Specially prepared quality control samples are tested daily. The results of these samples must be within a pre-established range before patient results can be reported.

265. **A** Afferent
RATIONALE: Afferent or sensory nerves transmit sensory information toward the brain. The impulses are interpreted in the brain, and transmitted away from the brain to an organ or body part by an efferent nerve.

266. **B** Sudoriferous glands
RATIONALE: Another name for a sweat gland is a sudoriferous gland. Sudoriferous glands are coiled, tube-like structures found in the dermis. They produce sweat and transport it to the surface of the skin. As it evaporates, it cools the body.

267. **B** Impetigo
RATIONALE: Impetigo is a highly infectious bacterial infection of the skin. It is caused by staphylococcus or streptococcus. It is characterized by vesicles that rupture and form a honey-colored crust. Lesions form primarily on the face, especially around the mouth and nose. Impetigo is treated with antibiotic ointment. Handwashing can help prevent its spread.

268. **C** Osteoporosis
RATIONALE: Osteoporosis is a disorder of the skeletal system characterized by porous, brittle bones. These bones then become susceptible to fractures. Osteoporosis occurs most frequently in postmenopausal women. It is treated with calcium supplements, hormone replacement therapy (estrogen), exercise, and medications.

269. **A** Cerebrum
RATIONALE: The cerebrum is the largest superior portion of the brain. It is divided into two hemispheres (halves). The hemispheres are further divided into lobes which are named for the skull bone that covers it.

270. **D** Presbyopia
RATIONALE: Presbyopia is a disorder of accommodation. It is due to the loss of elasticity of the lens of the eye due to aging. It can be corrected with bifocals or trifocals.

271. **A** Otitis media
RATIONALE: Otitis media is an inflammation/in-

fection of the middle ear. Fluid collects behind the tympanic membrane. Otitis media is often associated with an upper respiratory infection. The patient will experience pain and fever. The canal and eardrum will appear red and swollen. There may be a purulent discharge. It is treated with antibiotics and analgesics.

272. **A** Tricuspid

RATIONALE: The tricuspid valve is located between the right atrium and the right ventricle. It is made up of three flaps of tissue. It prevents the blood from flowing back into the atrium when the ventricle contracts.

273. **C** Pertussis

RATIONALE: Pertussis is a bacterial infection of the lung. It is caused by the *Bordetella pertussis* bacterium. It is characterized by a barking (whooping) cough. Pertussis can be prevented by immunization (DTP, DtaP).

274. **D** Mediastinum

RATIONALE: The mediastinum is the portion of the thoracic cavity in the middle of the chest. It extends from the sternum to vertebral column. It contains the heart, great vessels, esophagus, and trachea.

275. **A** Rhinitis

RATIONALE: Rhinitis is the inflammation of the mucous membranes of the nose, usually accompanied by swelling of the mucosa and nasal discharge It is also called coryza. *Rhin-* means nose; *-itis* means inflammation of.

276. **D** Parkinson's disease

RATIONALE: Parkinson's disease is a slowly progressive degenerative neurological disorder. It is characterized by tremors, pill rolling of the fingers, shuffling gait, and muscle rigidity and weakness. It is an idiopathic disease of patients over the age of 60.

277. **D** Gallbladder

RATIONALE: The gallbladder is a pear-shaped sac located on the inferior surface of the liver. It can store up to 50 ml of bile and concentrates it. The gallbladder releases bile into the duodenum where it helps in fat metabolism.

278. **A** Urination

RATIONALE: A main function of the urinary system is to eliminate liquid nitrogen-containing waste products from the body. This is accomplished through the formation of urine and the process of urination or micturition.

279. **C** Exacerbation

RATIONALE: Exacerbation is an increase in the seriousness of a disease. It is indicated by a greater intensity in the signs or symptoms.

280. **B** Multipara

RATIONALE: Multipara describes a female patient who has had two or more pregnancies. Parity refers to the number of live births or still births the patient has delivered after 28 weeks' gestation.

281. **A** Ovulation

RATIONALE: Ovulation is the spontaneous expulsion of an ovum (egg) from the ovary when the follicle ruptures. This happens on approximately the fourteenth day of the menstrual cycle. Ovulation is regulated by the female sex hormone estrogen.

282. **D** Vasectomy

RATIONALE: Vasectomy is a procedure for male sterilization. The procedure involves the bilateral surgical removal of a portion of the vas deferens to stop sperm from reaching the prostate the mixing with the semen. Sexual potency is not affected by the procedure.

283. **E** All of the above

RATIONALE: Pathogens are microorganisms that are capable of causing disease. Microorganisms are almost every place. They can be transmitted by either direct transmission (contact with an infected person or infected discharges) or indirect transmission (air droplets, insects, contaminated food or drink, contaminated objects).

284. **E** Iris

RATIONALE: The iris the pigmented (colored) part of the eye. It is made up of muscle fibers that dilate and constrict. This dilation and constriction causes the pupil (opening in the eye) to increase or decrease in order to control the amount of light entering the eye.

285. **B** Pinna

RATIONALE: The pinna is also known as the auricle. It is the portion of the ear that is attached to the head. The malleus, incus, and stapes are the ossicles or bones of the middle ear.

286. **B** Osteo-

RATIONALE: *Osteo-* is the combining form for bone. *Arthro-* is the combining form for joint, *uro-* is the combining form for urine, *onco-* is the combining form for cancer, and *adeno-* is the combining form for gland.

287. **E** Bradycardia

RATIONALE: Bradycardia is a slow heartbeat characterized by a pulse rate of less than 60 beats per minute. *Brady-* means slow; *-cardia* means heart.

288. **B** Apnea

RATIONALE: Apnea is an abnormal breathing pattern characterized by an absence of spontaneous respiration. *A-* means absence of, without. *-Pnea* means breathing.

289. **A** Hemothorax
RATIONALE: A hemothorax is an accumulation of blood and fluid in the pleural cavity. It is usually the result of trauma, but could also be caused from pneumonia, tuberculosis, or tumors.

290. **A** Sigmoidoscopy
RATIONALE: A sigmoidoscopy is the procedure performed to visualize, through a lighted scope, the mucous membrane lining of the rectum and sigmoid colon. It may be performed to confirm a diagnosis, or to obtain a specimen.

291. **A** Uvula
RATIONALE: The uvula is the fingerlike projection of the soft palate.

292. **C** Lip
RATIONALE: *Labio-* is the combining form meaning lip or lips.

293. **D** Urinary bladder
RATIONALE: The urinary bladder is a flexible muscular sac located posterior to the pubic symphysis in the pelvis. It functions to temporarily store urine until it is excreted from the body.

294. **B** Hormone
RATIONALE: A hormone is a chemical substance release directly into the bloodstream from an endocrine gland. The function of hormones on the body is to stimulate body cells, glands, or other hormones to function.

295. **A** Corpus luteum
RATIONALE: The corpus luteum is a structure left on the surface of the ovary after ovulation has occurred. It secretes progesterone which causes the uterine lining to thicken and further prepare for the implantation of the fertilized ovum.

296. **B** Perineum
RATIONALE: The perineum is the area between the vaginal opening and the rectum. It supports and surrounds the distal portions of the urogenital and gastrointestinal tracts of the body.

297. **A** Scapula
RATIONALE: The axial skeleton consists of the bones that form the skull (cranial bones), spine (vertebrae), and chest (ribs and sternum). The appendicular skeleton is made up of the bones of the extremities and pelvis.

298. **B** Superficial
RATIONALE: Superficial refers to anything close to a surface. A superficial wound would be close to the surface of the skin, and not serious.

299. **C** Myringotomy
RATIONALE: A myringotomy is a surgical incision into the eardrum. It is performed to relieve pressure and release fluid or pus from behind the eardrum.

300. **A** Fever
RATIONALE: An antipyretic agent reduces fever. These drugs work on the thermoregulation center in the hypothalamus. Examples of these drugs include aspirin and acetaminophen.

Pre-Test Answer Sheet

Name _____   **Date** _____

　　　　　Last　　　　　　　　　　First　　　　　　　　Middle

Directions　• Using a No. 2 pencil, fill in the circle that best represents the correct answer for each question.
　　　　　　　• Make sure you erase completely any answer you wish to change.
　　　　　　　• Do not make any stray marks on this answer sheet.
　　　　　　　• Mark only one answer for each question.

Correct　　　　　　　　　Incorrect
Ⓐ Ⓑ Ⓒ ● Ⓔ　　　　　Ⓐ Ⓑ Ⓒ Ⓓ Ⓔ

1	Ⓐ Ⓑ Ⓒ Ⓓ Ⓔ	32	Ⓐ Ⓑ Ⓒ Ⓓ Ⓔ	63	Ⓐ Ⓑ Ⓒ Ⓓ Ⓔ	94 Ⓐ Ⓑ Ⓒ Ⓓ Ⓔ
2	Ⓐ Ⓑ Ⓒ Ⓓ Ⓔ	33	Ⓐ Ⓑ Ⓒ Ⓓ Ⓔ	64	Ⓐ Ⓑ Ⓒ Ⓓ Ⓔ	95 Ⓐ Ⓑ Ⓒ Ⓓ Ⓔ
3	Ⓐ Ⓑ Ⓒ Ⓓ Ⓔ	34	Ⓐ Ⓑ Ⓒ Ⓓ Ⓔ	65	Ⓐ Ⓑ Ⓒ Ⓓ Ⓔ	96 Ⓐ Ⓑ Ⓒ Ⓓ Ⓔ
4	Ⓐ Ⓑ Ⓒ Ⓓ Ⓔ	35	Ⓐ Ⓑ Ⓒ Ⓓ Ⓔ	66	Ⓐ Ⓑ Ⓒ Ⓓ Ⓔ	97 Ⓐ Ⓑ Ⓒ Ⓓ Ⓔ
5	Ⓐ Ⓑ Ⓒ Ⓓ Ⓔ	36	Ⓐ Ⓑ Ⓒ Ⓓ Ⓔ	67	Ⓐ Ⓑ Ⓒ Ⓓ Ⓔ	98 Ⓐ Ⓑ Ⓒ Ⓓ Ⓔ
6	Ⓐ Ⓑ Ⓒ Ⓓ Ⓔ	37	Ⓐ Ⓑ Ⓒ Ⓓ Ⓔ	68	Ⓐ Ⓑ Ⓒ Ⓓ Ⓔ	99 Ⓐ Ⓑ Ⓒ Ⓓ Ⓔ
7	Ⓐ Ⓑ Ⓒ Ⓓ Ⓔ	38	Ⓐ Ⓑ Ⓒ Ⓓ Ⓔ	69	Ⓐ Ⓑ Ⓒ Ⓓ Ⓔ	100 Ⓐ Ⓑ Ⓒ Ⓓ Ⓔ
8	Ⓐ Ⓑ Ⓒ Ⓓ Ⓔ	39	Ⓐ Ⓑ Ⓒ Ⓓ Ⓔ	70	Ⓐ Ⓑ Ⓒ Ⓓ Ⓔ	101 Ⓐ Ⓑ Ⓒ Ⓓ Ⓔ
9	Ⓐ Ⓑ Ⓒ Ⓓ Ⓔ	40	Ⓐ Ⓑ Ⓒ Ⓓ Ⓔ	71	Ⓐ Ⓑ Ⓒ Ⓓ Ⓔ	102 Ⓐ Ⓑ Ⓒ Ⓓ Ⓔ
10	Ⓐ Ⓑ Ⓒ Ⓓ Ⓔ	41	Ⓐ Ⓑ Ⓒ Ⓓ Ⓔ	72	Ⓐ Ⓑ Ⓒ Ⓓ Ⓔ	103 Ⓐ Ⓑ Ⓒ Ⓓ Ⓔ
11	Ⓐ Ⓑ Ⓒ Ⓓ Ⓔ	42	Ⓐ Ⓑ Ⓒ Ⓓ Ⓔ	73	Ⓐ Ⓑ Ⓒ Ⓓ Ⓔ	104 Ⓐ Ⓑ Ⓒ Ⓓ Ⓔ
12	Ⓐ Ⓑ Ⓒ Ⓓ Ⓔ	43	Ⓐ Ⓑ Ⓒ Ⓓ Ⓔ	74	Ⓐ Ⓑ Ⓒ Ⓓ Ⓔ	105 Ⓐ Ⓑ Ⓒ Ⓓ Ⓔ
13	Ⓐ Ⓑ Ⓒ Ⓓ Ⓔ	44	Ⓐ Ⓑ Ⓒ Ⓓ Ⓔ	75	Ⓐ Ⓑ Ⓒ Ⓓ Ⓔ	106 Ⓐ Ⓑ Ⓒ Ⓓ Ⓔ
14	Ⓐ Ⓑ Ⓒ Ⓓ Ⓔ	45	Ⓐ Ⓑ Ⓒ Ⓓ Ⓔ	76	Ⓐ Ⓑ Ⓒ Ⓓ Ⓔ	107 Ⓐ Ⓑ Ⓒ Ⓓ Ⓔ
15	Ⓐ Ⓑ Ⓒ Ⓓ Ⓔ	46	Ⓐ Ⓑ Ⓒ Ⓓ Ⓔ	77	Ⓐ Ⓑ Ⓒ Ⓓ Ⓔ	108 Ⓐ Ⓑ Ⓒ Ⓓ Ⓔ
16	Ⓐ Ⓑ Ⓒ Ⓓ Ⓔ	47	Ⓐ Ⓑ Ⓒ Ⓓ Ⓔ	78	Ⓐ Ⓑ Ⓒ Ⓓ Ⓔ	109 Ⓐ Ⓑ Ⓒ Ⓓ Ⓔ
17	Ⓐ Ⓑ Ⓒ Ⓓ Ⓔ	48	Ⓐ Ⓑ Ⓒ Ⓓ Ⓔ	79	Ⓐ Ⓑ Ⓒ Ⓓ Ⓔ	110 Ⓐ Ⓑ Ⓒ Ⓓ Ⓔ
18	Ⓐ Ⓑ Ⓒ Ⓓ Ⓔ	49	Ⓐ Ⓑ Ⓒ Ⓓ Ⓔ	80	Ⓐ Ⓑ Ⓒ Ⓓ Ⓔ	111 Ⓐ Ⓑ Ⓒ Ⓓ Ⓔ
19	Ⓐ Ⓑ Ⓒ Ⓓ Ⓔ	50	Ⓐ Ⓑ Ⓒ Ⓓ Ⓔ	81	Ⓐ Ⓑ Ⓒ Ⓓ Ⓔ	112 Ⓐ Ⓑ Ⓒ Ⓓ Ⓔ
20	Ⓐ Ⓑ Ⓒ Ⓓ Ⓔ	51	Ⓐ Ⓑ Ⓒ Ⓓ Ⓔ	82	Ⓐ Ⓑ Ⓒ Ⓓ Ⓔ	113 Ⓐ Ⓑ Ⓒ Ⓓ Ⓔ
21	Ⓐ Ⓑ Ⓒ Ⓓ Ⓔ	52	Ⓐ Ⓑ Ⓒ Ⓓ Ⓔ	83	Ⓐ Ⓑ Ⓒ Ⓓ Ⓔ	114 Ⓐ Ⓑ Ⓒ Ⓓ Ⓔ
22	Ⓐ Ⓑ Ⓒ Ⓓ Ⓔ	53	Ⓐ Ⓑ Ⓒ Ⓓ Ⓔ	84	Ⓐ Ⓑ Ⓒ Ⓓ Ⓔ	115 Ⓐ Ⓑ Ⓒ Ⓓ Ⓔ
23	Ⓐ Ⓑ Ⓒ Ⓓ Ⓔ	54	Ⓐ Ⓑ Ⓒ Ⓓ Ⓔ	85	Ⓐ Ⓑ Ⓒ Ⓓ Ⓔ	116 Ⓐ Ⓑ Ⓒ Ⓓ Ⓔ
24	Ⓐ Ⓑ Ⓒ Ⓓ Ⓔ	55	Ⓐ Ⓑ Ⓒ Ⓓ Ⓔ	86	Ⓐ Ⓑ Ⓒ Ⓓ Ⓔ	117 Ⓐ Ⓑ Ⓒ Ⓓ Ⓔ
25	Ⓐ Ⓑ Ⓒ Ⓓ Ⓔ	56	Ⓐ Ⓑ Ⓒ Ⓓ Ⓔ	87	Ⓐ Ⓑ Ⓒ Ⓓ Ⓔ	118 Ⓐ Ⓑ Ⓒ Ⓓ Ⓔ
26	Ⓐ Ⓑ Ⓒ Ⓓ Ⓔ	57	Ⓐ Ⓑ Ⓒ Ⓓ Ⓔ	88	Ⓐ Ⓑ Ⓒ Ⓓ Ⓔ	119 Ⓐ Ⓑ Ⓒ Ⓓ Ⓔ
27	Ⓐ Ⓑ Ⓒ Ⓓ Ⓔ	58	Ⓐ Ⓑ Ⓒ Ⓓ Ⓔ	89	Ⓐ Ⓑ Ⓒ Ⓓ Ⓔ	120 Ⓐ Ⓑ Ⓒ Ⓓ Ⓔ
28	Ⓐ Ⓑ Ⓒ Ⓓ Ⓔ	59	Ⓐ Ⓑ Ⓒ Ⓓ Ⓔ	90	Ⓐ Ⓑ Ⓒ Ⓓ Ⓔ	121 Ⓐ Ⓑ Ⓒ Ⓓ Ⓔ
29	Ⓐ Ⓑ Ⓒ Ⓓ Ⓔ	60	Ⓐ Ⓑ Ⓒ Ⓓ Ⓔ	91	Ⓐ Ⓑ Ⓒ Ⓓ Ⓔ	122 Ⓐ Ⓑ Ⓒ Ⓓ Ⓔ
30	Ⓐ Ⓑ Ⓒ Ⓓ Ⓔ	61	Ⓐ Ⓑ Ⓒ Ⓓ Ⓔ	92	Ⓐ Ⓑ Ⓒ Ⓓ Ⓔ	123 Ⓐ Ⓑ Ⓒ Ⓓ Ⓔ
31	Ⓐ Ⓑ Ⓒ Ⓓ Ⓔ	62	Ⓐ Ⓑ Ⓒ Ⓓ Ⓔ	93	Ⓐ Ⓑ Ⓒ Ⓓ Ⓔ	124 Ⓐ Ⓑ Ⓒ Ⓓ Ⓔ

125	Ⓐ Ⓑ Ⓒ Ⓓ Ⓔ		169	Ⓐ Ⓑ Ⓒ Ⓓ Ⓔ		213	Ⓐ Ⓑ Ⓒ Ⓓ Ⓔ		257	Ⓐ Ⓑ Ⓒ Ⓓ Ⓔ
126	Ⓐ Ⓑ Ⓒ Ⓓ Ⓔ		170	Ⓐ Ⓑ Ⓒ Ⓓ Ⓔ		214	Ⓐ Ⓑ Ⓒ Ⓓ Ⓔ		258	Ⓐ Ⓑ Ⓒ Ⓓ Ⓔ
127	Ⓐ Ⓑ Ⓒ Ⓓ Ⓔ		171	Ⓐ Ⓑ Ⓒ Ⓓ Ⓔ		215	Ⓐ Ⓑ Ⓒ Ⓓ Ⓔ		259	Ⓐ Ⓑ Ⓒ Ⓓ Ⓔ
128	Ⓐ Ⓑ Ⓒ Ⓓ Ⓔ		172	Ⓐ Ⓑ Ⓒ Ⓓ Ⓔ		216	Ⓐ Ⓑ Ⓒ Ⓓ Ⓔ		260	Ⓐ Ⓑ Ⓒ Ⓓ Ⓔ
129	Ⓐ Ⓑ Ⓒ Ⓓ Ⓔ		173	Ⓐ Ⓑ Ⓒ Ⓓ Ⓔ		217	Ⓐ Ⓑ Ⓒ Ⓓ Ⓔ		261	Ⓐ Ⓑ Ⓒ Ⓓ Ⓔ
130	Ⓐ Ⓑ Ⓒ Ⓓ Ⓔ		174	Ⓐ Ⓑ Ⓒ Ⓓ Ⓔ		218	Ⓐ Ⓑ Ⓒ Ⓓ Ⓔ		262	Ⓐ Ⓑ Ⓒ Ⓓ Ⓔ
131	Ⓐ Ⓑ Ⓒ Ⓓ Ⓔ		175	Ⓐ Ⓑ Ⓒ Ⓓ Ⓔ		219	Ⓐ Ⓑ Ⓒ Ⓓ Ⓔ		263	Ⓐ Ⓑ Ⓒ Ⓓ Ⓔ
132	Ⓐ Ⓑ Ⓒ Ⓓ Ⓔ		176	Ⓐ Ⓑ Ⓒ Ⓓ Ⓔ		220	Ⓐ Ⓑ Ⓒ Ⓓ Ⓔ		264	Ⓐ Ⓑ Ⓒ Ⓓ Ⓔ
133	Ⓐ Ⓑ Ⓒ Ⓓ Ⓔ		177	Ⓐ Ⓑ Ⓒ Ⓓ Ⓔ		221	Ⓐ Ⓑ Ⓒ Ⓓ Ⓔ		265	Ⓐ Ⓑ Ⓒ Ⓓ Ⓔ
134	Ⓐ Ⓑ Ⓒ Ⓓ Ⓔ		178	Ⓐ Ⓑ Ⓒ Ⓓ Ⓔ		222	Ⓐ Ⓑ Ⓒ Ⓓ Ⓔ		266	Ⓐ Ⓑ Ⓒ Ⓓ Ⓔ
135	Ⓐ Ⓑ Ⓒ Ⓓ Ⓔ		179	Ⓐ Ⓑ Ⓒ Ⓓ Ⓔ		223	Ⓐ Ⓑ Ⓒ Ⓓ Ⓔ		267	Ⓐ Ⓑ Ⓒ Ⓓ Ⓔ
136	Ⓐ Ⓑ Ⓒ Ⓓ Ⓔ		180	Ⓐ Ⓑ Ⓒ Ⓓ Ⓔ		224	Ⓐ Ⓑ Ⓒ Ⓓ Ⓔ		268	Ⓐ Ⓑ Ⓒ Ⓓ Ⓔ
137	Ⓐ Ⓑ Ⓒ Ⓓ Ⓔ		181	Ⓐ Ⓑ Ⓒ Ⓓ Ⓔ		225	Ⓐ Ⓑ Ⓒ Ⓓ Ⓔ		269	Ⓐ Ⓑ Ⓒ Ⓓ Ⓔ
138	Ⓐ Ⓑ Ⓒ Ⓓ Ⓔ		182	Ⓐ Ⓑ Ⓒ Ⓓ Ⓔ		226	Ⓐ Ⓑ Ⓒ Ⓓ Ⓔ		270	Ⓐ Ⓑ Ⓒ Ⓓ Ⓔ
139	Ⓐ Ⓑ Ⓒ Ⓓ Ⓔ		183	Ⓐ Ⓑ Ⓒ Ⓓ Ⓔ		227	Ⓐ Ⓑ Ⓒ Ⓓ Ⓔ		271	Ⓐ Ⓑ Ⓒ Ⓓ Ⓔ
140	Ⓐ Ⓑ Ⓒ Ⓓ Ⓔ		184	Ⓐ Ⓑ Ⓒ Ⓓ Ⓔ		228	Ⓐ Ⓑ Ⓒ Ⓓ Ⓔ		272	Ⓐ Ⓑ Ⓒ Ⓓ Ⓔ
141	Ⓐ Ⓑ Ⓒ Ⓓ Ⓔ		185	Ⓐ Ⓑ Ⓒ Ⓓ Ⓔ		229	Ⓐ Ⓑ Ⓒ Ⓓ Ⓔ		273	Ⓐ Ⓑ Ⓒ Ⓓ Ⓔ
142	Ⓐ Ⓑ Ⓒ Ⓓ Ⓔ		186	Ⓐ Ⓑ Ⓒ Ⓓ Ⓔ		230	Ⓐ Ⓑ Ⓒ Ⓓ Ⓔ		274	Ⓐ Ⓑ Ⓒ Ⓓ Ⓔ
143	Ⓐ Ⓑ Ⓒ Ⓓ Ⓔ		187	Ⓐ Ⓑ Ⓒ Ⓓ Ⓔ		231	Ⓐ Ⓑ Ⓒ Ⓓ Ⓔ		275	Ⓐ Ⓑ Ⓒ Ⓓ Ⓔ
144	Ⓐ Ⓑ Ⓒ Ⓓ Ⓔ		188	Ⓐ Ⓑ Ⓒ Ⓓ Ⓔ		232	Ⓐ Ⓑ Ⓒ Ⓓ Ⓔ		276	Ⓐ Ⓑ Ⓒ Ⓓ Ⓔ
145	Ⓐ Ⓑ Ⓒ Ⓓ Ⓔ		189	Ⓐ Ⓑ Ⓒ Ⓓ Ⓔ		233	Ⓐ Ⓑ Ⓒ Ⓓ Ⓔ		277	Ⓐ Ⓑ Ⓒ Ⓓ Ⓔ
146	Ⓐ Ⓑ Ⓒ Ⓓ Ⓔ		190	Ⓐ Ⓑ Ⓒ Ⓓ Ⓔ		234	Ⓐ Ⓑ Ⓒ Ⓓ Ⓔ		278	Ⓐ Ⓑ Ⓒ Ⓓ Ⓔ
147	Ⓐ Ⓑ Ⓒ Ⓓ Ⓔ		191	Ⓐ Ⓑ Ⓒ Ⓓ Ⓔ		235	Ⓐ Ⓑ Ⓒ Ⓓ Ⓔ		279	Ⓐ Ⓑ Ⓒ Ⓓ Ⓔ
148	Ⓐ Ⓑ Ⓒ Ⓓ Ⓔ		192	Ⓐ Ⓑ Ⓒ Ⓓ Ⓔ		236	Ⓐ Ⓑ Ⓒ Ⓓ Ⓔ		280	Ⓐ Ⓑ Ⓒ Ⓓ Ⓔ
149	Ⓐ Ⓑ Ⓒ Ⓓ Ⓔ		193	Ⓐ Ⓑ Ⓒ Ⓓ Ⓔ		237	Ⓐ Ⓑ Ⓒ Ⓓ Ⓔ		281	Ⓐ Ⓑ Ⓒ Ⓓ Ⓔ
150	Ⓐ Ⓑ Ⓒ Ⓓ Ⓔ		194	Ⓐ Ⓑ Ⓒ Ⓓ Ⓔ		238	Ⓐ Ⓑ Ⓒ Ⓓ Ⓔ		282	Ⓐ Ⓑ Ⓒ Ⓓ Ⓔ
151	Ⓐ Ⓑ Ⓒ Ⓓ Ⓔ		195	Ⓐ Ⓑ Ⓒ Ⓓ Ⓔ		239	Ⓐ Ⓑ Ⓒ Ⓓ Ⓔ		283	Ⓐ Ⓑ Ⓒ Ⓓ Ⓔ
152	Ⓐ Ⓑ Ⓒ Ⓓ Ⓔ		196	Ⓐ Ⓑ Ⓒ Ⓓ Ⓔ		240	Ⓐ Ⓑ Ⓒ Ⓓ Ⓔ		284	Ⓐ Ⓑ Ⓒ Ⓓ Ⓔ
153	Ⓐ Ⓑ Ⓒ Ⓓ Ⓔ		197	Ⓐ Ⓑ Ⓒ Ⓓ Ⓔ		241	Ⓐ Ⓑ Ⓒ Ⓓ Ⓔ		285	Ⓐ Ⓑ Ⓒ Ⓓ Ⓔ
154	Ⓐ Ⓑ Ⓒ Ⓓ Ⓔ		198	Ⓐ Ⓑ Ⓒ Ⓓ Ⓔ		242	Ⓐ Ⓑ Ⓒ Ⓓ Ⓔ		286	Ⓐ Ⓑ Ⓒ Ⓓ Ⓔ
155	Ⓐ Ⓑ Ⓒ Ⓓ Ⓔ		199	Ⓐ Ⓑ Ⓒ Ⓓ Ⓔ		243	Ⓐ Ⓑ Ⓒ Ⓓ Ⓔ		287	Ⓐ Ⓑ Ⓒ Ⓓ Ⓔ
156	Ⓐ Ⓑ Ⓒ Ⓓ Ⓔ		200	Ⓐ Ⓑ Ⓒ Ⓓ Ⓔ		244	Ⓐ Ⓑ Ⓒ Ⓓ Ⓔ		288	Ⓐ Ⓑ Ⓒ Ⓓ Ⓔ
157	Ⓐ Ⓑ Ⓒ Ⓓ Ⓔ		201	Ⓐ Ⓑ Ⓒ Ⓓ Ⓔ		245	Ⓐ Ⓑ Ⓒ Ⓓ Ⓔ		289	Ⓐ Ⓑ Ⓒ Ⓓ Ⓔ
158	Ⓐ Ⓑ Ⓒ Ⓓ Ⓔ		202	Ⓐ Ⓑ Ⓒ Ⓓ Ⓔ		246	Ⓐ Ⓑ Ⓒ Ⓓ Ⓔ		290	Ⓐ Ⓑ Ⓒ Ⓓ Ⓔ
159	Ⓐ Ⓑ Ⓒ Ⓓ Ⓔ		203	Ⓐ Ⓑ Ⓒ Ⓓ Ⓔ		247	Ⓐ Ⓑ Ⓒ Ⓓ Ⓔ		291	Ⓐ Ⓑ Ⓒ Ⓓ Ⓔ
160	Ⓐ Ⓑ Ⓒ Ⓓ Ⓔ		204	Ⓐ Ⓑ Ⓒ Ⓓ Ⓔ		248	Ⓐ Ⓑ Ⓒ Ⓓ Ⓔ		292	Ⓐ Ⓑ Ⓒ Ⓓ Ⓔ
161	Ⓐ Ⓑ Ⓒ Ⓓ Ⓔ		205	Ⓐ Ⓑ Ⓒ Ⓓ Ⓔ		249	Ⓐ Ⓑ Ⓒ Ⓓ Ⓔ		293	Ⓐ Ⓑ Ⓒ Ⓓ Ⓔ
162	Ⓐ Ⓑ Ⓒ Ⓓ Ⓔ		206	Ⓐ Ⓑ Ⓒ Ⓓ Ⓔ		250	Ⓐ Ⓑ Ⓒ Ⓓ Ⓔ		294	Ⓐ Ⓑ Ⓒ Ⓓ Ⓔ
163	Ⓐ Ⓑ Ⓒ Ⓓ Ⓔ		207	Ⓐ Ⓑ Ⓒ Ⓓ Ⓔ		251	Ⓐ Ⓑ Ⓒ Ⓓ Ⓔ		295	Ⓐ Ⓑ Ⓒ Ⓓ Ⓔ
164	Ⓐ Ⓑ Ⓒ Ⓓ Ⓔ		208	Ⓐ Ⓑ Ⓒ Ⓓ Ⓔ		252	Ⓐ Ⓑ Ⓒ Ⓓ Ⓔ		296	Ⓐ Ⓑ Ⓒ Ⓓ Ⓔ
165	Ⓐ Ⓑ Ⓒ Ⓓ Ⓔ		209	Ⓐ Ⓑ Ⓒ Ⓓ Ⓔ		253	Ⓐ Ⓑ Ⓒ Ⓓ Ⓔ		297	Ⓐ Ⓑ Ⓒ Ⓓ Ⓔ
166	Ⓐ Ⓑ Ⓒ Ⓓ Ⓔ		210	Ⓐ Ⓑ Ⓒ Ⓓ Ⓔ		254	Ⓐ Ⓑ Ⓒ Ⓓ Ⓔ		298	Ⓐ Ⓑ Ⓒ Ⓓ Ⓔ
167	Ⓐ Ⓑ Ⓒ Ⓓ Ⓔ		211	Ⓐ Ⓑ Ⓒ Ⓓ Ⓔ		255	Ⓐ Ⓑ Ⓒ Ⓓ Ⓔ		299	Ⓐ Ⓑ Ⓒ Ⓓ Ⓔ
168	Ⓐ Ⓑ Ⓒ Ⓓ Ⓔ		212	Ⓐ Ⓑ Ⓒ Ⓓ Ⓔ		256	Ⓐ Ⓑ Ⓒ Ⓓ Ⓔ		300	Ⓐ Ⓑ Ⓒ Ⓓ Ⓔ

Post-Test Answer Sheet

Name _____   **Date** _____
Last   First   Middle

Directions
- Using a No. 2 pencil, fill in the circle that best represents the correct answer for each question.
- Make sure you erase completely any answer you wish to change.
- Do not make any stray marks on this answer sheet.
- Mark only one answer for each question.

Correct   Incorrect
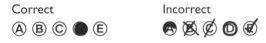

1	Ⓐ Ⓑ Ⓒ Ⓓ Ⓔ	32	Ⓐ Ⓑ Ⓒ Ⓓ Ⓔ	63	Ⓐ Ⓑ Ⓒ Ⓓ Ⓔ	94	Ⓐ Ⓑ Ⓒ Ⓓ Ⓔ
2	Ⓐ Ⓑ Ⓒ Ⓓ Ⓔ	33	Ⓐ Ⓑ Ⓒ Ⓓ Ⓔ	64	Ⓐ Ⓑ Ⓒ Ⓓ Ⓔ	95	Ⓐ Ⓑ Ⓒ Ⓓ Ⓔ
3	Ⓐ Ⓑ Ⓒ Ⓓ Ⓔ	34	Ⓐ Ⓑ Ⓒ Ⓓ Ⓔ	65	Ⓐ Ⓑ Ⓒ Ⓓ Ⓔ	96	Ⓐ Ⓑ Ⓒ Ⓓ Ⓔ
4	Ⓐ Ⓑ Ⓒ Ⓓ Ⓔ	35	Ⓐ Ⓑ Ⓒ Ⓓ Ⓔ	66	Ⓐ Ⓑ Ⓒ Ⓓ Ⓔ	97	Ⓐ Ⓑ Ⓒ Ⓓ Ⓔ
5	Ⓐ Ⓑ Ⓒ Ⓓ Ⓔ	36	Ⓐ Ⓑ Ⓒ Ⓓ Ⓔ	67	Ⓐ Ⓑ Ⓒ Ⓓ Ⓔ	98	Ⓐ Ⓑ Ⓒ Ⓓ Ⓔ
6	Ⓐ Ⓑ Ⓒ Ⓓ Ⓔ	37	Ⓐ Ⓑ Ⓒ Ⓓ Ⓔ	68	Ⓐ Ⓑ Ⓒ Ⓓ Ⓔ	99	Ⓐ Ⓑ Ⓒ Ⓓ Ⓔ
7	Ⓐ Ⓑ Ⓒ Ⓓ Ⓔ	38	Ⓐ Ⓑ Ⓒ Ⓓ Ⓔ	69	Ⓐ Ⓑ Ⓒ Ⓓ Ⓔ	100	Ⓐ Ⓑ Ⓒ Ⓓ Ⓔ
8	Ⓐ Ⓑ Ⓒ Ⓓ Ⓔ	39	Ⓐ Ⓑ Ⓒ Ⓓ Ⓔ	70	Ⓐ Ⓑ Ⓒ Ⓓ Ⓔ	101	Ⓐ Ⓑ Ⓒ Ⓓ Ⓔ
9	Ⓐ Ⓑ Ⓒ Ⓓ Ⓔ	40	Ⓐ Ⓑ Ⓒ Ⓓ Ⓔ	71	Ⓐ Ⓑ Ⓒ Ⓓ Ⓔ	102	Ⓐ Ⓑ Ⓒ Ⓓ Ⓔ
10	Ⓐ Ⓑ Ⓒ Ⓓ Ⓔ	41	Ⓐ Ⓑ Ⓒ Ⓓ Ⓔ	72	Ⓐ Ⓑ Ⓒ Ⓓ Ⓔ	103	Ⓐ Ⓑ Ⓒ Ⓓ Ⓔ
11	Ⓐ Ⓑ Ⓒ Ⓓ Ⓔ	42	Ⓐ Ⓑ Ⓒ Ⓓ Ⓔ	73	Ⓐ Ⓑ Ⓒ Ⓓ Ⓔ	104	Ⓐ Ⓑ Ⓒ Ⓓ Ⓔ
12	Ⓐ Ⓑ Ⓒ Ⓓ Ⓔ	43	Ⓐ Ⓑ Ⓒ Ⓓ Ⓔ	74	Ⓐ Ⓑ Ⓒ Ⓓ Ⓔ	105	Ⓐ Ⓑ Ⓒ Ⓓ Ⓔ
13	Ⓐ Ⓑ Ⓒ Ⓓ Ⓔ	44	Ⓐ Ⓑ Ⓒ Ⓓ Ⓔ	75	Ⓐ Ⓑ Ⓒ Ⓓ Ⓔ	106	Ⓐ Ⓑ Ⓒ Ⓓ Ⓔ
14	Ⓐ Ⓑ Ⓒ Ⓓ Ⓔ	45	Ⓐ Ⓑ Ⓒ Ⓓ Ⓔ	76	Ⓐ Ⓑ Ⓒ Ⓓ Ⓔ	107	Ⓐ Ⓑ Ⓒ Ⓓ Ⓔ
15	Ⓐ Ⓑ Ⓒ Ⓓ Ⓔ	46	Ⓐ Ⓑ Ⓒ Ⓓ Ⓔ	77	Ⓐ Ⓑ Ⓒ Ⓓ Ⓔ	108	Ⓐ Ⓑ Ⓒ Ⓓ Ⓔ
16	Ⓐ Ⓑ Ⓒ Ⓓ Ⓔ	47	Ⓐ Ⓑ Ⓒ Ⓓ Ⓔ	78	Ⓐ Ⓑ Ⓒ Ⓓ Ⓔ	109	Ⓐ Ⓑ Ⓒ Ⓓ Ⓔ
17	Ⓐ Ⓑ Ⓒ Ⓓ Ⓔ	48	Ⓐ Ⓑ Ⓒ Ⓓ Ⓔ	79	Ⓐ Ⓑ Ⓒ Ⓓ Ⓔ	110	Ⓐ Ⓑ Ⓒ Ⓓ Ⓔ
18	Ⓐ Ⓑ Ⓒ Ⓓ Ⓔ	49	Ⓐ Ⓑ Ⓒ Ⓓ Ⓔ	80	Ⓐ Ⓑ Ⓒ Ⓓ Ⓔ	111	Ⓐ Ⓑ Ⓒ Ⓓ Ⓔ
19	Ⓐ Ⓑ Ⓒ Ⓓ Ⓔ	50	Ⓐ Ⓑ Ⓒ Ⓓ Ⓔ	81	Ⓐ Ⓑ Ⓒ Ⓓ Ⓔ	112	Ⓐ Ⓑ Ⓒ Ⓓ Ⓔ
20	Ⓐ Ⓑ Ⓒ Ⓓ Ⓔ	51	Ⓐ Ⓑ Ⓒ Ⓓ Ⓔ	82	Ⓐ Ⓑ Ⓒ Ⓓ Ⓔ	113	Ⓐ Ⓑ Ⓒ Ⓓ Ⓔ
21	Ⓐ Ⓑ Ⓒ Ⓓ Ⓔ	52	Ⓐ Ⓑ Ⓒ Ⓓ Ⓔ	83	Ⓐ Ⓑ Ⓒ Ⓓ Ⓔ	114	Ⓐ Ⓑ Ⓒ Ⓓ Ⓔ
22	Ⓐ Ⓑ Ⓒ Ⓓ Ⓔ	53	Ⓐ Ⓑ Ⓒ Ⓓ Ⓔ	84	Ⓐ Ⓑ Ⓒ Ⓓ Ⓔ	115	Ⓐ Ⓑ Ⓒ Ⓓ Ⓔ
23	Ⓐ Ⓑ Ⓒ Ⓓ Ⓔ	54	Ⓐ Ⓑ Ⓒ Ⓓ Ⓔ	85	Ⓐ Ⓑ Ⓒ Ⓓ Ⓔ	116	Ⓐ Ⓑ Ⓒ Ⓓ Ⓔ
24	Ⓐ Ⓑ Ⓒ Ⓓ Ⓔ	55	Ⓐ Ⓑ Ⓒ Ⓓ Ⓔ	86	Ⓐ Ⓑ Ⓒ Ⓓ Ⓔ	117	Ⓐ Ⓑ Ⓒ Ⓓ Ⓔ
25	Ⓐ Ⓑ Ⓒ Ⓓ Ⓔ	56	Ⓐ Ⓑ Ⓒ Ⓓ Ⓔ	87	Ⓐ Ⓑ Ⓒ Ⓓ Ⓔ	118	Ⓐ Ⓑ Ⓒ Ⓓ Ⓔ
26	Ⓐ Ⓑ Ⓒ Ⓓ Ⓔ	57	Ⓐ Ⓑ Ⓒ Ⓓ Ⓔ	88	Ⓐ Ⓑ Ⓒ Ⓓ Ⓔ	119	Ⓐ Ⓑ Ⓒ Ⓓ Ⓔ
27	Ⓐ Ⓑ Ⓒ Ⓓ Ⓔ	58	Ⓐ Ⓑ Ⓒ Ⓓ Ⓔ	89	Ⓐ Ⓑ Ⓒ Ⓓ Ⓔ	120	Ⓐ Ⓑ Ⓒ Ⓓ Ⓔ
28	Ⓐ Ⓑ Ⓒ Ⓓ Ⓔ	59	Ⓐ Ⓑ Ⓒ Ⓓ Ⓔ	90	Ⓐ Ⓑ Ⓒ Ⓓ Ⓔ	121	Ⓐ Ⓑ Ⓒ Ⓓ Ⓔ
29	Ⓐ Ⓑ Ⓒ Ⓓ Ⓔ	60	Ⓐ Ⓑ Ⓒ Ⓓ Ⓔ	91	Ⓐ Ⓑ Ⓒ Ⓓ Ⓔ	122	Ⓐ Ⓑ Ⓒ Ⓓ Ⓔ
30	Ⓐ Ⓑ Ⓒ Ⓓ Ⓔ	61	Ⓐ Ⓑ Ⓒ Ⓓ Ⓔ	92	Ⓐ Ⓑ Ⓒ Ⓓ Ⓔ	123	Ⓐ Ⓑ Ⓒ Ⓓ Ⓔ
31	Ⓐ Ⓑ Ⓒ Ⓓ Ⓔ	62	Ⓐ Ⓑ Ⓒ Ⓓ Ⓔ	93	Ⓐ Ⓑ Ⓒ Ⓓ Ⓔ	124	Ⓐ Ⓑ Ⓒ Ⓓ Ⓔ

125 Ⓐ Ⓑ Ⓒ Ⓓ Ⓔ	169 Ⓐ Ⓑ Ⓒ Ⓓ Ⓔ	213 Ⓐ Ⓑ Ⓒ Ⓓ Ⓔ	257 Ⓐ Ⓑ Ⓒ Ⓓ Ⓔ
126 Ⓐ Ⓑ Ⓒ Ⓓ Ⓔ	170 Ⓐ Ⓑ Ⓒ Ⓓ Ⓔ	214 Ⓐ Ⓑ Ⓒ Ⓓ Ⓔ	258 Ⓐ Ⓑ Ⓒ Ⓓ Ⓔ
127 Ⓐ Ⓑ Ⓒ Ⓓ Ⓔ	171 Ⓐ Ⓑ Ⓒ Ⓓ Ⓔ	215 Ⓐ Ⓑ Ⓒ Ⓓ Ⓔ	259 Ⓐ Ⓑ Ⓒ Ⓓ Ⓔ
128 Ⓐ Ⓑ Ⓒ Ⓓ Ⓔ	172 Ⓐ Ⓑ Ⓒ Ⓓ Ⓔ	216 Ⓐ Ⓑ Ⓒ Ⓓ Ⓔ	260 Ⓐ Ⓑ Ⓒ Ⓓ Ⓔ
129 Ⓐ Ⓑ Ⓒ Ⓓ Ⓔ	173 Ⓐ Ⓑ Ⓒ Ⓓ Ⓔ	217 Ⓐ Ⓑ Ⓒ Ⓓ Ⓔ	261 Ⓐ Ⓑ Ⓒ Ⓓ Ⓔ
130 Ⓐ Ⓑ Ⓒ Ⓓ Ⓔ	174 Ⓐ Ⓑ Ⓒ Ⓓ Ⓔ	218 Ⓐ Ⓑ Ⓒ Ⓓ Ⓔ	262 Ⓐ Ⓑ Ⓒ Ⓓ Ⓔ
131 Ⓐ Ⓑ Ⓒ Ⓓ Ⓔ	175 Ⓐ Ⓑ Ⓒ Ⓓ Ⓔ	219 Ⓐ Ⓑ Ⓒ Ⓓ Ⓔ	263 Ⓐ Ⓑ Ⓒ Ⓓ Ⓔ
132 Ⓐ Ⓑ Ⓒ Ⓓ Ⓔ	176 Ⓐ Ⓑ Ⓒ Ⓓ Ⓔ	220 Ⓐ Ⓑ Ⓒ Ⓓ Ⓔ	264 Ⓐ Ⓑ Ⓒ Ⓓ Ⓔ
133 Ⓐ Ⓑ Ⓒ Ⓓ Ⓔ	177 Ⓐ Ⓑ Ⓒ Ⓓ Ⓔ	221 Ⓐ Ⓑ Ⓒ Ⓓ Ⓔ	265 Ⓐ Ⓑ Ⓒ Ⓓ Ⓔ
134 Ⓐ Ⓑ Ⓒ Ⓓ Ⓔ	178 Ⓐ Ⓑ Ⓒ Ⓓ Ⓔ	222 Ⓐ Ⓑ Ⓒ Ⓓ Ⓔ	266 Ⓐ Ⓑ Ⓒ Ⓓ Ⓔ
135 Ⓐ Ⓑ Ⓒ Ⓓ Ⓔ	179 Ⓐ Ⓑ Ⓒ Ⓓ Ⓔ	223 Ⓐ Ⓑ Ⓒ Ⓓ Ⓔ	267 Ⓐ Ⓑ Ⓒ Ⓓ Ⓔ
136 Ⓐ Ⓑ Ⓒ Ⓓ Ⓔ	180 Ⓐ Ⓑ Ⓒ Ⓓ Ⓔ	224 Ⓐ Ⓑ Ⓒ Ⓓ Ⓔ	268 Ⓐ Ⓑ Ⓒ Ⓓ Ⓔ
137 Ⓐ Ⓑ Ⓒ Ⓓ Ⓔ	181 Ⓐ Ⓑ Ⓒ Ⓓ Ⓔ	225 Ⓐ Ⓑ Ⓒ Ⓓ Ⓔ	269 Ⓐ Ⓑ Ⓒ Ⓓ Ⓔ
138 Ⓐ Ⓑ Ⓒ Ⓓ Ⓔ	182 Ⓐ Ⓑ Ⓒ Ⓓ Ⓔ	226 Ⓐ Ⓑ Ⓒ Ⓓ Ⓔ	270 Ⓐ Ⓑ Ⓒ Ⓓ Ⓔ
139 Ⓐ Ⓑ Ⓒ Ⓓ Ⓔ	183 Ⓐ Ⓑ Ⓒ Ⓓ Ⓔ	227 Ⓐ Ⓑ Ⓒ Ⓓ Ⓔ	271 Ⓐ Ⓑ Ⓒ Ⓓ Ⓔ
140 Ⓐ Ⓑ Ⓒ Ⓓ Ⓔ	184 Ⓐ Ⓑ Ⓒ Ⓓ Ⓔ	228 Ⓐ Ⓑ Ⓒ Ⓓ Ⓔ	272 Ⓐ Ⓑ Ⓒ Ⓓ Ⓔ
141 Ⓐ Ⓑ Ⓒ Ⓓ Ⓔ	185 Ⓐ Ⓑ Ⓒ Ⓓ Ⓔ	229 Ⓐ Ⓑ Ⓒ Ⓓ Ⓔ	273 Ⓐ Ⓑ Ⓒ Ⓓ Ⓔ
142 Ⓐ Ⓑ Ⓒ Ⓓ Ⓔ	186 Ⓐ Ⓑ Ⓒ Ⓓ Ⓔ	230 Ⓐ Ⓑ Ⓒ Ⓓ Ⓔ	274 Ⓐ Ⓑ Ⓒ Ⓓ Ⓔ
143 Ⓐ Ⓑ Ⓒ Ⓓ Ⓔ	187 Ⓐ Ⓑ Ⓒ Ⓓ Ⓔ	231 Ⓐ Ⓑ Ⓒ Ⓓ Ⓔ	275 Ⓐ Ⓑ Ⓒ Ⓓ Ⓔ
144 Ⓐ Ⓑ Ⓒ Ⓓ Ⓔ	188 Ⓐ Ⓑ Ⓒ Ⓓ Ⓔ	232 Ⓐ Ⓑ Ⓒ Ⓓ Ⓔ	276 Ⓐ Ⓑ Ⓒ Ⓓ Ⓔ
145 Ⓐ Ⓑ Ⓒ Ⓓ Ⓔ	189 Ⓐ Ⓑ Ⓒ Ⓓ Ⓔ	233 Ⓐ Ⓑ Ⓒ Ⓓ Ⓔ	277 Ⓐ Ⓑ Ⓒ Ⓓ Ⓔ
146 Ⓐ Ⓑ Ⓒ Ⓓ Ⓔ	190 Ⓐ Ⓑ Ⓒ Ⓓ Ⓔ	234 Ⓐ Ⓑ Ⓒ Ⓓ Ⓔ	278 Ⓐ Ⓑ Ⓒ Ⓓ Ⓔ
147 Ⓐ Ⓑ Ⓒ Ⓓ Ⓔ	191 Ⓐ Ⓑ Ⓒ Ⓓ Ⓔ	235 Ⓐ Ⓑ Ⓒ Ⓓ Ⓔ	279 Ⓐ Ⓑ Ⓒ Ⓓ Ⓔ
148 Ⓐ Ⓑ Ⓒ Ⓓ Ⓔ	192 Ⓐ Ⓑ Ⓒ Ⓓ Ⓔ	236 Ⓐ Ⓑ Ⓒ Ⓓ Ⓔ	280 Ⓐ Ⓑ Ⓒ Ⓓ Ⓔ
149 Ⓐ Ⓑ Ⓒ Ⓓ Ⓔ	193 Ⓐ Ⓑ Ⓒ Ⓓ Ⓔ	237 Ⓐ Ⓑ Ⓒ Ⓓ Ⓔ	281 Ⓐ Ⓑ Ⓒ Ⓓ Ⓔ
150 Ⓐ Ⓑ Ⓒ Ⓓ Ⓔ	194 Ⓐ Ⓑ Ⓒ Ⓓ Ⓔ	238 Ⓐ Ⓑ Ⓒ Ⓓ Ⓔ	282 Ⓐ Ⓑ Ⓒ Ⓓ Ⓔ
151 Ⓐ Ⓑ Ⓒ Ⓓ Ⓔ	195 Ⓐ Ⓑ Ⓒ Ⓓ Ⓔ	239 Ⓐ Ⓑ Ⓒ Ⓓ Ⓔ	283 Ⓐ Ⓑ Ⓒ Ⓓ Ⓔ
152 Ⓐ Ⓑ Ⓒ Ⓓ Ⓔ	196 Ⓐ Ⓑ Ⓒ Ⓓ Ⓔ	240 Ⓐ Ⓑ Ⓒ Ⓓ Ⓔ	284 Ⓐ Ⓑ Ⓒ Ⓓ Ⓔ
153 Ⓐ Ⓑ Ⓒ Ⓓ Ⓔ	197 Ⓐ Ⓑ Ⓒ Ⓓ Ⓔ	241 Ⓐ Ⓑ Ⓒ Ⓓ Ⓔ	285 Ⓐ Ⓑ Ⓒ Ⓓ Ⓔ
154 Ⓐ Ⓑ Ⓒ Ⓓ Ⓔ	198 Ⓐ Ⓑ Ⓒ Ⓓ Ⓔ	242 Ⓐ Ⓑ Ⓒ Ⓓ Ⓔ	286 Ⓐ Ⓑ Ⓒ Ⓓ Ⓔ
155 Ⓐ Ⓑ Ⓒ Ⓓ Ⓔ	199 Ⓐ Ⓑ Ⓒ Ⓓ Ⓔ	243 Ⓐ Ⓑ Ⓒ Ⓓ Ⓔ	287 Ⓐ Ⓑ Ⓒ Ⓓ Ⓔ
156 Ⓐ Ⓑ Ⓒ Ⓓ Ⓔ	200 Ⓐ Ⓑ Ⓒ Ⓓ Ⓔ	244 Ⓐ Ⓑ Ⓒ Ⓓ Ⓔ	288 Ⓐ Ⓑ Ⓒ Ⓓ Ⓔ
157 Ⓐ Ⓑ Ⓒ Ⓓ Ⓔ	201 Ⓐ Ⓑ Ⓒ Ⓓ Ⓔ	245 Ⓐ Ⓑ Ⓒ Ⓓ Ⓔ	289 Ⓐ Ⓑ Ⓒ Ⓓ Ⓔ
158 Ⓐ Ⓑ Ⓒ Ⓓ Ⓔ	202 Ⓐ Ⓑ Ⓒ Ⓓ Ⓔ	246 Ⓐ Ⓑ Ⓒ Ⓓ Ⓔ	290 Ⓐ Ⓑ Ⓒ Ⓓ Ⓔ
159 Ⓐ Ⓑ Ⓒ Ⓓ Ⓔ	203 Ⓐ Ⓑ Ⓒ Ⓓ Ⓔ	247 Ⓐ Ⓑ Ⓒ Ⓓ Ⓔ	291 Ⓐ Ⓑ Ⓒ Ⓓ Ⓔ
160 Ⓐ Ⓑ Ⓒ Ⓓ Ⓔ	204 Ⓐ Ⓑ Ⓒ Ⓓ Ⓔ	248 Ⓐ Ⓑ Ⓒ Ⓓ Ⓔ	292 Ⓐ Ⓑ Ⓒ Ⓓ Ⓔ
161 Ⓐ Ⓑ Ⓒ Ⓓ Ⓔ	205 Ⓐ Ⓑ Ⓒ Ⓓ Ⓔ	249 Ⓐ Ⓑ Ⓒ Ⓓ Ⓔ	293 Ⓐ Ⓑ Ⓒ Ⓓ Ⓔ
162 Ⓐ Ⓑ Ⓒ Ⓓ Ⓔ	206 Ⓐ Ⓑ Ⓒ Ⓓ Ⓔ	250 Ⓐ Ⓑ Ⓒ Ⓓ Ⓔ	294 Ⓐ Ⓑ Ⓒ Ⓓ Ⓔ
163 Ⓐ Ⓑ Ⓒ Ⓓ Ⓔ	207 Ⓐ Ⓑ Ⓒ Ⓓ Ⓔ	251 Ⓐ Ⓑ Ⓒ Ⓓ Ⓔ	295 Ⓐ Ⓑ Ⓒ Ⓓ Ⓔ
164 Ⓐ Ⓑ Ⓒ Ⓓ Ⓔ	208 Ⓐ Ⓑ Ⓒ Ⓓ Ⓔ	252 Ⓐ Ⓑ Ⓒ Ⓓ Ⓔ	296 Ⓐ Ⓑ Ⓒ Ⓓ Ⓔ
165 Ⓐ Ⓑ Ⓒ Ⓓ Ⓔ	209 Ⓐ Ⓑ Ⓒ Ⓓ Ⓔ	253 Ⓐ Ⓑ Ⓒ Ⓓ Ⓔ	297 Ⓐ Ⓑ Ⓒ Ⓓ Ⓔ
166 Ⓐ Ⓑ Ⓒ Ⓓ Ⓔ	210 Ⓐ Ⓑ Ⓒ Ⓓ Ⓔ	254 Ⓐ Ⓑ Ⓒ Ⓓ Ⓔ	298 Ⓐ Ⓑ Ⓒ Ⓓ Ⓔ
167 Ⓐ Ⓑ Ⓒ Ⓓ Ⓔ	211 Ⓐ Ⓑ Ⓒ Ⓓ Ⓔ	255 Ⓐ Ⓑ Ⓒ Ⓓ Ⓔ	299 Ⓐ Ⓑ Ⓒ Ⓓ Ⓔ
168 Ⓐ Ⓑ Ⓒ Ⓓ Ⓔ	212 Ⓐ Ⓑ Ⓒ Ⓓ Ⓔ	256 Ⓐ Ⓑ Ⓒ Ⓓ Ⓔ	300 Ⓐ Ⓑ Ⓒ Ⓓ Ⓔ